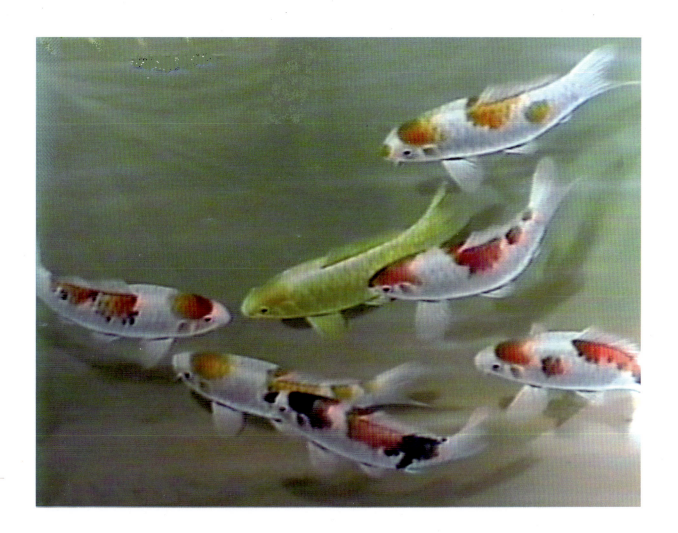

Advanced Koi Care

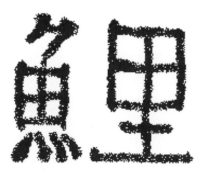

Advanced Koi Care for Veterinarians and Professional Koi Keepers

Nicholas Saint-Erne, DVM

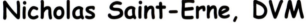

Published by

Erne Enterprises

3845 West Calle Lejos
Glendale, Arizona, USA
85310

All photographs are by the author except some of the photographs of the koi varieties in Chapter 1, which were courteously provided by Joel Burkard, PanIntercorp - Kenmore, Washington, who can be reached at koi.com.

Back cover photograph by Judy Saint-Erne.

Cover illustration and design by Tiffany Nicole Miller Las Vegas, Nevada.

(C) Copyright MMII, MMX

Nicholas de Saint-Erne

All rights reserved.

No part of this publication may be reproduced or stored by any means without prior written permission from the copyright holder. The author and publisher have made extensive efforts to ensure that treatments, drug dosages, and other data are accurate and conform to the standards accepted at the time of publication. However, the reader is advised to exercise individual judgement when making a clinical decision and, if necessary, consult and compare with information from other sources. The reader assumes all responsibility for misuse or misapplication of treatment modalities or other information in this book.

Printed in the United States of America

SECOND PRINTING, REVISED 2010

This book is dedicated
to the veterinarians
who influenced my choice
of Fish Medicine
as a career goal:

Dr. Mark Dulin

Dr. Donald M. Trotter

Dr. Donald Abt

Dr. John B. Gratzek

Dr. Ruth Francis-Floyd

Dr. Greg Lewbart

The author gratefully acknowledges
the patience and support of his wife,

Judy,

and daughters,

Victoria, Alexandra and Rachel

during the protracted production of this work.

TABLE OF CONTENTS

FOREWORD	1
BY DR. GREG LEWBART	
PREFACE	2
KOI ART	3
CHAPTER 1: INTRODUCTION TO KOI	4
WHAT ARE KOI?	5
TAXONOMY OF KOI	5
THE STORY OF CARP	7
KOI COLORS	12
KOI BREEDING AND GENETICS	18
KOI WEIGHT VERSUS TOTAL LENGTH	25
ANATOMY OF KOI	27
RADIOGRAPHIC ANATOMY	35
CHAPTER 2: CLINICAL PROCEDURES	**38**
DISEASE PRECURSORS	39
OFFICE VISIT OR HOUSE CALL?	39
PATIENT HISTORY	40
DIAGNOSTIC METHODS	40
HEMATOLOGY	45
RADIOLOGY	47
SONOGRAPHY	49
ENDOSCOPY	49
ANESTHESIA	50
SURGERY	53
ELECTROCARDIOGRAM	57
PULSE OXIMETER	57
INJECTIONS	58
MICROCHIP IDENTIFICATION	59
EUTHANASIA	59
CHAPTER 3: INFECTIOUS DISEASES	**62**
VIRAL DISEASES	63
BACTERIAL DISEASES	65
FUNGAL DISEASES	69
CHAPTER 4: PARASITIC DISEASES	**72**
PROTOZOAL PARASITES	73
HELMINTH PARASITES	79
CRUSTACEAN PARASITES	83
MOLLUSC PARASITES	85
CHAPTER 5: ENVIRONMENTAL MANAGEMENT	**88**
KOI NUTRITION	89
WATER QUALITY IN THE KOI POND	94
FILTRATION SYSTEMS	110
SEASONAL VARIATIONS OF THE KOI POND	118
TRAUMATIC INJURIES AND TOXICITY	121

CHAPTER 6: DISEASE PREVENTION — 128
STRESS AND DISEASE IN KOI — 129
DISEASE PREVENTION — 129
KOI ACQUISITION — 129
TRANSPORTATION — 130
QUARANTINE — 131
KOI SHOWS — 131
DISEASE PREVENTION SUMMARY — 132

CHAPTER 7: CASE STUDIES — 134
NEOPLASIA IN KOI — 135
BACTERIAL INFECTIONS — 139
ENVIRONMENTAL PROBLEMS — 141
PARASITE INFESTATIONS — 142

CHAPTER 8: FORMULARY — 146
APPLICATION OF CHEMICALS TO THE POND — 147
CHLORAMINE-T — 149
COPPER SULFATE — 150
FORMALIN SOLUTION — 151
FORMALIN/MALACHITE GREEN SOLUTION — 152
HYDROGEN PEROXIDE — 153
IODINE SOLUTION — 154
METRONIDAZOLE — 155
POTASSIUM PERMANGANATE — 156
SIMAZINE, 0.60% SOLUTION — 157
SIMAZINE GRANULES, 90% — 158
SODIUM CHLORIDE — 159
SODIUM THIOSULFATE, 20% — 160
TETRACYCLINE HYDROCHLORIDE, USP — 161
TRICHLORFON, 80% ACTIVE — 162
QUICK REFERENCE GUIDE TO CHEMOTHERAPEUTICS FOR KOI — 163

GLOSSARY — 166
MEDICAL TERMINOLOGY — 166
JAPANESE TERMINOLOGY USED WITH KOI — 168

BIBLIOGRAPHY — 172
KOI BOOKS — 172
POND AND WATER GARDEN BOOKS — 175
KOI AND WATER GARDENING MAGAZINES — 181
AQUARIUM FISH MAGAZINES — 182

APPENDIX — 184
PERIODIC TABLE OF THE ELEMENTS — 183-184
POND CONSTRUCTION — 185

INDEX — 190

FOREWORD

It is a privilege to write the introduction for what I feel is the most complete and state-of-the-science medical text pertaining to the Nishikigoi (*Cyprinus carpio*). And it couldn't come at a better time. In the past 10 years the water garden and koi keeping hobbies have exploded here in the United States and abroad. Farmers, wholesalers, and retailers are reporting record sales of koi including the higher end or "premium" fish. Many koi owners are well educated, sophisticated, and dedicated to their koi. Along with this commitment to their koi charges comes the need and desire for qualified veterinary assistance. The number of veterinarians treating koi has probably increased by an order of magnitude during the past decade. Nearly every major veterinary conference offers lectures and laboratory sessions dealing with ornamental fish, and it would be unusual not to find koi medicine included as a major topic. Most practitioners I speak with say that koi comprise at least 50 percent of their fish practice. This is a pretty remarkable statistic considering that several hundred species of fish are commonly kept as pets in the home aquarium or garden pond.

While there are certainly some excellent fish medicine textbooks on the market, none deal with koi at the exhaustive level that Dr. Saint-Erne achieves in this book. All of the major medical and surgical topics pertinent to the koi are covered. Whether dealing with a straightforward water quality problem or a complicated abdominal surgery, all of the "need to know" information is contained within these pages. The images and illustrations are clear, accurate, and adequately descriptive. The variety and breadth of the photographs and drawings help make this the most comprehensive text on koi medicine available today. The reader is also treated to a detailed history of koi and koi keeping as well as a complete description of the natural history of this magnificent fish.

Advanced Koi Care is a one-stop reference for the veterinary practitioner, veterinary student, fisheries biologist, public aquarist, and advanced koi keeping hobbyist. It is written in an orderly, easy to follow, and concise format that the reader will bond to immediately.

Dr. Saint-Erne should be commended and congratulated for bringing to our bookshelves an invaluable resource to better the lives of the world's koi and their owners.

Gregory A. Lewbart MS, VMD
Diplomate ACZM
Raleigh, North Carolina
September 2, 2001

PREFACE

As a young aquarist, while still in grade school, I first read about Japanese colored carp, or koi, in the December 1969 issue of *Tropical Fish Hobbyist* magazine. The pictures of the fish were beautiful and their history fascinating. I knew then that koi would become popular in the fish-keeping hobby and important to me in my life. Now, 32 years later, I have spent the first half of the ensuing time as a hobbyist myself, and the last half professionally, dealing with koi and koi ponds in my practice as a veterinarian.

Originally there were few veterinarians aware of the need for veterinary involvement in fish keeping. Most of the work on fish diseases that had been done was with trout, salmon, and catfish aquaculture for the food industry. Little thought was given by veterinarians and fish scientists to "pet fish" and their needs. But as a dedicated hobbyist, I used my veterinary skills on fish, in addition to the dogs and cats and exotic pets seen in my practice. I found there was a steady demand by concerned owners who wanted the same high quality of medical attention for their koi as for their other pets.

It is due to the support of all my "exotic" clients, and to the veterinarians who promoted pet fish medicine as a legitimate field of clinical medicine, that I ultimately wrote this book. I owe many thanks to them for encouragement over the years of my medical practice. It is my wish, as a form of repayment to these supporters, to make the going easier for fellow veterinarians, aquaculturists, koi breeders and dealers, and advanced koi hobbyists. By following the information in this book, they will benefit from the experiences I had as both a hobbyist and a veterinarian. The reader will also benefit from my review of over one hundred veterinary and koi hobbyist texts in order to compare treatments, confirm dosages, and ensure the best and most current information is at hand. All the needed information is gathered here in one source.

Fish have long been among the most popular household pets. According to the 2000 survey by the American Pet Products Manufacturer's Association, 12% of U.S. households keep freshwater fish as pets, making it the third most popular type of pet after dogs, then cats. In total numbers, the largest number of pets kept in U.S. households are fish, with an estimated 159 million freshwater fish kept in aquariums. Now, hobbyists are rapidly expanding their fish keeping to outdoor ponds in addition to aquariums. The 2000 APPMA survey estimates that there are 1.9 million households in the U.S. with fish ponds in their backyard. The National Pond Society, based in Roswell, Georgia, reports that the number of homes having an ornamental pond (a water garden or a fish pond) has increased from 1 million in 1989 to 5.6 million in 1999, and will continue to increase by 35% each year. The value of koi in these ponds goes beyond their initial cost, as each fish becomes a pet to the pond keeper, often eating out of the owner's hand. These koi owners are in need of professionals to help them with their koi care and deserve the most advanced care possible for maintaining the health of their koi fish, the aquatic living jewels.

Nicholas Saint-Erne, DVM
Phoenix, Arizona
September, 2001

KOI ART

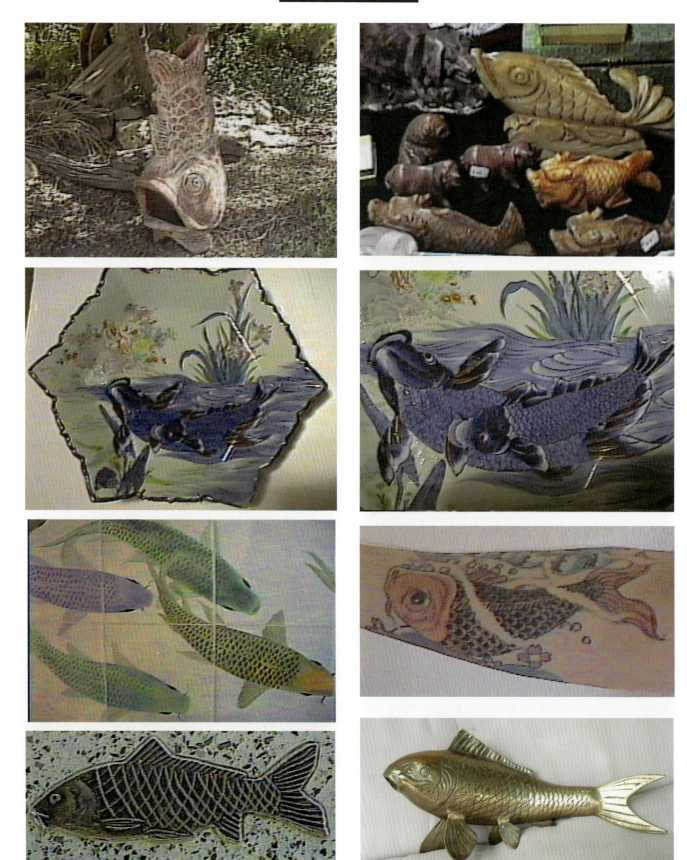

CHAPTER 1: INTRODUCTION TO KOI

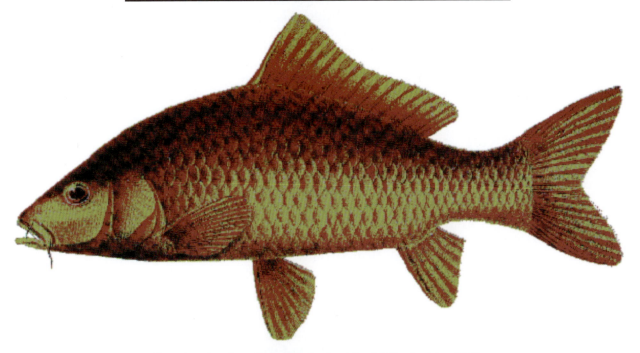

Carp drawing from Peter Bleeker's *Atlas Ichthyologique*, 1863.

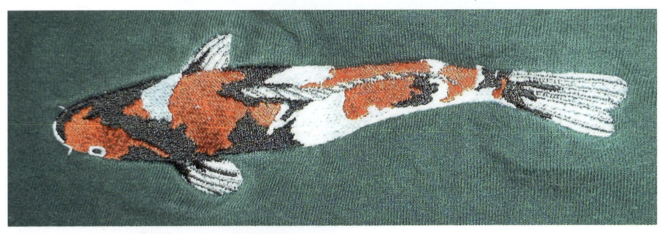

Showa Sanshoku koi embroidered on a shirt

FACING PAGE (left to right, top to bottom):
A chimnea (small outside fireplace) in the shape of a koi
Koi carvings for sale at a koi show
Antique Chinese porcelain plate
Close-up of spawning carp on the Chinese porcelain plate
Hand painted koi on kitchen ceramic tiles
Tattoo of a koi on a forearm
Brass carp by artists Judith and Daniel Caldwell in the floor of the Seattle, Washington airport
Brass koi statue

WHAT ARE KOI?

Koi are fast becoming one of the most popular pets in the United States and the world. They are brightly colored pond fish that grow quite large, live for 60 or more years, and can be tame enough to eat out of the owner's hand or be petted in the water. They breed readily and prolifically under proper conditions, which adds another dimension to the koi keeping hobby. And if one of those koi seems to be perfectly colored, it can be entered into koi shows, much like professional dog breeders strive to reach the annual Westminster Dog Show with their prize pooch. But with koi the stakes can be outstanding, with a Grand Champion koi selling for tens and even hundreds of thousands of dollars! But what exactly is a koi? Well, it is a domesticated color variety of the common carp!

TAXONOMY OF KOI

Kingdom - Animalia (animals) - approximately 1.1 million species of animals
Phylum - Chordata (chordates) - having a spinal cord (notochord)
Subphylum - Vertebrata (vertebrates) - having a vertebral column - about 55,000 species
Superclass - Gnathostomata (jawed mouth) - fish, amphibian, reptile, bird, mammal
Grade - Osteichthyes (bony fishes) "Teleostomi" - over 28,000 fish species
Class - Actinopterygii (spiny finned fishes) - about 27,000 species
Subclass - Neopterygii (new finned) "Teleostei" (whole bones)
Superorder - Ostariophysi (bone air bladder) - having Weber's ossicles
Order - Cypriniformes (carp-shaped) - over 3200 species divided into 6 families
Suborder - Cyprinoidei (carp-like) - over 2000 species, all freshwater
Family - Cyprinidae (carps and minnows) - the largest family of freshwater fishes
Genus - *Cyprinus* - Latin for carp, from the Greek "kyprinos," which may refer to their copper coloration ("kupros" is Greek for copper)
Species - *carpio* Linnaeus 1758 - common carp

The name and date after the species indicates that the *Cyprinus carpio* was first named and described by Carolus Linnaeus [Karl von Linne - a Swedish botanist who was the creator of the binomial nomenclature or scientific names for plants and animals, who also Latinized his own name] in the 1758 edition of his book *Systema Naturae*.

Variety - Japanese colored carp, or koi, from "Nishikigoi" which is Japanese for "brocaded carp," a domesticated color variety of the common carp.

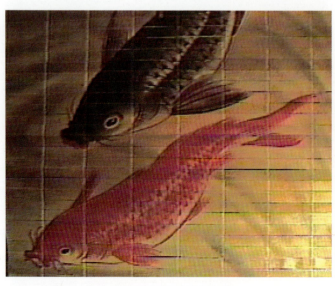

Japanese bamboo screen painting of a Higoi (red carp), the earliest color mutation of the common carp (top fish pictured), which is the foundation stock of all the Nishikigoi, or Japanese colored carp.

Other closely related carp:

Common (wild) carp - *Cyprinus carpio*
Mirror carp - common carp with fewer scales (also called German carp)
Leather carp - common carp with no scales (also known as Israeli carp)
Crucian carp - *Carassius carassius*
Prussian carp (Europe) - *Carassius gibelio*
Goldfish (Asia) - *Carassius auratus*
Bighead carp - *Aristichthys nobilis*
Grass carp - *Ctenopharyngodon idellus*
Silver carp - *Hypophthalmichthys molitrix*
Mrigal carp - *Cirrhinus mrigala*
Mud carp - *Cirrhinus mulitorella*
Black Amur carp - *Mylopharyngodon piceus*
Milem carp - *Osteochilus hasselti*
Hoven carp - *Leptobarbus hoeveni*
Indian carp - *Catla catla*

Carp in the genus *Cyprinus* have two pairs of barbels on the upper lip (maxilla).
Carp in the genus *Carassius* do not have barbels.
Koi can be easily distinguished from goldfish by the lack of barbels in goldfish.

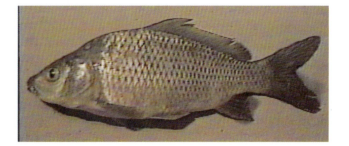

Common carp (*Cyprinus carpio*)

RIGHT:
World record common carp caught fishing,
82 pounds.   (Photo from the internet)

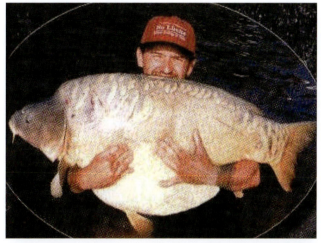

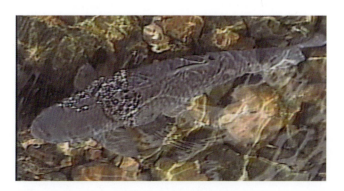

The shark-like grass carp
(*Ctenopharyngodon idellus*)

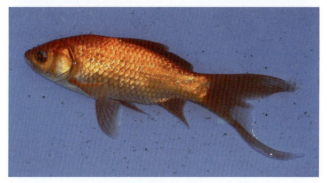

Comet (longtail) goldfish
(*Carassius auratus*)

THE STORY OF CARP

The story of the carp is a long one, not in words, but in years. It starts over 500 million years ago (MYA), during the Cambrian Period of the Paleozoic Era, when the first fish-like animals appeared. They were the Ostracoderms (shell-skinned fish), all of which are now extinct, but most similar to the extant (living) lampreys and hagfish. From the Ostracoderms came the Placoderms (armored fish) during the Silurian Period, 415 MYA. The Chondrichthyes (sharks and rays) are their closest living descendents. The next period, the Devonian (360-408 MYA), was the true "Age of Fishes" when the fish were the most highly evolved species and their numbers were greatly increasing. This is when the Osteichthyes (bony fish) first developed.

A long time passed before what are considered "modern" fish appeared. The first Neopterygian (new finned) fish evolved 255 MYA, near the end of the Permian Period. The main period of evolution for these completely boned (Teleosts) fish was the Jurassic Period (144-208 MYA). Only 70 MYA, during the end of the Cretaceous Period, did the first Ostariophysans appear. Now we're getting closer, these are the carps, minnows, and catfishes! The early Cypriniformes were well established in the lakes of Europe in the Oligocene Epoch (23-36 MYA) of the Tertiary Period. The actual *Cyprinus carpio* species probably evolved in the area around the Black and Caspian Seas near the end of the Pliocene Epoch (2 MYA). From this time on it's a matter of fine-tuning, evolving, and diversifying.

Finally hominids appeared, beginning over 1 MYA during the Pleistocene Epoch of the Quaternary Period (1.6 million years ago to the present). It was just over 100,000 years ago when the Neanderthal Man was the dominant species. Finally about 30,000 years ago, *Homo sapiens sapiens* was the main man. By 14,000 years ago, man had his first domesticated animal, the dog. As civilization and agriculture progressed, the number of animals domesticated increased. Keeping and breeding food animals was much easier than hunting and gathering, so cultures that had a readily obtainable food supply tended to flourish. Eventually, about 4000 years ago in China, wild-caught riverine carp were kept in ponds as an easily accessible source of food.

Carp belong to the family Cyprinidae – which was named after the Latin word for carp (*cyprinus*). This includes the carps and minnows.

Fish in this family have a forked (emarginate) caudal fin and no adipose fin. The jaws are protractile (able to extend out) and have no teeth. All Cyprinids do have one to three rows of teeth on the lower pharyngeal bones, which rub against a thick pad on the roof of the pharynx. Cyprinids may have one or two pairs of barbels on the upper lip – or none at all. The head is scaleless and the body is evenly scaled. The early fish of this family originated in southern Eurasia, and spread in fresh waters throughout Europe, Asia, India, Africa, and North America. No Cyprinids are native to South America or Australia.

The common carp (*Cyprinus carpio*) from the Danube River has now been introduced by human transplantation worldwide. These have two pairs of barbels on the upper lip – one large and one small. They have large cycloid scales numbering 35-39 along the lateral line. The wild riverine carp has an elongated body, but the cultured variety of common carp has a high arched back with a notch in its nape. The body color is yellowish brown to olive-green. In the wild they can attain weights of over 50 pounds, with the world record weighing just over 82 pounds, but they average much less, about 5-15 pounds. They commonly grow 2 to 3 feet (61-91.5 centimeters) in length, occasionally 3½ feet (106.7 cm).

Sexual maturity is reached around 3 years old. The female common carp lays hundreds of thousands of adhesive eggs on aquatic plants. The males follow the spawning females frantically fertilizing the eggs as they are laid. The eggs hatch in 3-6 days, depending on water temperature, untended by either parent. Newly hatched fry are 5-6 millimeters (mm) long, and become free-swimming 2-3 days after hatching.

The culture of carp occurred in China as long ago as 2000 BC. A Chinese treatise on how to spawn carp, entitled *Yogyokyo,* was produced in 533 BC, and another on fish breeding was written in 475 BC. The Greek philosopher Aristotle (384-322 BC) recorded carp (*Kyprianos*) in his list of 540 animal species in his *Historia Animalium.* Pliny the Elder (AD 23-79) mentioned carp (*Cyprinus*) in his book *Naturalis Historia.* The Romans kept carp in ponds, as a ready source of food, and transported them from the Danube River to the western Roman provinces in the first few centuries AD. Carp were a favorite food of the Ostrogoth king, Theodoric of Ravenna (AD 455-526), ruler of Italy. His Roman administrator, Cassiodorus (AD 490-585), wrote of the "rare delicacies of the Carp which lives in the Danube." Charlemagne (AD 768-814), the first Holy Roman

Emperor, ordered his tenant farmers to maintain fishponds; likely these were stocked with carp.

Pondfish culture spread through Europe near the end of the Middle Ages (AD 476-1453), perhaps as a result of the return of the crusaders (11th–15th centuries). Albertus Magnus (AD 1193-1280) wrote about breeding common carp in ponds in 1260. Carp ponds were built in Wittingau (Czechoslovakia) in 1358. Carp were introduced to Poland by 1466, England in 1512, Denmark in 1560, Prussia in 1585, and St. Petersburg, Russia in 1729. Izaak Walton, in *The Compleat Angler* published in England in 1653, calls the carp "...the Queen of Rivers: a stately, a good, and a very subtle fish." The Germans, in the late 1700s, bred a strain of carp that had almost no scales (the leather carp), or had large scales only along the back (mirror carp). These were easier for cooks to prepare for dinner.

In America, immigrants from Germany longed for their favorite food fish, the carp. Captain Henry M. Robinson brought carp to North America in 1832, keeping them in a pond near Newburgh, New York. In 1872, J.A. Poppe brought carp over from Holstein, Germany to stock private ponds in Sonoma County, California.

A fish culturist for the United States government, Rudolph Hessel, was sent to Hochst, near Frankfurt, Germany to procure these wonderful fish. On May 26, 1877 he returned to New York Harbor with a cargo of 345 German carp – 227 of them mirror carp and 118 normal scaled carp. These were transported to ponds in Druid Hill Park, Baltimore, Maryland. The following year, 65 mirror carp and 48 scaled carp were transferred to Babcock Lake in Monument Park, Washington, DC. By 1879 there were enough carp in these ponds to spread across America. Some 12,265 carp were spread to 25 states and territories. In 1883 another 260,000 carp were disseminated across America. The rest is history. By 1895 the carp had overpopulated native waters and were regarded with alarm and disgust. They were muddying lakes and streams and eliminating the native fishes. Since then, extreme efforts have been made to remove the alien carp from native waters, with limited success. What was once considered to be a delicacy is now considered to be a pest!

Notice that this is titled "The Story of Carp," not koi. The history of koi is as muddy as the water in which they originated. Carp were imported from China into Japan around AD 1500. The rice farmers in Niigata prefecture on the northwestern coast of Japan started raising carp (Magoi) in the irrigation reservoirs above their rice paddies. The fish would spawn in the spring and by fall the babies would be about 4 inches (10 cm) long. These would be dried and salted and eaten during the winter months. The parent stock would be brought indoors and kept in water-filled depressions dug in the dirt floors of the house until the following spring. Family members would take turns stirring the water to provide oxygen to keep the fish alive through the winter.

Color mutations in the young fish were first noticed in 1803, and these reddish carp (Higoi) were kept and added to the breeding stock. By cross-breeding the different mutations, early Kohaku, Asagi, Higoi, and Bekko strains were stabilized between 1830 and 1850. By the late 1880s many current varieties had been established. In 1904, eight German mirror carp were brought to Japan. Crossing these with the Asagi resulted in the first Shusui in 1909.

Colored carp (then called Irogoi) were mostly unknown outside of Niigata until Hikosaburo Hirasawa, the Mayor of Higashiyama Mura, sent 27 koi to the 1914 Tokyo Taisho Exhibition as unique products of his prefecture. These fish were awarded the second prize at the exhibition, and eight of them were presented to Emperor Yoshihito's son, Hirohito. These were placed in the moat around the emperor's palace.

Soon all of Japan wanted to keep koi, and the rest of the world followed. Koi were first exported to San Francisco in 1938, to Hawaii in 1947, to Canada in 1949, to Brazil in 1953, England in 1966, and to South Africa in 1971. Herbert R. Axelrod, owner of Gulf Fish Farms in Palmetto, Florida, imported breeding stock koi in January 1969 from the Yoshida family koi farm in Japan, winners of the grand champion trophy at the first All-Japan Nishikigoi Show for their Taisho Sanke in 1968. From these fish were bred millions of koi which were sold in petshops throughout the United States, introducing aquarists to koi. Now koi are regularly imported into this country from Japanese koi farms, and from Taiwan, Hong Kong, South Africa, and Israel, as well as being bred in koi farms all over the United States.

The Deputy Commissioner of Fisheries, Hugh M. Smith, stated in 1907 (30 years after carp were imported into America) "...the introduction of the carp into the United States will remain the leading achievement in fish acclimatization in recent times, and, with the exception of the original introduction of the same fish into Europe from Asia, the most important the world has known." He was right. And now, the recent introduction of

GEOLOGIC TIME SCALE

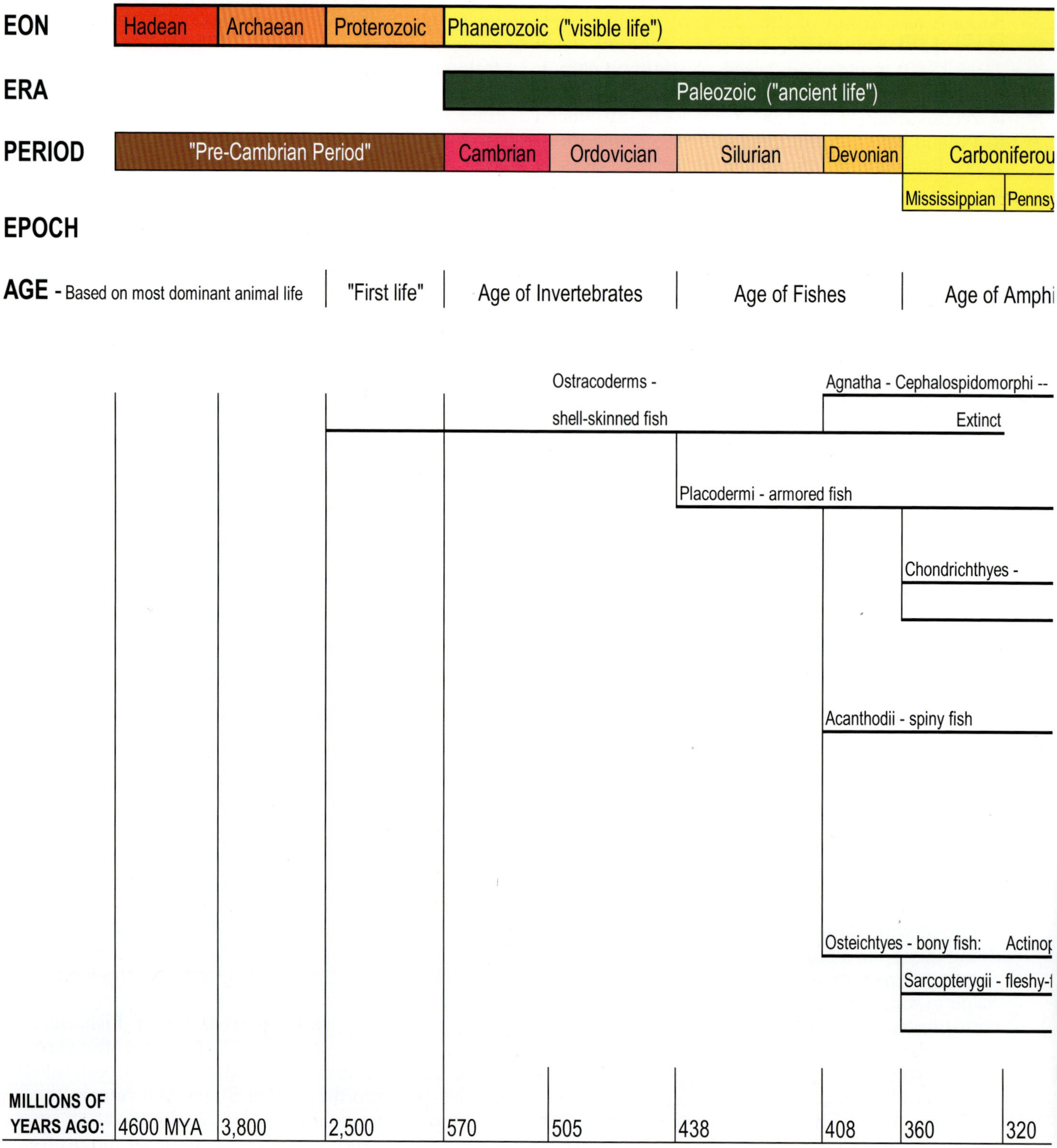

EON			
Hadean	Archaean	Proterozoic	Phanerozoic ("visible life")

ERA — Paleozoic ("ancient life")

PERIOD							
"Pre-Cambrian Period"			Cambrian	Ordovician	Silurian	Devonian	Carboniferou...

| | | | | | | | Mississippian | Pennsy... |

EPOCH

AGE - Based on most dominant animal life | "First life" | Age of Invertebrates | Age of Fishes | Age of Amphi...

Ostracoderms -
shell-skinned fish

Agnatha - Cephalospidomorphi --
Extinct

Placodermi - armored fish

Chondrichthyes -

Acanthodii - spiny fish

Osteichtyes - bony fish: Actinop...
Sarcopterygii - fleshy-...

MILLIONS OF YEARS AGO:	4600 MYA	3,800	2,500	570	505	438	408	360	320

NSE 2002

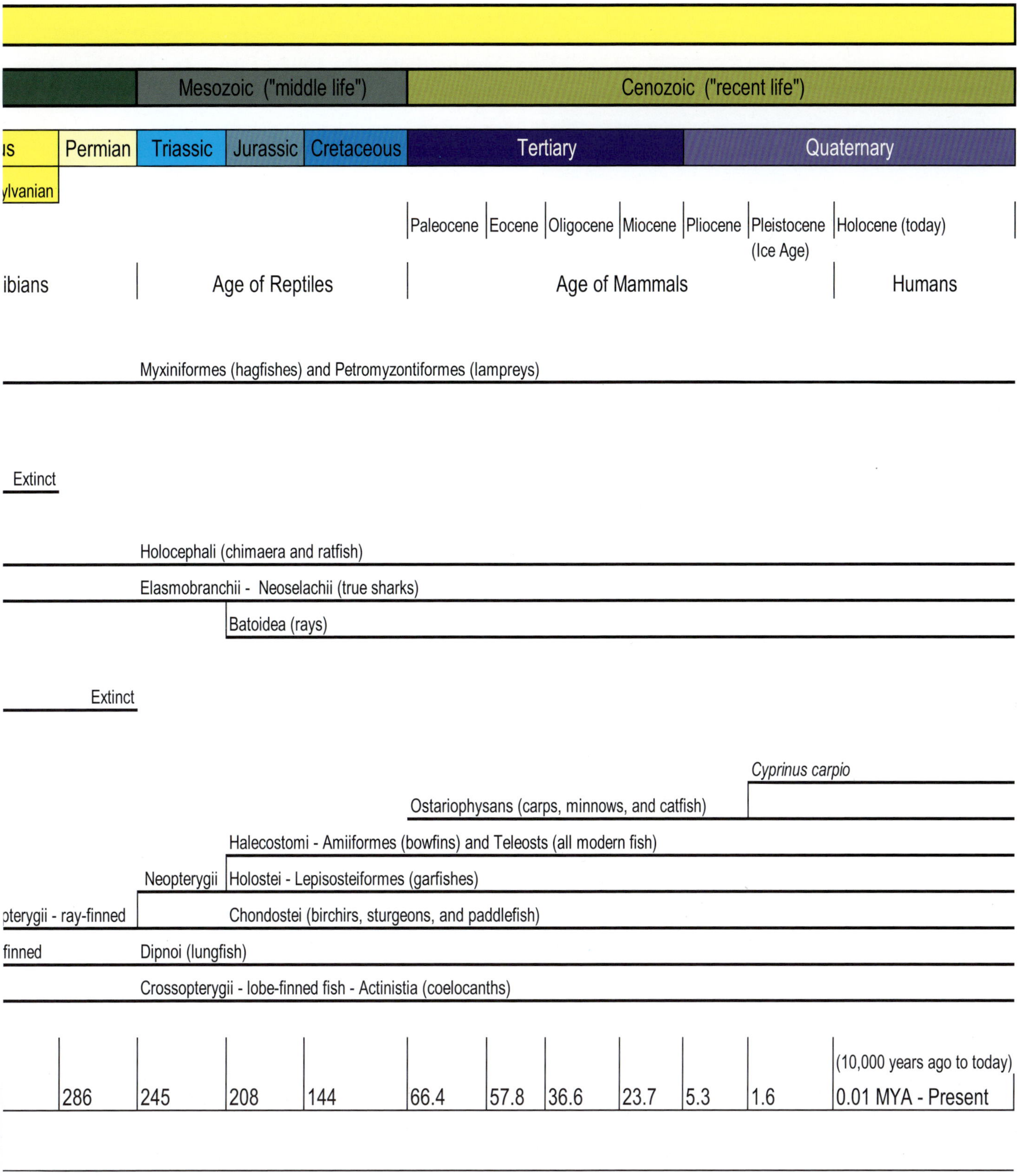

	Mesozoic ("middle life")	Cenozoic ("recent life")	

...s	Permian	Triassic	Jurassic	Cretaceous	Tertiary	Quaternary

...ylvanian

	Paleocene	Eocene	Oligocene	Miocene	Pliocene	Pleistocene (Ice Age)	Holocene (today)	

...ibians | Age of Reptiles | Age of Mammals | Humans

Myxiniformes (hagfishes) and Petromyzontiformes (lampreys)

Extinct

Holocephali (chimaera and ratfish)

Elasmobranchii - Neoselachii (true sharks)

Batoidea (rays)

Extinct

Cyprinus carpio

Ostariophysans (carps, minnows, and catfish)

Halecostomi - Amiiformes (bowfins) and Teleosts (all modern fish)

Neopterygii | Holostei - Lepisosteiformes (garfishes)

...pterygii - ray-finned | Chondostei (birchirs, sturgeons, and paddlefish)

...finned | Dipnoi (lungfish)

Crossopterygii - lobe-finned fish - Actinistia (coelocanths)

286	245	208	144	66.4	57.8	36.6	23.7	5.3	1.6	(10,000 years ago to today) 0.01 MYA - Present

high quality domestic-bred koi carp into the pet fish market (30 years since koi were first commercially bred in America) will probably be just as significant a contribution to the pet trade of the future.

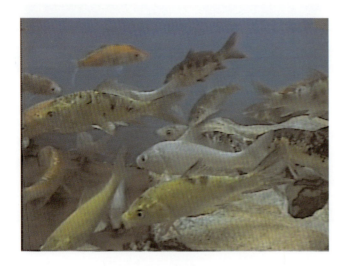

Domestic-bred baby koi for sale in an aquarium at a pet store.

REFERENCES:

Axelrod, Herbert R. 1969. "Koi, Japanese Imperial Colored Carp," *Tropical Fish Hobbyist,* vol. XVIII, no. 4, December 1969, T.F.H. Publications, Neptune, NJ.

Axelrod, Herbert R. 1973. *Koi of the World: Japanese Colored Carp*, T.F.H. Publications, Neptune, NJ.

Axelrod, Herbert R., Eugene Balon, Richard C. Hoffman, Shmuel Rothbard, and Giora W. Wohlfarth. 1996. *The Completely Illustrated Guide to Koi for Your Pond,* T.F.H. Publications, Neptune, NJ.

Evanoff, Vlad. 1964. *The Fresh-Water Fisherman's Bible,* Doubleday, Garden City, NY.

Laycock, George. 1966. *The Alien Animals,* The Natural History Press, Garden City, NY.

Limburg, Peter R. 1980. *Farming the Waters,* Beaufort Books, New York.

Long, John A. 1995. *The Rise of Fishes,* Johns Hopkins University Press, Baltimore.

Maisey, John G. 1996. *Discovering Fossil Fishes*, Henry Holt, New York.

Moyle, Peter B. 1993. *Fish: An Enthusiast's Guide,* University of California Press, Berkeley, CA.

Nelson, Joseph S. 2006. *Fishes of the World*, 4th ed., John Wiley & Sons, Hoboken, NJ.

Paxton, John R. and William N. Eschmeyer. 1998. *Encyclopedia of Fishes,* 2nd ed., Academic Press, San Diego, CA.

Saint-Erne, Nicholas. 1986. *Taxonomy Basics for Aquarists,* Las Vegas Aquarium Society Monthly Bulletin, November 1986, Las Vegas, NV.

Smith, Hugh M. 1907. "Our Fish Immigrants," *National Geographic Magazine,* June 1907, National Geographic Society, Washington, DC.

Sperling, Alan. 1999. "Report On the Pond Market" from *Pondscapes*, National Pond Society, Roswell, GA.

Sterba, Gunther. 1959. *Freshwater Fishes of the World,* The Pet Library, LTD, New York. Revised English language edition, 1966.

Tamadachi, Michugo. 1994. *The Cult of the Koi,* 2nd ed., T.F.H. Publications, Neptune, NJ.

Waddington, Peter. 1995. *Koi Kichi,* Infiltration, Golborne, Warrington, Cheshire, UK.

Walden, Howard T. 1964. *Familiar Freshwater Fishes of America,* Harper & Row, New York.

Watt, Ronnie and Servaas de Kock. 1996. *Living Jewels - Koi Keeping in South Africa,* Delta Books, Johannesburg, South Africa.

Wise, J. Karl. 1997. *U.S. Pet Ownership & Demographics Sourcebook,* American Veterinary Medical Association, Schaumburg, IL.

KOI COLORS

Koi are classified by the colors and patterns on their back (dorsum). The 15 major classifications of koi listed below are based on color (13 classes) and scalation (2 types). There can be many variations within each major classification. For judging koi competitions, similar-colored koi are grouped together according to their sizes. Judges compare each fish's body conformation, quality of colors, and pattern to determine the best of each classification. The best quality koi will have deep pigmentation of each color, with distinct edges. Many pet koi do not meet the exact criteria of the perfect show koi color patterns, but will be identifiable as similar to one of the following classes.

Kohaku – This is the classic koi color pattern. It is a snow-white (shiro) fish with a red (hi) patched pattern along its body. The red should start at the head and make interesting patterns down to the caudal peduncle. The fins should be all-white.

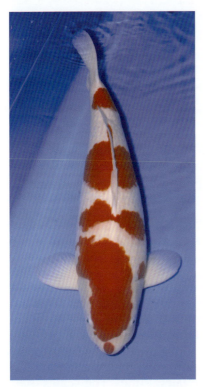

Yon Dan (four-step) color pattern on a Kohaku koi.

Photograph courtesy of Pan Intercorp - koi.com

Taisho Sanke (or Sanshoku) – This is the classic three-color koi, presented to Emperor Yoshihito (Taisho era 1912-1926) at the Tokyo Taisho Exhibition held in 1914. It is a snow-white (shiro) koi with red patches (hi) – like the Kohaku – plus smaller glossy black (sumi) spots. The sumi preferably should not occur on the head. The fins may be all-white or have a few black stripes.

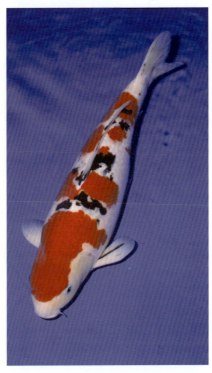

Taisho Sanke

Photograph courtesy of Pan Intercorp- koi.com

Showa Sanshoku – First produced in 1927, during the Showa era (1926-1989) of Emperor Hirohito, this tricolor koi has predominant black (sumi) areas that extend from the nose or head to the tail, and onto the pectoral and caudal fins. The red (hi) and white (shiro) markings blend with the black along the body. The amount of white is less and the black is more than on the Sanke. A new-style Showa called Kindai has less black on the body, similar to a Sanke, but the black extends onto the head.

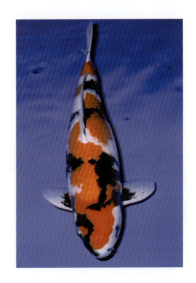

Showa Sanshoku

Photograph courtesy of Pan Intercorp - koi.com

Tancho – These are Kohaku, Sanke, or Showa koi that have a single red mark (hi) on the head only. It is named after the Tancho crane (*Grus japonensis*), the national bird of Japan, which is black and white with a round red mark on its head. Tancho koi with the Kinginrin and Doitsu scale patterns are also included in this class.

Kinginrin (golden silvery scales) – This describes a sparkling or pearly pattern of the scales. It gives each individual scale an iridescence, rather than a uniform shine as in the Hikari (metallic) color patterns. This category is divided into two classes. Class A contains only Kinginrin Kohaku, Sanke, and Showa koi (the Gosanke, or "Big Three Families"). Other colors of koi with this type of scales are judged in class B.

Doitsu (Japanese for "Deutsche," meaning German) – This scale pattern developed from crossing scaleless German carp sent to Japan in 1904 with koi. Doitsu koi have only two rows of scales along the dorsum or may also have some scales along the lateral line. Some judges include only Doitsu Kohaku, Sanke, and Showa in this class. Others include all color patterns with Doitsu scales except for Shusui, which have their own class.

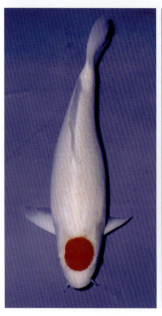
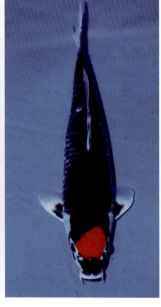

Tancho Kohaku   Tancho Showa

Photographs courtesy of
Pan Intercorp - koi.com

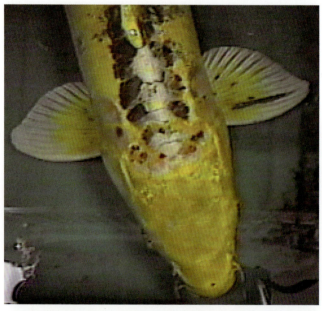

This Doitsu koi has a dark pigmented double row of scales down its dorsum, while the rest of the body is scaleless.

Bekko (tortoise-shell) – The name comes from the black markings on tortoise shells. These are non-metallic white body (shiro), red body (aka), or yellow body (ki) koi with small black marks (sumi) along the dorsum. There should be no sumi on the head or ventral to the lateral line. The scales may be normal, Kinginrin, or Doitsu patterns, although only the normal-scaled (wagoi) Bekko are judged in this class. Metallic Bekkos are part of the Hikari Moyo class.

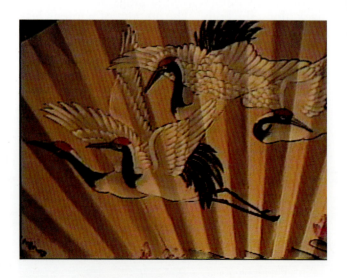

Japanese fan painted with Tancho Cranes.

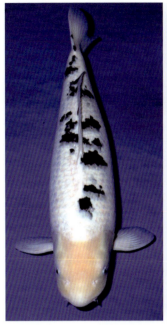
Shiro Bekko

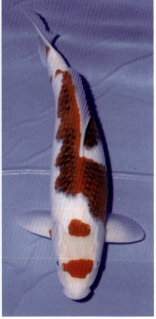
Sumigoromo

Photographs courtesy of
Pan Intercorp - koi.com

Utsuri (reflection) – Like the Bekko, these are two-color koi: black with either white, red, or yellow as the second color. The difference is that in Utsuri the black is the base color, extending onto the head and around the sides of the body. The bases of the pectoral fins should be black (motogoro). The other color (the reflected color) is white in Shiro Utsuri, red in Hi Utsuri, and yellow in Ki Utsuri. Normal-scaled (wagoi) and Kinginrin Utsuri are judged in this class. Metallic Usturi have their own class, Hikari Utsuri.

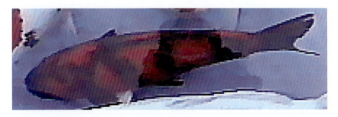
Hi Utsuri

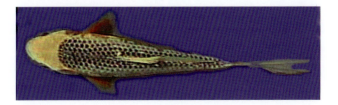
Asagi

Asagi (light blue) – This is one of the earliest color patterns developed from the original Japanese black carp (Magoi). They are nonmetallic light blue or blue-gray color, with each scale lighter-colored along its edge. This gives the dorsum a netlike pattern. The sides of the head and body should be red (hi) below the lateral line. The hi should extend onto the base of the fins.

Shusui (autumn water) – This is the Doitsu-scaled Asagi. It was first produced by Professor Yoshigoro Akiyama of the Japanese National Fisheries Institute in 1909 by crossing an Asagi koi with the German-scaled common carp. It is the only Doitsu koi to be classed by itself. The scaleless head and sides are pale blue, with the row of scales along the dorsum and lateral lines a darker blue color. The jaw and sides below the lateral lines are red, as are the bases of the fins. If red spots occur above the lateral line they are called Hana (flowery) Shusui, or Hi Shusui if the red extends up to the dorsal row of blue scales.

Koromo or Goromo (robed) – These koi were bred from Kohaku crossed with Asagi. The pattern is the Kohaku white body with red patches. The difference from Kohaku is that the red scales are edged with a darker color (robed). The Aigoromo (blue-robed) has red scales edged in indigo blue (ai). The Sumigoromo has red scales edged with black (sumi). Budogoromo (grape-robed) have red scales that are both edged with a grape color and look like a bunch of burgundy grapes. Koromo koi with sumi markings on the white areas also are called Budo Sanke, Koromo Sanke, or Koromo Showa depending on the extent of the black. These are judged in the Kawarigoi class, however. Metallic Koromo are classed with the Hikari Moyo.

Kawarigoi (different koi) – Non-metallic koi that do not fit into any of the above classifications are lumped into this group. There are a great number of koi varieties in this class, but the most common are: Karasugoi (crow carp) which are entirely ebony black; Hajiro which are black except for white on the edges of the fins; Benigoi, pure red koi, Shiro Muji, pure white koi, Kigoi, yellow koi, Chagoi, tea-colored koi, Soragoi, gray-blue koi, and Midorigoi, green koi; Matsubagoi (pinecone carp) which are single-color koi that have darker centers to each scale giving them a pinecone pattern; and Kage (shadow) patterns which have a black shaded pattern over the shiro or hi markings of Utsuri or Showa koi.

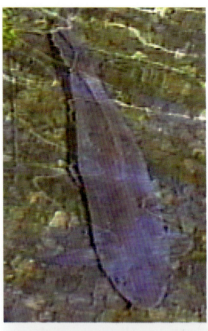

Having a Karasugoi in the koi pond is considered to be good luck by many koi enthusiasts, maybe because you are lucky if you see it!

Goshiki

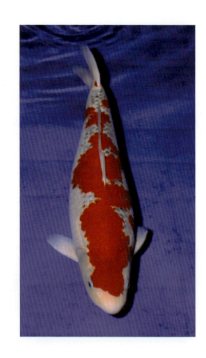

Photograph courtesy of Pan Intercorp - koi.com

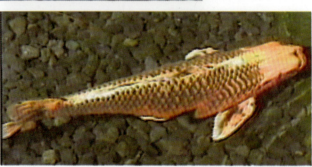

Kin Matsubagoi

Hikari Muji (metallic, single color) – This category includes all solid-color koi with a metallic luster. They are fully scaled and can have the Matsuba (pinecone) coloration to the scales. The head and fins should have the same hue as the body. Some of the colors are Platinum Ogon, a bright white; Yamabuki Ogon, yellow-gold; Orenji Ogon, metallic orange; Kin (gold) Matsuba; and Gin (silver) Matsuba.

The Kumonryu (dragon fish) is a Doitsu black and white Kawarigoi, often having a black body with a white head and white on the fins. The Goshiki, the only five-color koi (red, white, black, blue, and indigo) is included in this class, but in Japan it is judged separately.

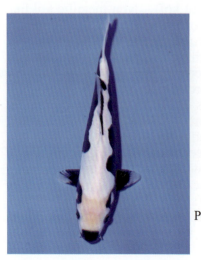

Kumonryu Dragon Fish

Photograph courtesy of Pan Intercorp - koi.com

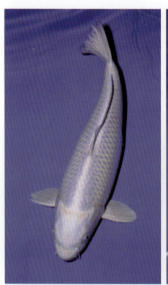
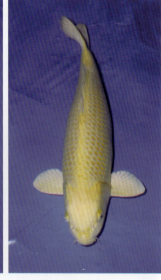

Platinum Ogon   Yamabuki Ogon

Photographs courtesy of Pan Intercorp - koi.com

Hikari Utsuri (metallic, reflection) – These are the metallic varieties of the Utsuri and Showa koi, which all have prominent sumi markings. They are called Kin Showa, Gin Shiro Utsuri, Kin Hi Utsuri, and Kin Ki Utsuri.

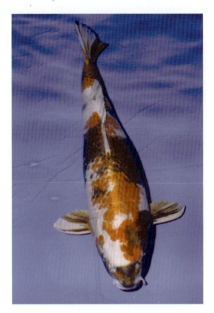

Kin Showa

Photograph courtesy of Pan Intercorp - koi.com

Hikari Moyo (metallic, patterns) – Any multicolored koi with a metallic sheen except for Showa and Utsuri fall into this category. Some of these colors are Yamato-Nishiki, a metallic Taisho Sanke; Hariwake, a metallic white with metallic ki pattern; Sakura (cherry blossom) Ogon, a metallic white with metallic hi pattern; Kikusui (chrysanthemum water), a metallic Doitsu Kohaku; and Kujaku (peacock) Ogon, which is platinum white with hi markings and Matsuba scales.

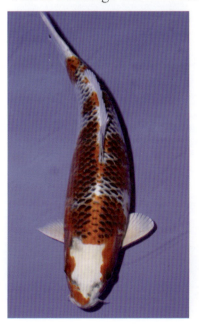

Kujaku

Photograph courtesy of Pan Intercorp - koi.com

This is a simplified listing of the koi varieties most commonly seen. Undoubtedly there will be new color varieties in the future. A new koi variety has been developed for the current emperor of Japan, Hirohito's son Akahito. It is a Doitsu metallic three-color (Taisho Sanke pattern) koi named for the Heisei era of Akahito's reign (since 1989), "Heisei-Nishiki."

Koi popularity is steadily increasing all over the world, and koi production continuously increases to meet the demand. In the early 1980s the long-finned Butterfly Koi was developed. While not allowed to enter into koi shows in Japan yet, it is very popular with American hobbyists. Many US koi shows have separate judging categories for the long-finned Butterfly Koi. Who could resist the beautiful sight of the mix of Kohaku, Sanke, Kin Showa, Ki Bekko, Aigoromo, Butterfly Ogon, Shusui, and Doitsu Hariwake swimming gracefully in a crystal clear koi pond?

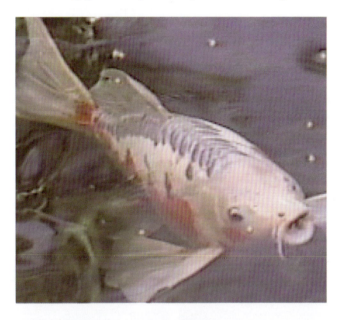

Butterfly Shusui

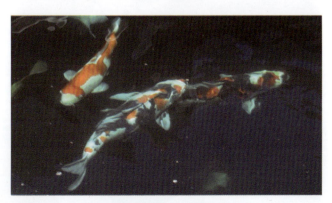

Kohaku and a pair of Showa koi

REFERENCES:

Associated Koi Clubs of America. 1998. *AKCA Koi Identification Poster,* Koi USA, Midway City, CA.

Axelrod, Herbert R. 1973. *Koi of the World: Japanese Colored Carp,* T.F.H. Publications, Neptune, NJ.

Axelrod, Herbert R. 1988. *Koi Varieties: Japanese Colored Carp - Nishikigoi,* T.F.H. Publications, Neptune, NJ.

Axelrod, Herbert R., Eugene Balon, Richard C. Hoffman, Shmuel Rothbard, and Giora W. Wohlfarth. 1996. *The Completely Illustrated Guide to Koi for Your Pond,* T.F.H. Publications, Neptune, NJ.

Fletcher, Nick. 1999. *The Ultimate Koi,* Howell Book House, New York.

James, Barry. 1985. *A Fishkeeper's Guide to Koi,* Tetra Press, Morris Plains, NJ.

Koi USA. 1995. *Practical Koi Keeping, volume III,* Koi USA, Midway City, CA.

McDowell, Anne (editor). 1989. *The Tetra Encyclopedia of Koi,* Tetra Press, Morris Plains, NJ.

Tamadachi, Michugo. 1994. *The Cult of the Koi,* 2nd ed., T.F.H. Publications, Neptune, NJ.

Waddington, Peter. 1995. *Koi Kichi,* Infiltration, Golborne, Warrington, Cheshire, UK.

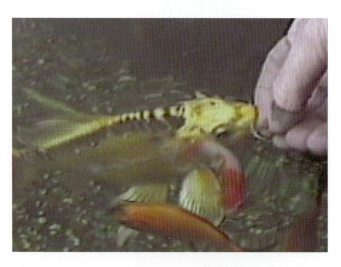

Koi can be tame enough to eat out of a person's hand, and even be petted!

Koi will often swim in school formation in a large pond.

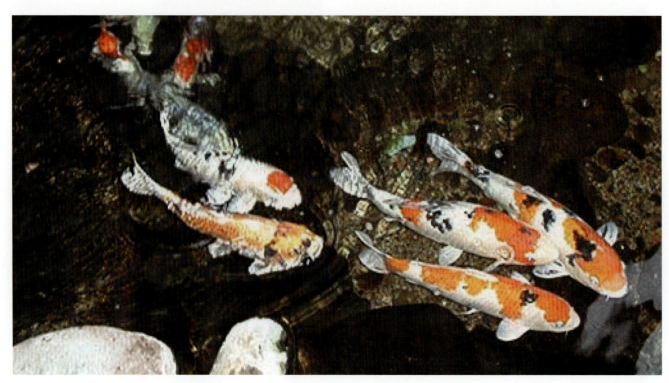

KOI BREEDING AND GENETICS

BREEDING

In outdoor ponds in temperate climates, koi grow about 6-8 inches (15-20 cm) per year when young, much slower when mature. Males usually are sexually mature at 2 years of age, females at 3 years. Both the growth and maturation rates are temperature-dependent, so the rates will increase in tropical areas or with koi kept in warm water year-around. In these cases koi will grow 10-14 inches (25-36 cm) in a year.

When the females become sexually mature, at about 12-18 inches (30-46 cm) in length, their abdomens become visibly distended with ova, making them appear stockier than the slimmer, tapered-bodied males. The female may also have a visibly enlarged genital papilla. The males of all Cyprinid fish get nuptial tubercles (small raised bumps) on the surface of the operculum and pectoral fins during breeding season. In koi, these may be very slight and hardly noticeable.

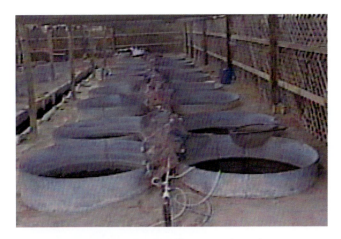

Breeding containers at a koi farm. Each vat has a water inlet and bottom drain. They are covered with shade cloth, and have netting that can be pulled over them to prevent predation and keep the fish from jumping out.

studies more difficult. Add floating spawning mats on which the female will lay the adhesive eggs. These can be made from floating aquatic plants or synthetic fiber mats. Several types are available commercially. The female will swim around under the spawning material when ready to lay. The male will push against her side with his body, expressing her eggs. The female may lay 50,000-100,000 beige eggs per pound of body weight on the spawning mats. The male follows her closely, spraying the eggs with milt. The eggs are 2-3 millimeters (mm) diameter, and will hatch in about 7 days at 63°F / 17°C, in 5 days at 70°F / 21°C, in 4 days at 75°F / 24°C, and in 3 days at 80°F / 26.7°C.

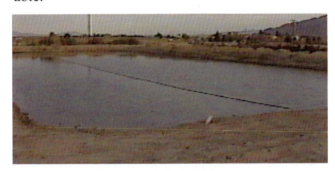

Grow-out pond at a California koi farm. An airline runs across the center of the pond providing aeration through airstones in the pond.

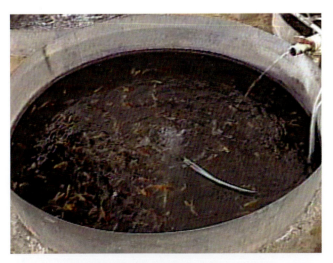

Koi fry in the breeding container. Each container has an airstone for aeration as well as a constant fresh water inflow, and a bottom drain for water circulation.

Prior to breeding, the koi should be prophylacticly treated against diseases (e.g., 2% salt dips, 0.3% salt in the pond, and formalin/malachite green treatments). Feed the breeders a high-protein diet (35-45% protein content) to ensure they are in good condition for spawning. Separate the best-colored pairs of koi into well-aerated breeding containers or ponds containing 300-500 gallons of water each. Use one or two males for each female. Multiple males increase egg fertilization rates, but make genetic

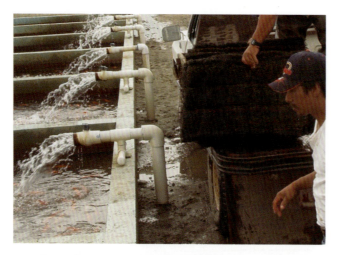

Spawning mats with eggs are being removed from shallow breeding ponds and placed on a truck bed to be transferred into a large grow-out pond.

Koi spawn when cooler water temperature is slowly raised above 63°F / 17°C. Usually the spawning occurs in the morning. After the eggs are laid and fertilized, the spawning media should be removed to hatching ponds or tanks, or if the mating occurred in fry-rearing tanks, then the adults are removed and the spawning mats left for the eggs to hatch. Adults will eat the eggs and fry (baby fish) as they forage for food if left together.

Change 25-50% of the water in the breeding pond or tank after the parents are removed to dilute out the excess milt. The added water should be of the same temperature and pH as in the breeding pond, and previously dechlorinated and aerated. The water temperature in the fry-rearing pond must stay fairly constant at all times.

Some of the eggs may not be fertilized and will turn opaque white within a day. These eggs are highly prone to saprophytic fungal infection by *Saprolegnia* or *Achlya*. Once these fungi start growing on dead eggs, they will rapidly spread and will affect even healthy fertilized eggs. Methylene blue (4 milligrams [mg] per gallon of pond water daily for 3 days), malachite green (0.38 mg per gallon of water), or hydrogen peroxide 3% (1 milliliter [ml] per gallon of water) can be added to the fry rearing pond to prevent fungal infection of the eggs.

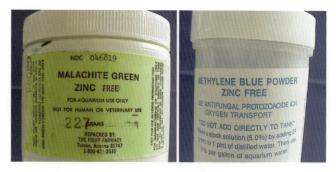

Malachite green and methylene blue, as well as hydrogen peroxide, are effective antifungal medications that can be added to koi ponds.

After the eggs hatch, the fry are 6 mm long and will attach themselves to a solid surface and hang vertically for 2 or 3 days to continue their development. At this stage the mouth, gills, and swim bladder still have not fully developed. They have a yolk sac to sustain them during this time. When the yolk sac is absorbed, they become free-swimming and search for their first meal.

Live foods such as microscopic protozoa known as infusoria, plus rotifers, or small crustacea like brine shrimp nauplii and daphnia can be used as first foods. Other fry foods consist of commercial liquid fry food, finely powdered flake fish foods, powdered milk, yolk of a hard-boiled

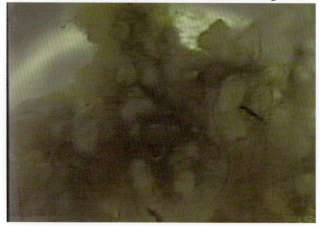

Mass of koi eggs infected with fungus.

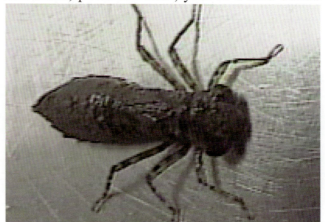

Koi fry are vulnerable to aquatic insects such as this dragonfly larva. Ponds should be preventively treated to ensure fry safety.

egg, and planktonic algae. Food is given frequently throughout the day, every 2-3 hours, but care must be taken not to overfeed and pollute the water.

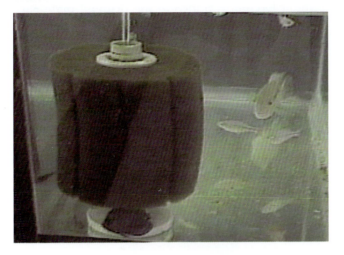

Foam filters are safe to use with fish fry.

Foam filters run by air pumps can be placed in the fry tank to aid biological filtration, as these tend not to suck baby fish into the filter media. Keep water agitation to a minimum initially because the fry are not very strong swimmers. Increase filtration as the fry grow stronger. Perform gradual water changes daily or every other day. Use netting over the drain tube to prevent fry getting sucked out, and remove some of the old water as fresh dechlorinated water is added, maintaining a constant water level.

It is always advisable to keep records of each spawning: the date, water temperature, which fish were bred, their age and size, and expected color of progeny. Photographs of the parents can be kept for comparison to the offspring. Referring back to the parent stock after seeing the offspring can tell more about the genetics (genotype) of the parents. Implanting microchip transponders into the adult koi provides a permanent means of identification of each breeder fish.

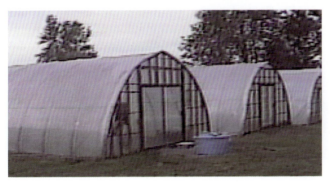

ARTIFICIAL BREEDING

Several techniques have been tried to stimulate koi to breed at a certain time. One is to inject the mature parent koi with carp pituitary extract (CPE), a substance that is taken from the pituitary portion of the brain and contains a gonadotropic hormone (GtH) that will stimulate reproduction. This is injected intramuscularly into the female koi at a dose of 2-5 milligrams (mg) per kilogram (kg) of body weight. The injection is repeated in 9 hours at 75°F / 24°C, or 12 hours at 68°F / 20°C. The male is injected one time, at 2 mg/kg. Spawning should commence within 1-2 days after the injections, assuming other environmental conditions are right. The eggs can also be manually removed by hand-stripping 24 hours after the first injection is given.

Gonadotropin Releasing Hormone (GnRH) has also been used to stimulate an increase in endogenous GtH production. It is given at 10-15 micrograms (µg) per kg 14 hours prior to desired spawning time. Human Chorionic Gonadotropin (HCG) at 20-30 IU/kg, given twice, 6 hours apart, has been used extensively in other fish species to induce spawning, and may be effective in koi. It is best to tranquilize the koi when handling and injecting them to reduce possible trauma.

Hand-stripping of eggs and milt by gentle abdominal pressure has been used by some koi breeders. It is best to withhold food for 24 hours prior to hand-stripping koi to prevent fecal contamination of the eggs or milt. An anesthetic can be used to allow safe handling of the fish. Once anesthetized, the koi is gently blotted dry (without removing the slime coat) to avoid pre-activation of the eggs by water contamination.

Hold the koi along the body with the right arm, the right hand under the belly, and the left hand holding onto the caudal peduncle. Then the ripe female fish is held over a plastic container and the eggs (roe) are carefully milked out by gently squeezing the abdomen and stroking toward the vent. Be sure the eggs do not become contaminated with water or feces. Then the selected male has his milt expressed into a separate sterilized glass container. Some 0.9% physiologic saline solution is added to the milt at a ratio of 1 part milt to 3 parts saline. There should be 2-5 ml of milt for

Covered grow-out ponds can extend the growing season through the winter in colder climates, allowing young koi to grow by as much as 10-14" per year.

every liter of roe, or at least 8 ml of the diluted milt solution per liter of roe. One liter (1 kilogram) of eggs contains about 600,000-800,000 eggs.

The expressed eggs can be stored for up to 8 hours at 66-70°F / 19-21°C prior to being fertilized. Expressed milt can be stored for 8-10 hours at 66-70°F / 19-21°C or for 24 hours if refrigerated at 39-43°F / 4-6°C. The eggs and milt are gently mixed together with a plastic spoon, then the fertilized eggs are placed into a prepared rearing pond, or into fry vats.

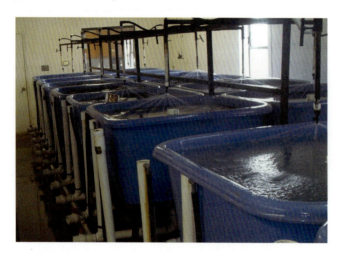

A measured quantity of fertilized eggs is added to each fry vat. Fresh water is continuously added from overhead sprays, and the overflow tube has fine screen mesh over it. Fry remain here until large enough to transfer to an outdoor grow-out pond.

If the eggs are to be hatched in glass or plastic jar incubators, they can be rendered nonadhesive by using Woynarovich's solution (1 liter [L] water, 3 grams [g] non-iodized salt, and 4 g of urea). Gently stir 100 ml of this solution per liter of eggs into the fertilized eggs, slowly adding more solution until the eggs are separate and suspended. Stir gently for 3-5 minutes, then let the eggs soak and swell for an hour, stirring every 10 minutes. After the soaking period, the eggs are rinsed in a 0.1% solution of tannic acid in water, for a few seconds. Then pour off the solution and rinse the eggs with clean water. Place these eggs in jar incubators at a temperature of 68-77°F / 20-25°C. The eggs are kept circulating by gentle air flow from an airstone on the bottom of the jar. When the eggs have hatched (4-5 days), transfer the fry to the rearing pond, vat or aquarium.

Once a male koi is identified as having both an exceptional phenotype and genotype, by monitoring the growth and color of its progeny, its milt can be manually stripped and stored frozen in liquid nitrogen canisters to be used for future breeding. The frozen sperm could also be traded or sold to other breeders to mix with their eggs, without having to transport the original male parent fish.

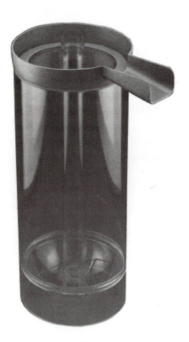

Catalog photograph of an egg incubating jar. Fresh water and air flow down center tube to aerate the water and keep eggs suspended.

CULLING

The process known as culling is to remove deformed, weak, or poorly colored fry, to make more room for the best fry. Overcrowded fry will resort to cannibalism, with the stronger koi (called "tobi" by Japanese breeders) eating their smaller cohorts. Baby koi should be separated by size and color, starting at about 2 weeks of age. Use a small shallow net to hold and view each baby koi. Remove poor quality or deformed koi, and separate the others into groups based on color and size. Plastic bowls or boxes filled with fry pond water can be floated in the pond and the sorted fry are placed into these. Then the selected fry are transferred into grow-out ponds with fry of similar size and color. After a period of repeated thinning by culling, professional koi breeders will have kept only about 7-10% of the initial number of fry.

Colors develop at different ages in fry. Showa Sanshoku are separated as predominantly black fry at 14 days of age. Ogon koi are selected as entirely metallic fry by 50 days of age. Taisho

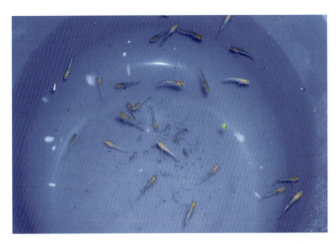

At a few weeks, koi fry are culled, separating the black, black and white, all white, and metallic colorations.

Sanke are white with red and black dots, and Kohaku are red or red and white, by 60 days of age. At this age they will be 2-3 inches (5-7.5 cm) long. By the time the fry are 4 months old, they should be 4-6 inches (10-15 cm) long, and their future color type can be determined. Tategoi are koi that pass through the culling process as having potential for good color development.

GENETICS

Molecules of deoxyribonucleic acid (DNA) contained in units called genes determine the physical characteristics of an organism. These visible physical characteristics are called the phenotype, while the unseen gene makeup is the genotype. Long twisted strands of genes form chromosomes, of which each species of organism has a specific number and type. The chromosomes are arranged in matched pairs in the cell nucleus. In sexual reproduction, one of each pair of chromosomes comes from the mother (egg) and the other half from the father (sperm). Therefore the haploid number of chromosomes (n) is equal to the number of chromosomes contributed by each parent, and the diploid number of chromosomes (2n) is equal to the total number of chromosomes.

Koi have a diploid (2n) number of 100, or 50 pairs of chromosomes. Each pair of chromosomes is identical except for the sex chromosomes. In this pair of chromosomes, the female has two identical chromosomes called XX; the male has two different chromosomes, one X and one Y. When the chromosome pairs split, half of the male's sperm will carry the X chromosome, and half will carry the Y chromosome. Each of the female's eggs will have one haploid X chromosome. If a sperm with the X chromosome fertilizes the egg, the embryo will be diploid XX and will develop into a female. If the Y sperm fertilizes the egg, it will be diploid XY and will become a male.

Inbreeding is the mating of closely related individuals: brother to sister, or offspring to parent. It is done in domesticated animals in order to strengthen desirable characteristics. However some undesirable inheritable traits may be increased at the same time. Inbreeding is necessary to some extent in selective breeding programs, but "outbreeding" of unrelated individuals should be encouraged as much as possible.

The genetics of koi coloration and scalation are rather complicated, and not fully understood. Breeding two Kohaku parents will not produce all Kohaku babies. In one study by Mr. Z. Kulikovski of Mag-Noy in Israel, sample breedings of two Kohaku produced about 10% Kohaku, 51% tricolor (Sanke and Showa), 16% Shiro Bekko, 4% orange (Orenji) koi, and 18% white or pale koi. These results are based on phenotypes without knowing the actual genotypes.

Two koi of similar phenotypes (Kohaku for example) may have different genotypes – one could be homozygous for Kohaku, the other heterozygous, carrying tricolor genes. Until enough detailed study is done to identify actual genotype, rather than just the phenotype of each individual, it will be difficult to predict offspring colors from any given fish. In order for this to happen, individual fish would need to be permanently identified by a dependable method, such as microchip transponder implantation. Then records would be kept of the matings between two identified koi. All of the offspring would need to be raised to a sufficient size to accurately determine their phenotype. If this were impossible to do, a random sampling of a statistically sufficient number of fry could then be raised until large enough to determine phenotype. Deformed fry and fry that have unexplained mortalities must also be taken into account, as there may be a genetic basis for this.

With enough matings, the genetic code could be determined for the parents. This is unlikely to occur by professional breeders, as economics will not allow them to keep all the offspring, but only the desirable color patterns. It would be an excellent project, however, for the advanced hobbyist or university student. If data were published in koi magazines, geneticists could compile enough information to predict possible genotypes for each phenotype.

SCALE GENETICS IN KOI

Koi scalation is controlled by two genes: **S** (scales) and **N** (abnormal-scales). The diploid pairing of genes will have two of each type of gene, one allele from each parent. A capital letter represents a dominant gene and a lower case letter represents a recessive gene. If the alleles of the genes are the same (both dominant or both recessive) the gene is termed homozygous. If they are different (one dominant and one recessive allele), the gene is heterozygous. Recessive genes only affect the physical appearance (phenotype) when they are homozygous. Heterozygous genotypes will have the phenotype of the dominant gene.

Normally scaled koi (Wagoi) have the scale gene turned on, and the abnormal-scales gene turned off. A normally scaled fish phenotype would have genotype of **SS nn** or **Ss nn**. Since the **S** is dominant, it will show up in the phenotype (visible appearance) whether the genotype is homozygous **SS** or heterozygous **Ss**. The **nn** genotype indicates the lack of abnormal scales (i.e., normal scales).

Koi with abnormal scales would therefore have **NN** or **Nn** genotype, however it is believed that the **NN** genotype is so abnormal that these fish don't survive embryonic development. So, all abnormal scaled koi will have an **Nn** genotype.

There are nine possible genotypes with the two genes controlling scale type. These produce four different phenotypes: normal scales (Wagoi); normal-sized scales only down the back and down the lateral line (Doitsu); enlarged mirror-like scales down the back and possibly on the sides (Kagamigoi); and scaleless or leather skinned koi (Kawagoi) that may sometimes have a few small scales only by the dorsal fin.

Genotype – Phenotype

SS nn – homozygous genotype; normal scaled (Wagoi) phenotype
SS NN – lethal homozygous genotype; does not survive embryonic development
SS Nn – scales only down the dorsum and lateral line (Doitsu)
Ss nn – normal scaled (wagoi) phenotype
Ss NN – lethal genotype; does not survive embryonic development
Ss Nn – heterozygous genotype; scales only down the dorsum and lateral line (Doitsu)
ss nn – homozygous recessive genotype; mirror scaled (Kagamigoi) phenotype
ss NN – lethal homozygous genotype; does not survive embryonic development
ss Nn – leather skinned (Kawagoi) phenotype

Using the Punnet Square method, the probabilities of the genotypes of the progeny can be determined if the parents' genotypes are known. Analyzing the offspring's phenotypes can also help to determine the parent's genotype as well. Each parent's possible combinations of alleles are placed on one side of the square. The offspring's possible genotypes from each of the parent's possible alleles are within the squares, and the frequency of occurrence determines their probability.

Parents	Male S n	S n	s n	s n
Female s N	Progeny Ss Nn	Ss Nn	ss Nn	ss Nn
s N	Ss Nn	Ss Nn	ss Nn	ss Nn
s n	Ss nn	Ss nn	ss nn	ss nn
s n	Ss nn	Ss nn	ss nn	ss nn

> This example shows all the probable results of a crossbreeding between a male heterozygous normally scaled wagoi (Ss nn) crossed with a female leather kawagoi (ss Nn). This should produce offspring that are 25% Doitsu koi (Ss Nn), 25% leather kawagoi (ss Nn), 25% heterozygous wagoi (Ss nn), and 25% homozygous kagamigoi (ss nn).

REFERENCES:

Argent Chemical Laboratory. 1985. *A Guide to Induced Spawning, Maturation and Sex Reversal in Aquaculture*, Argent Chemical Laboratory, Redmond, WA.

Axelrod, Herbert R. 1988. *Koi Varieties: Japanese Colored Carp - Nishikigoi*, T.F.H. Publications, Neptune, NJ.

Axelrod, Herbert R., Eugene Balon, Richard C. Hoffman, Shmuel Rothbard, and Giora W. Wohlfarth. 1996. *The Completely Illustrated Guide to Koi For Your Pond*, T.F.H. Publications, Neptune, NJ.

Caswell, Bertrelle. 1979. *Spawning of Koi*, Ventura County Koi Society Lecture, Ventura, CA.

Fujita, Grant. 1989. *Koi,* 2nd ed., AKCA, Midway City, CA.

Gratzek, John B. (editor). 1992. *Aquariology: Fish Breeding and Genetics,* Tetra Press, Morris Plains, NJ.

McDowall, Anne. 1989. *The Tetra Encyclopedia of Koi*, Tetra Press, Morris Plains, NJ.

Nelson, Joseph S. 2006. *Fishes of the World*, John Wiley & Sons, Hoboken, NJ.

Penzes, Bethen and Istvan Tolg. 1983. *Goldfish and Ornamental Carp*, Barron's Educational Series, Woodbury, NY.

Rothbard, Schmuel. 1997. *Koi Breeding,* T.F.H. Publications, Neptune, NJ.

Schroder, J. 1976. *Genetics for the Aquarist*, T.F.H. Publications, Neptune, NJ.

Stoskopf, Michael K. 1993. *Fish Medicine,* W.B. Saunders, Philadelphia.

Tamadachi, Michugo. 1994. *The Cult of the Koi*, T.F.H. Publications, Neptune, NJ.

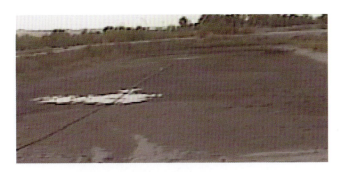

Typical shallow, earthen grow-out pond. These are drained and allowed to dry out between batches of fry in order to reduce disease transmission and aquatic insects.

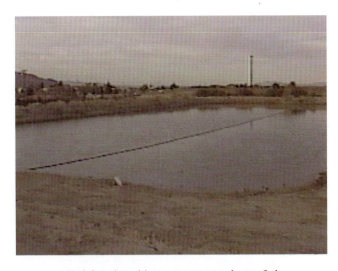

Koi fry placed in grow-out ponds are fed commercial foods regularly to increase growth rate and prevent cannibalism.

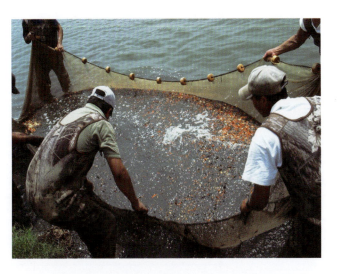

Fry are seined from the grow-out pond on a regular basis to cull and sort by size and color.

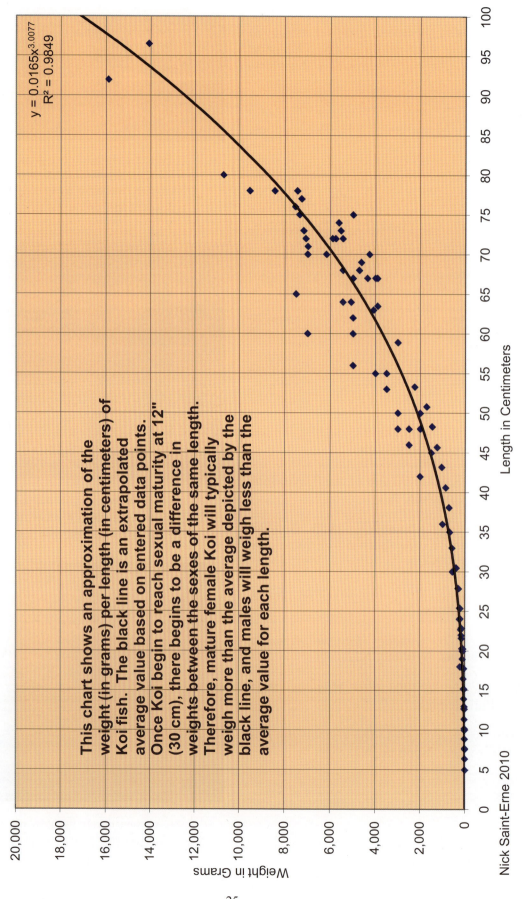

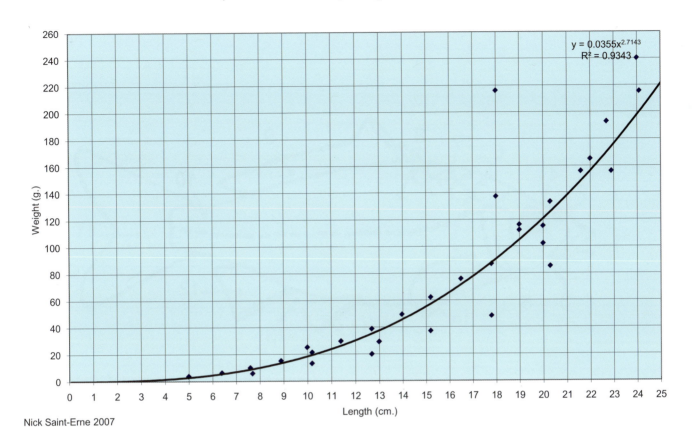

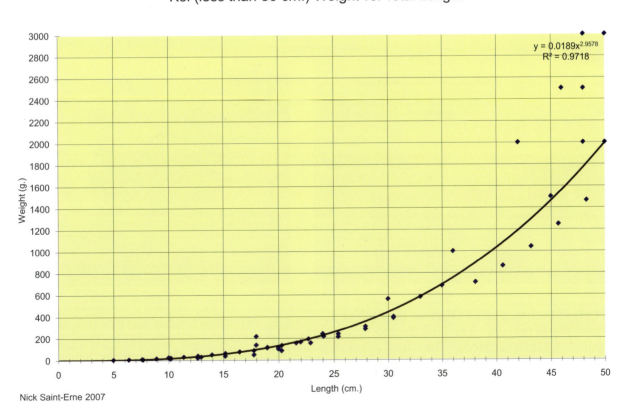

ANATOMY OF KOI

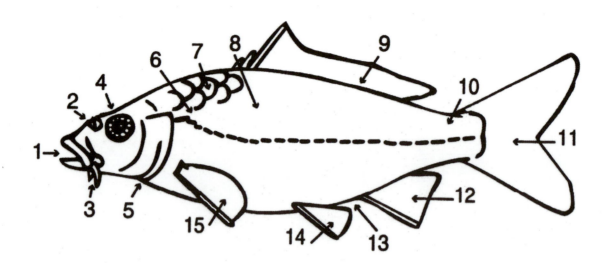

EXTERNAL ANATOMY

Mouth (1) - Koi have no teeth in their jaws. The upper jaw consists of the premaxilla and maxilla bones, and the lower jaw bone is the mandible. Their mouth is protrusible, with fleshy lips.

Nostrils (2) - Each nostril or naris is divided by a septum into an anterior inlet and posterior outlet. Water enters into an olfactory sac filled with scent-detector cells. Butterfly koi may have a very large fleshy median septum rotruding from the nostril.

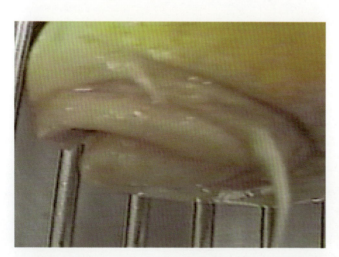

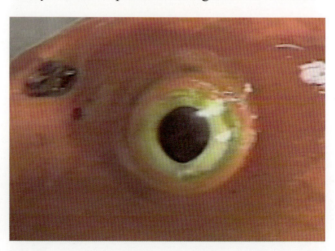

Barbels (3) - Two pairs of barbels extend ventrally from the upper lip. The barbels and lips have taste buds on their surfaces. The front (upper) barbel is half as long as the second (lower) barbel.

Eye (4) - The lens of the eye is spherical, giving fish a wide angle of vision. They have both rod and cone cells in the retina, so they can see colors. Fish have no eyelids.

27

Operculum (5) - This is a hinged bony plate covered with epithelium that opens and closes to pull water from the mouth and across the gills, and out the gill slit. It consists of the preopercle, interopercle, opercle, and subopercle bones, and the branchiostegal membrane.

Lateral line (6) - This is a groove on each side of the fish lined with neuromast receptors that can detect low-frequency vibrations (1-200 Hertz) in water, caused by sound or motion. This vibration detection allows the fish to be aware of objects in the water even if it is too dark or muddy to see.

Scales (7) - Calcified flexible cycloid plates, consisting of collagen fibers, albuminoid materials, and hydroxyapatite crystals. Growth rings are added frequently as the fish grows, and are not an indicator of age. The scales come from the dermis layer of the skin and are covered with a thin layer of epidermis. Koi do not have scales on the head. There are usually 37-39 scales along body at the lateral line, and 6 rows of scales above that and 6 below. The scales over the lateral line have holes through them to allow vibrations to pass through to the neuromast receptors. There is a total of about 800-900 scales on the body of a koi.

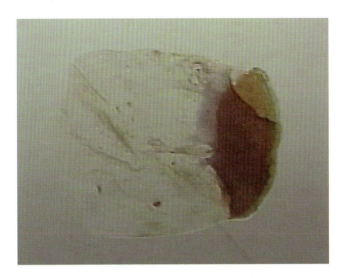

The above scale shows the posterior exposed section (right edge) covered with pigmented epidermis. The clear anterior part of the scale is embedded in the dermis.

Below is a microscopic photograph of an edge of a koi scale that shows the many growth rings that encircle the scale. The rings are added at the periphery as the scale grows. If a scale is lost, it will regrow if the dermis is not damaged, and may not have rings in the center as it will grow continuously to its original size, not leaving rings that normally mark pauses in growth rate.

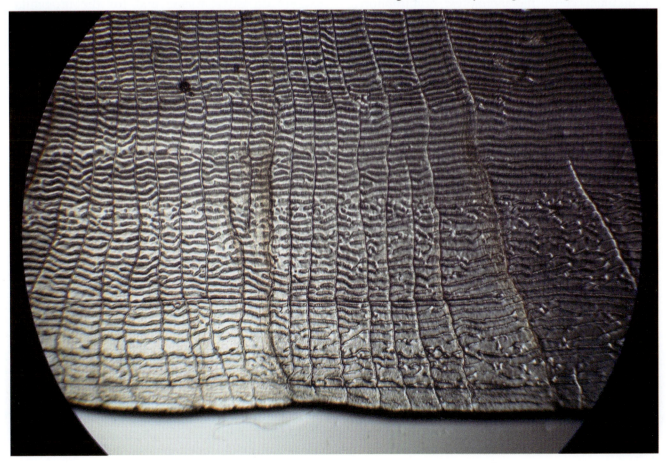

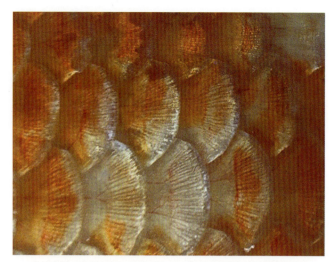

Section of skin showing orange and white pigmented epidermis covering the exposed portion of the overlapping scales. Each scale extends below 6 others.

Skin (8) - The skin is made of 3 layers: hypodermis, dermis, and epidermis. The hypodermis, or subcutaneous tissue, is a vascularized fatty layer covering the muscles. The dermis consists of fibrous connective tissue, blood vessels, nerves, osteogenic cells for scale production, scales, and chromatophores (pigment cells). There are 4 types of pigment cells: melanophores, erythrophores, xanthophores, and iridophores. The melanophores contain black melanin pigment, and can expand or contract under neurological control to darken or lighten the skin color. Erythrophores contain red and orange carotenoid and pteridine pigments that are obtained from the diet. Xanthophores contain yellow carotenoid pigments. The iridophores (also called iridocytes, or guanophores) contain crystalline deposits of guanine that produce the silvery glitter by reflecting light. The thin epidermis consists of a basal cell layer, fibrous epithelial cells, mucus-secreting goblet cells, leukocytes in the intracellular spaces, and some pigment cells. The skin is coated with a cuticle, or glycocalyx, which is a slimy mucus layer of mucopolysaccharide and sloughed epidermal cells. It protects the skin from pathogens, aids osmoregulation by reducing permeability of the skin, and helps the fish glide through the water by reducing friction.

Dorsal fin (9) - A single median fin having 3 stiff spines (2 small and 1 large), with 18-22 softer branched fin rays. It stabilizes the fish during forward motion. It can be held erect or fold down caudally against the dorsum by voluntary control.

Caudal peduncle (10) - The tail base contains the dorsal epural and ventral hypural bones, flat articulated plates that support the caudal fin.

Caudal fin (11) - Tail fin consisting of 17-19 soft fin rays, forked with equal lobes. It functions in rapid forward propulsion of the fish by strong side-to-side motions.

Anal fin (12) - Single median fin behind the vent, having 3 spines and 5 soft rays. It serves as a stabilizer during forward motion.

Vent (13) - External opening for the rectum to excrete digestive waste, and for the urogenital papilla, which is posterior to the rectum.

Pelvic (ventral) fins (14) - Paired fins having 2 spines and 8-9 soft rays. They stabilize the body against pitch and are used to counterbalance lift.

Pectoral fins (15) - Paired fins behind the gill plates having 1 spine and 15-18 soft rays. The multifunctional pectoral fins stabilize and steer the body when swimming forward, moving it up and down. They are also used for braking, and to swim backward, and can propel the fish forward slowly when searching for food.

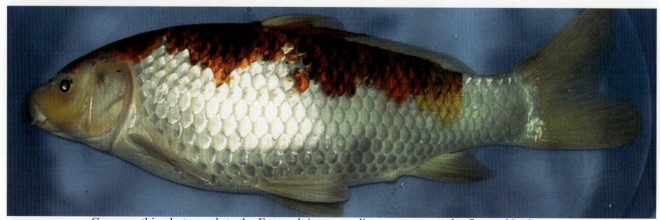

Compare this photograph to the External Anatomy diagram to name the fins and body areas.

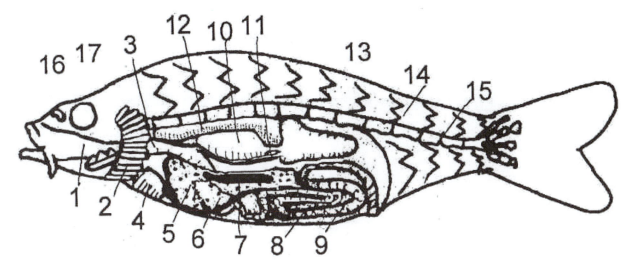

INTERNAL ANATOMY

Pharynx (1) - There are 3 rows of pharyngeal teeth in each of the lower pharyngeal ceratobranchial bones (modified 5th gill arches). These teeth grind against a thick masticating plate on the roof of the pharynx, attached to the basioccipital bone. The teeth are periodically shed and can often be found at the bottom of a koi pond.

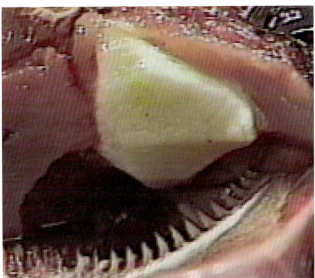

Masticating plate visible above the gill rakers.

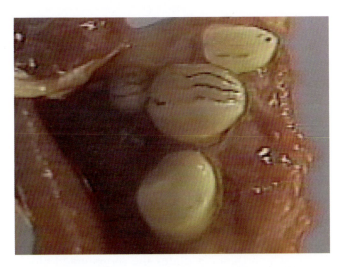
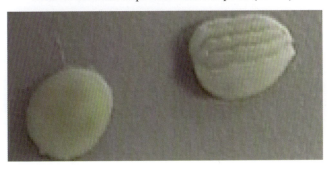

Teeth rows in ceratobranchial bone (above) and shed teeth found in plastic-lined koi pond (below).

Gills (2) - Gill filaments project in pairs from 4 bony gill arches on each side of the pharynx. The gill arches also have short, sharp gill rakers that extend into the pharynx. Each gill filament contains 2 rows of semicircular lamellae through which blood flows in short lamellar arteries. These small "leaves" have a very high surface area across which the water passes in a countercurrent direction to the blood flow. Oxygen diffuses from the water into the blood as the water passes over the gill lamellae. The red blood cells in the blood are very efficient oxygen transporters and 1 ml of blood will be able to carry the amount of oxygen contained in 15-25 ml of water. The gills also release carbon dioxide and ammonia from the blood into the water. In fish the gills are the main sites of ammonia and urea excretion, rather than through the kidneys.

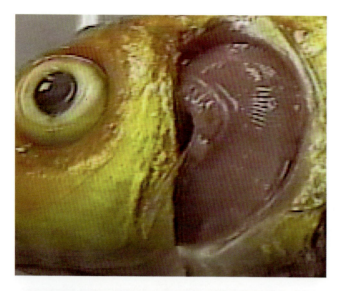

Necropsy on a koi showing position of the gills after removal of the operculum plate.

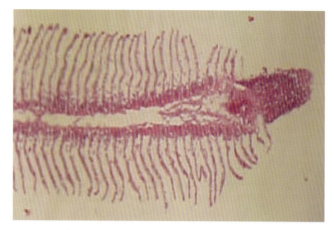

A microscopic photograph of an H&E Stained histology section of a normal gill filament. Note the thinness and separation of the lamellae extending from the filament.

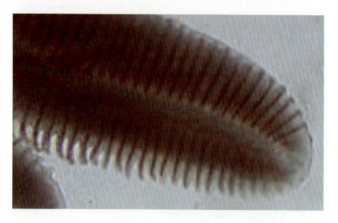

Microscopic photograph showing the clear central cartilage of a gill filament and the lamellae extending out on each side.

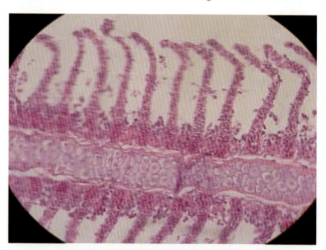

A microscopic photograph of an H&E Stained histology section of a normal gill filament. The cells of the cartilage are visible down the center of the filament.

Esophagus (3) - Food passes down the muscular esophagus directly into the intestines; koi have no glandular stomach and do not secrete digestive acids. The pneumatic duct arises from the dorsal surface of the anterior esophagus.

Heart (4) - The heart is below and just caudal to the gills in the pericardial cavity. It consists of the sinus venosus, atrium, ventricle, and bulbus arteriosus. Blood flows through paired sinoatrial valves from the sinus venosus into the atrium. Diastolic contraction of the thin-walled atrium forces blood through atrioventricular valves into the muscular ventricle. Systolic contraction of the ventricle pushes blood through a pair of semilunar ventriculobulbar valves into the bulbus arteriosus. Blood leaves the elastic bulbus arteriosus through the ventral aorta and goes to the gills to get oxygen and release carbon dioxide and ammonia. The blood passes up through the afferent branchial arteries to the gill lamellae to get oxygenated. The efferent branchial arteries join to form the dorsal aorta, which then circulates the oxygenated blood through the body via lateral arteries. The blood returns to the heart through the hepatic and cardinal veins and enters into the sinus venosus.

Liver (5) - There are 2 main liver lobes, united cranially, and 2 smaller accessory liver lobes. The liver is closely attached to the loops of the intestines. The liver produces bile, which is stored in the gallbladder. It also has some hematopoietic (blood forming) tissues, and stores glycogen.

Gallbladder (6) - The greenish colored gallbladder is within the right liver lobe. It stores bile produced by the liver, and empties it into the intestines through the common bile duct.

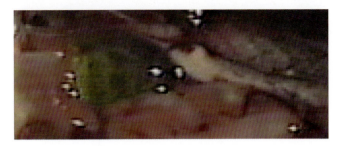

The gallbladder is the transparent green sac filled with bile that is embedded within the liver tissues.

Spleen (7) - The spleen is on the left side of the abdomen, covered by the left liver lobe. It is elongate and dark red in color in koi. It contains phagocytic and hematopoietic tissues.

Pancreas (8) - The pancreatic tissue is diffused within the liver tissue (hepatopancreas) and mesentery. It produces exocrine digestive enzymes and endocrine hormones.

Intestine (9) - The intestine of a koi runs from the esophagus to the vent. The intestine coils back on itself 6 times. A long recurving intestine allows better digestion of a herbivorous diet. It is normally light pink in color.

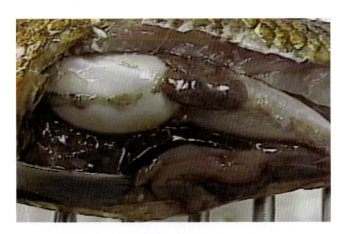

The liver is the dark mass in the anterior abdomen (under the pectoral fin); the spleen is the elongated dark red organ that runs above the pink intestines and below the silver swim bladder; the anterior kidneys are above the swim bladder near the spine, but the posterior kidney is the brownish-red mass over the swim bladder isthmus separating the cranial and caudal chambers.

Swim bladder (10) - The koi's physostomous swim bladder has 2 chambers, connected by an isthmus. Air can pass from the caudal chamber into the cranial chamber through the isthmus. The caudal chamber is connected to the esophagus by the pneumatic duct. The swim badder displaces about 7% of the koi's body with air, providing neutral buoyancy. Guanine crystals impart a silvery appearance to the swim bladder. The surface of the swim bladder contains blood capillaries.

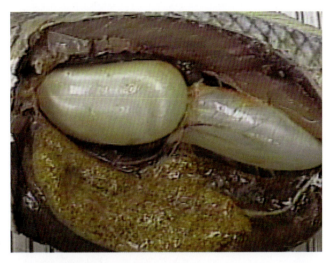

The gas or swim bladder is visible after the egg-filled ovary is reflected downward within the abdomen. The cranial chamber is an oval cylinder and the caudal chamber is a tapered cylinder. They connect through a small ventral tube called the isthmus, and the pneumatic duct attaches to the caudal swim bladder below the isthmus.

Pneumatic duct (11) - Air tube connecting the lower front end of the caudal swim bladder to the esophagus. Swallowed air is forced into the caudal bladder to increase buoyancy, or air can be released from the bladder through this tube.

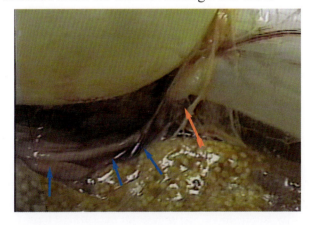

Red arrow points to pneumatic duct's attachment site to the caudal chamber. Blue arrows point to the duct.

Kidney (12) - There is a right and a left kidney, closely attached ventral to the backbone, each divided into an anterior hematopoietic (blood-forming) and a posterior excretory (urine-producing) kidney. The ureter ducts carry the urine from the kidneys to the urinary papilla that is in the vent caudal to the anus. Creatine is the main nitrogenous waste excreted through the posterior kidneys of fish, and in lesser amounts ammonia, uric acid, and creatinine. The major site of nitrogenous waste elimination in freshwater fish is the gills. Urine production in freshwater fish is primarily for osmoregulation, as it removes excess water from the body as dilute urine. The glomeruli of freshwater fish kidneys retain salts to maintain the body's osmotic pressure. Freshwater fish are hyperosmotic (greater salt concentration) compared to the surrounding water, so are constantly needing to conserve salt and eliminate water.

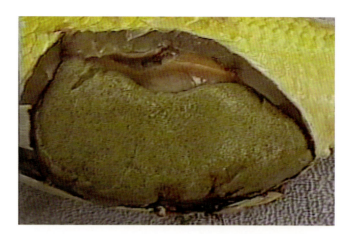

The female koi in breeding season carries a tremendous quantity of eggs (roe). Immature koi will have small testes or ovaries on each side of the abdomen above the caudal chamber of the swim bladder, but in mature koi, a significant portion of the abdomen is filled with gonads.

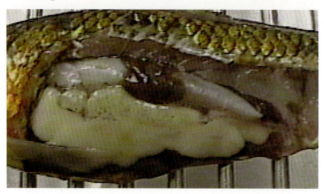

The dark red posterior kidney is pendulous in koi and hangs down between the chambers of the swim bladder. Male koi have cream-colored testes on each side of the abdomen, against the body wall.

Gonads (13) - The male's cream-colored testes are paired and attached to mesentary below the kidneys. Each vas deferens carries spermatozoa from the testis to an excretory meatus at the urinary papilla in the vent. The female's paired ovaries are suspended in mesentary lateral to the kidneys and viscera, and contain brownish orange ova. The eggs pass through the oviduct and out the genital opening in the vent. In addition to gametogenesis, the gonads produce androgen and estrogen hormones.

Muscles (14) - The muscle myomeres are separated into right and left sides by the median septum, and into upper (epaxial) and lower (hypaxial) muscle by the transverse horizontal septum. There are 2 types of muscle fibers: the red muscle fibers that run superficially along the side of the muscle mass, and the white muscle fibers making up the rest of the muscle mass. The red fibers are aerobic, slow-contracting fibers capable of slow, sustained activity. The white muscle fibers are anaerobic, fast-contracting fibers for short-term, rapid swimming. The red muscles have greater vascularization and a higher lipid content than do the white muscles.

Spine (15) - The cylindrical vertebral bodies or centra are connected to each other by longitudinal elastic ligaments, and have a cushioning intervertebral pad between them. Each centrum has a neural arch and neural spine dorsally. The spinal cord runs through the neural canal formed by the arch. The anterior (abdominal) vertebrae have 15 paired ventral pleural ribs, starting at the third vertebra, and the posterior (caudal) vertebrae have ventral hemal arches and spines. The caudal artery, which is the continuation of the dorsal aorta, along with the caudal vein run through the hemal canal formed by the hemal arches. There are a total of 38 vertebrae in the koi spine. The first 3 vertebrae have small ventral parts that connect the inner ear to the swim bladder to aid in sound perception. The first vertebra produces the claustrum and scaphium, the second the intercalarium, and the third the tripus. These are interconnected by ligaments, and together are called the Weberian apparatus, or Weber's ossicles.

Skull (16) - Koi are teleost fish with skeletons made of true bone (osteocytes). There is no hematopoietic tissue (marrow) in the bones of fish. The skull of teleost fish has 185 bones, more than in any other vertebrate.

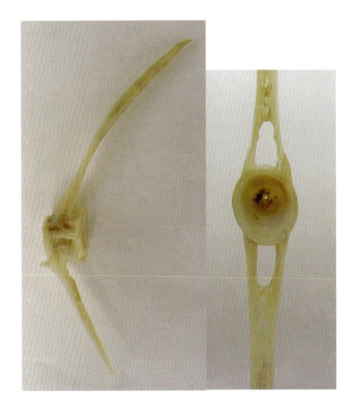

A koi vertebra from the spine caudal to the abdomen. The neural arch forms the upper canal through which the spinal cord runs. The ventral hemal arch forms the hemal canal for the caudal artery and vein.

Internal Ear - Fish have no external ears, but have an inner ear in each side of the skull consisting of 3 semicircular canals, plus the pars superior (utriculus), and a pars inferior (sacculus and lagena). There is a calcareous otolith in each of the utriculus, sacculus, and lagena chambers. The pars superior functions in maintaining equilibrium, while the pars inferior functions in sound detection. In koi, this inner ear is connected to the air bladder by a series of bones called Weber's ossicles that increases the ability to hear. The range of tone perception for carp is 8-22,000 cycles per second (Hertz).

REFERENCES:

Butcher, Ray L. 1992. *Manual of Ornamental Fish,* British Small Animal Veterinary Association, Gloucestershire, UK.

Gratzek, John B. (editor). 1992. *Aquariology: Fish Anatomy, Physiology, and Nutrition,* Tetra Press, Morris Plains, NJ.

Roberts, Ronald J. 1989. *Fish Pathology,* 2nd ed., Bailliere Tindall, London, UK.

Saint-Erne, Nicholas. 1984. *A Veterinarian's Guide to the Diseases of Freshwater Aquarium Fishes,* Kansas State University College of Veterinary Medicine, Manhattan, KS.

Smith, Lynwood S. 1982. *Introduction to Fish Physiology,* T.F.H. Publications, Neptune, NJ.

Stoskopf, Michael K. 1993. *Fish Medicine,* W.B. Saunders, Philadelphia.

Brain (17) - The brain is divided into the olfactory lobe, optic lobe, pituitary, inferior lobe, cerebellum, facial lobe, vagal lobe, and the medulla that attaches to the spinal cord. Fish have 10 pairs of cranial nerves: the olfactory, optic, oculomotor, trochlear, trigeminal, abducens, facial, acoustic, glossopharyngeal, and vagus nerves.

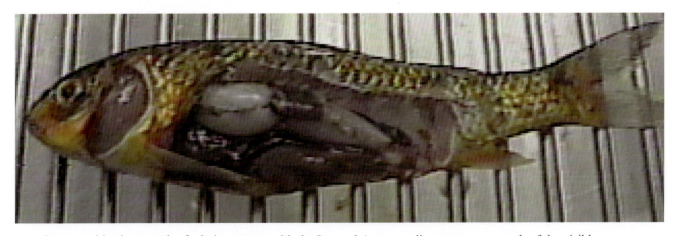

Compare this photograph of a koi necropsy with the Internal Anatomy diagram to name each of the visible organs.

RADIOGRAPHIC ANATOMY

Normal radiographs of koi will show the bone structure and the swim (gas) bladder. Abdominal organs are not readily visualized. Gonadal tumors of increased density can sometimes be seen on radiographs. The koi below was given barium solution by an oral tube so that its intestines would be visible.

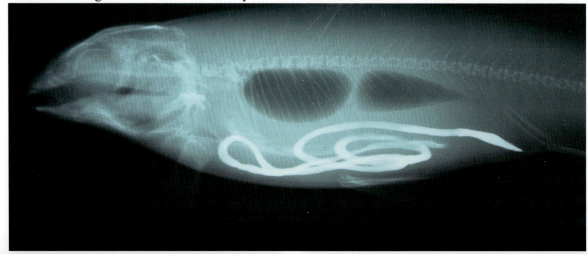

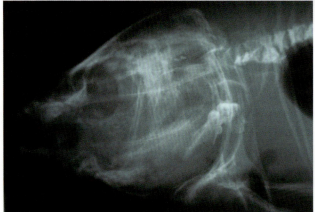

Radiograph of a koi skull showing the opercular bones, the molars, and the Weberian apparatus below the spine.

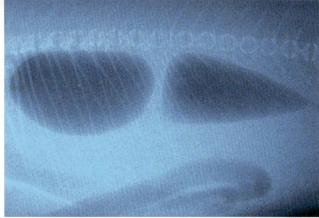

Close-up view of the swim bladder chambers at the dorsal aspect of the abdominal cavity, within the rib cage.

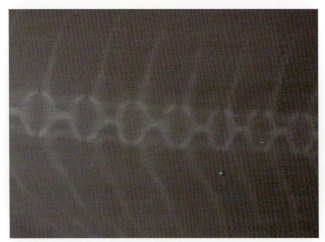

Close-up view of the caudal peduncle portion of the spine. The vertebral bodies (centra) are visible along with the dorsal neural spines and ventral hemal spines.

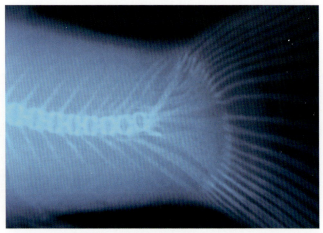

Radiograph of the caudal peduncle showing the epural and hypural plates going to the caudal fin.

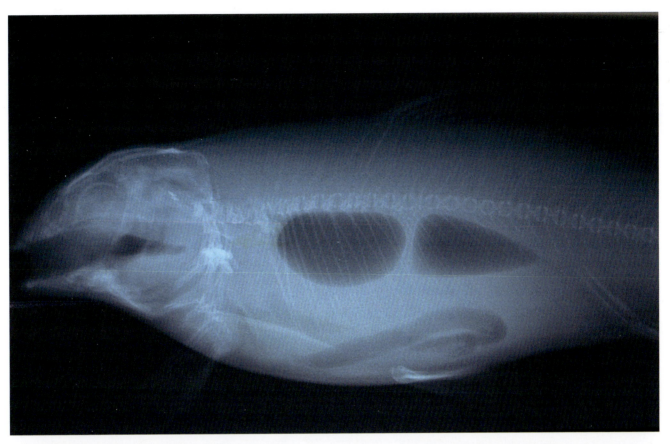

This radiograph of a koi shows the skull outline, the dense molars in the pharynx, the operculum, the spine with its Weberian apparatus ventral to the first three vertebrae, the abdominal ribs ventral to the spine, the cranial and caudal chambers of the swim bladder, the attachment site of the pneumatic duct on the cranioventral portion of the caudal chamber, the pectoral and pelvic fins, and the bony spines at the anterior end of the dorsal fin and the anal fin. The abdominal organs all blend together due to their similar densities, but gas in the proximal intestinal loop makes it visible. The more dense bones show up lighter, and the less dense gas in the swim bladder is darker.

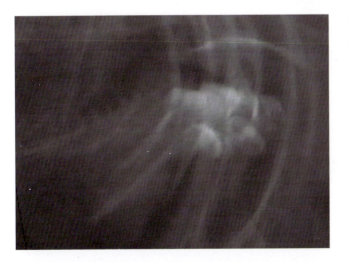

This radiograph shows a close-up view of the molars in the pharynx. The horizontal line above the molars is the masticating plate. Gill rakers are visible on the gill arch to the left of the molars. The operclulum plate (opercle) bones are visible over the molars.

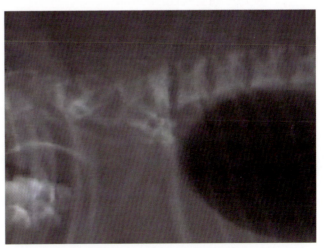

This radiograph shows a close-up view of the Weberian apparatus. The first three vertebrae have ventral ossicles that connect the cranial swim bladder (on the right) with the inner ear in the skull (to the left) in order to transmit vibrations, thus increasing the sensitivity of hearing.

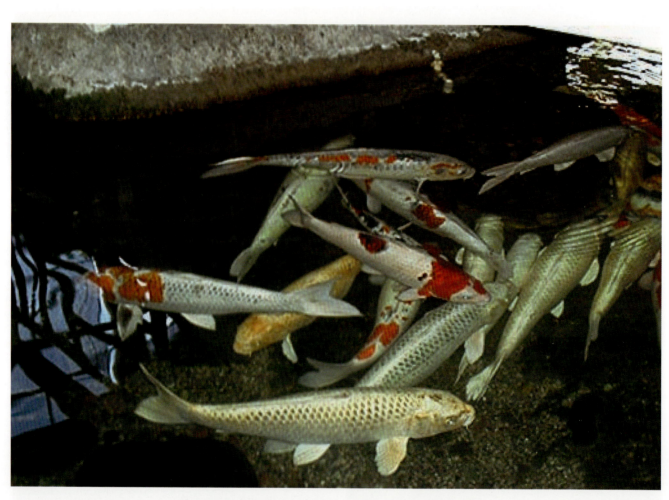
Koi pond at the Embassy Suites Hotel, Scottsdale, Arizona.

CHAPTER 2:
CLINICAL PROCEDURES

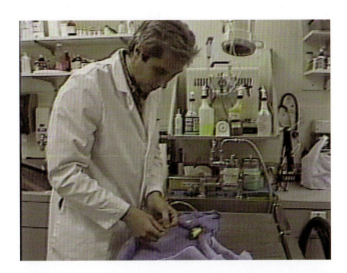

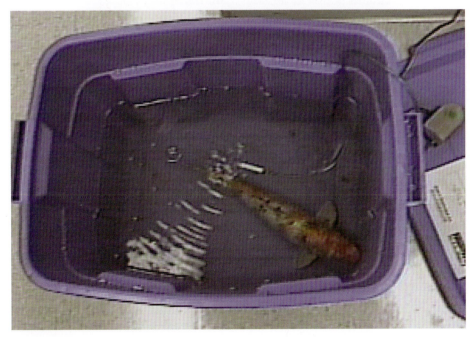

Koi may be brought to the veterinary clinic for diagnosis or treatment in a variety of ways. Be sure to have an air pump and airline tubing with an air stone on it to aerate the container of water. The best transportation method is to use strong plastic bags filled 1/3 with water and 2/3 with oxygen, then placed in an insulated cardboard box for ease of carrying. It is beneficial to have a 20 gallon or larger glass aquarium for use as a hospital tank for holding small koi, and a 100 gallon or larger plastic vat for hospitalizing large koi. These should have aeration and water filtration and be emptied and thoroughly disinfected between patients. Monitor water quality daily and change part of the water each day to prevent toxic waste accumulation, as the filter will not develop biological denitrification of ammonia in these conditions and with medications in the water.

CLINICAL PROCEDURES

Disease Precursors

Fish diseases can be very perplexing and frustrating for the koi pond keeper. So many things can affect the pond and make the fish go belly up. Many times there are not any obvious signs of disease when the fish die.

The most important aspect in maintaining fish health is proper water quality. This depends on such things as pH, temperature, alkalinity, hardness, ammonia, nitrite, nitrate, oxygen concentration, population density, and biological, chemical, and mechanical filtration systems. When all of these parameters are within their proper ranges, the fish will have less stress and be more immune to disease.

Infectious and parasitic diseases occur more easily in fish stressed from improper environmental conditions. In the wild, fish may harbor a variety of parasites without incurring problems; but, the artificial environments in ponds or aquaria are more likely to be abnormal, therefore parasites can then cause serious diseases.

A combination of the environment, nutrition, genetics, and the presence of pathogens or parasites is involved in the development of disease. Anything we can do to improve these will improve the health of the fish.

Office Visit or House Call?

There are pros and cons for each answer to this question. Having a client bring a sick fish into the veterinary hospital allows treatment in a quarantine tank where all the conditions can be controlled and properly maintained. Regular daily observations can be made, and appropriate diagnostic tests and treatments performed. Sick fish are isolated from the remaining fish in the pond. Once a diagnosis is made, the owner can treat the pond as necessary, and the sick fish can be cared for until it is well enough to return home.

Disadvantages include the lack of examination of the remaining fish and the pond itself; having the owner transport the sick fish in plastic bags or ice chests to the clinic; and in many cases the unwillingness of the owner to bring in one of their koi for fear of it dying on the way to the clinic, or while there. To most owners, these are their pets, and need to be treated carefully and compassionately.

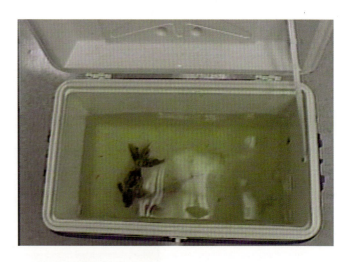

Koi owners will bring fish into the clinic transported in ice chests, buckets, trash bags, and other inventive conveyances. It is important that the fish are given aeration and protected from temperature extremes.

By making a house call, the fish can be examined in its own environment. Pond filtration units can be examined, and water tests performed on the spot. Apparently healthy fish can be biopsied and checked for early signs of lesions that the owner might have missed. Suggestions on improving pond design and fish husbandry are easier to make when the facilities have been visited, rather than having just the owner's descriptions. One very important factor is the ability to measure the pond and calculate the size in gallons. Many times the owner can only guess as to how much water the pond holds, and this can lead to inaccurate dosing of medications, making them less effective on one hand, or toxic on the other.

Making a house call does require more time than an office visit, though. Transportation time must be taken into account. Portable diagnostic equipment including microscopes, slides and coverslips, bacterial culturettes, and water test kits must be brought along. A "Doctor's Bag" of

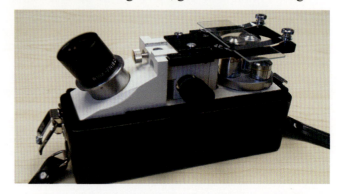

A Swift brand portable field microscope is an excellent investment for making house calls to the koi pond.

common medications and antibiotics can be made up for house calls. Even Mobile Veterinary Clinics (Dodgen Industries, Bowie Manufacturing, La Boit, or Porta-Vet) could be used to bring all the needs of the clinic to the client's pond. Some very important pieces of equipment to bring are your own quality long-handled koi nets (many pond owners have only pool skimmer nets!), a plastic container for holding the koi for examination, and chest-high waders!

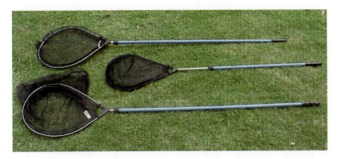

A quality koi net is a necessity. These koi nets have telescoping handles for ease of use in all sizes of ponds. The different sizes of mesh bags are useful for various koi handling tasks. The mesh is small enough to prevent fin damage. Nets used for fishing have mesh that is too large and rough for handling koi.

Patient History

Prior to the actual examination of the fish, some information should be gathered. What is the fish's name? How old is it? What sex is it? What color is it? How big is it? How long has it been in the pond? Where was it obtained? What abnormal signs does the fish exhibit? Which fish are sick (all or a few or only one)? How long have they appeared to be ill? Are they still eating? What are they being fed? What type of filtration system is used? When was it last cleaned? When was the last water change? How frequently are the water changes made? When was the water tested and what were the results? Were any new fish or plants introduced recently?

Many times the answers to these questions will provide significant clues to the type of disease process affecting the fish. If many fish are affected quickly, water quality problems are frequently the cause. If some fish are affected initially and then others become sick later, this suggests a contagious disease. Always check the water, filtration, and fish to be sure that there are not multiple conditions causing the fish stress.

Diagnostic Methods

Examining tissue samples taken from a living patient in order to obtain diagnostic information is the field of clinical pathology. These samples may be blood, tissues taken by skin scrapes, fin and gill biopsies, needle aspirations of masses or abdominal fluids, surgical biopsy of tissues, or urine and fecal samples. The samples are then examined under the microscope or analyzed by biochemical tests to determine their components. Abnormal findings can lead to diagnosing the cause of the disease.

A live moribund fish should be examined when possible, or a freshly dead specimen. If the fish has been dead for more than a few hours, even if refrigerated, the chance of accurate diagnosis is diminished.

If the fish is alive, observe its respiration by watching its mouth movements and the motion of the operculum (gill cover). Note how it positions itself in the water. Is it neutrally buoyant (normal) or does it float or sink? Does it list to one side, or float with its head down? Are there lesions on the head, body, or fins? Are the fins congested or eroded? Are any scales missing? Are the cornea and lenses clear? Fluorescein stain can be used to check for corneal ulcers. Lift the operculum and examine the gills for hemorrhage, discoloration, or necrosis. Always wet the hands first before handling koi, or wear smooth latex gloves, to prevent damage to the slime coating the skin of the fish.

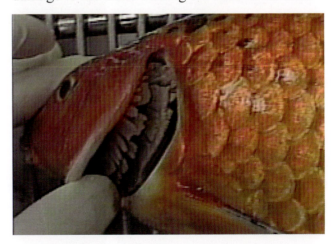

An examination of the gills can reveal clues about the etiology of the problem. Pale gills can be due to a lack of oxygen in the water, brownish gill color results from nitrite toxicity, deep red indicates inflammation, and excess mucus on the gills occurs with both water quality problems such as ammonia or chlorine toxicity or from external parasitism.

After the initial physical examination, biopsy samples should be taken. Place the fish on a wet towel or chamois cloth, and wrap it to keep it from jumping. The cloth can be coated with artificial mucus (e.g., Stress Coat) to protect the fish's slime coat (cuticle). Be sure to keep the fish wet and handle it gently. Uncover sections of the fish as necessary to take biopsy samples. If anesthetic is available, add it to fresh dechlorinated water to anesthetize the fish prior to the biopsy. Have another container of dechlorinated water without anesthetic available in which to awaken the fish.

Using a blunt blade or spatula, or even a plastic microscope coverslip, gently scrape a small sample of mucus off the body of the fish. Place this in a drop of water on a microscope slide and cover it with a coverslip. If there are skin or fin lesions, take a sample from the margin of the lesion and prepare it the same way. Next snip a small section of the caudal or other fin rays using small sharp scissors, such as iris or suture scissors. Also take a sample of one or two gill filament tips. Place these on a slide and prepare as with the skin scraping. Examine these samples microscopically at 40-400X magnifications.

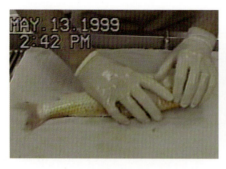

Skin and gill biopsies can often be obtained without anesthesia. Lay the koi on a wet towel and wrap it around the fish as necessary.

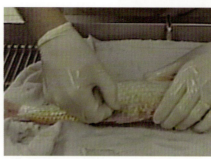

Use a microscope coverslip to scrape a small sample of mucus (glycocalyx) from the skin surface, moving from the head toward the tail.

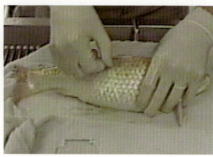

Several different areas of the skin or fins may be scraped to get samples for external parasite examinations.

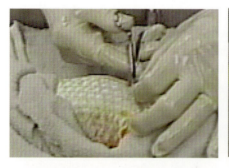

A small section of the margin of the pectoral fin, or other fin, is collected for a microscopic examination.

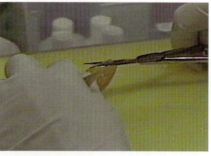

A small section of the margin of the caudal fin is being removed for microscopic examination for parasites.

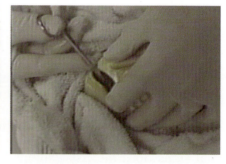

Wrap a conscious koi in the wet towel to restrain it for taking a gill biopsy.

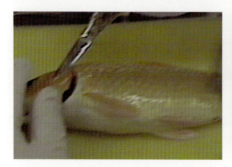

Taking a gill biopsy sample on an anesthetized koi is easy and reduces the risk of injury to the koi.

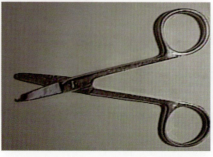

The notch in one blade of small suture removal scissors is useful in gill biopsies.

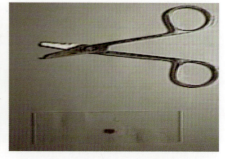

The gill tip biopsy is placed on a glass microscope slide in a drop of water and covered with a coverslip.

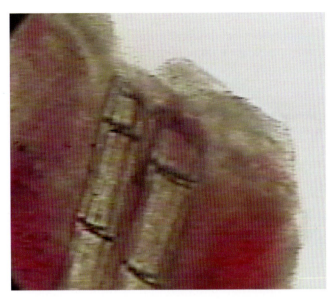

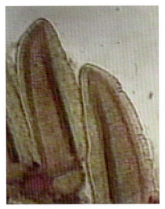 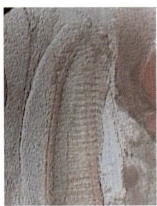

Gill tip biopsies showing severe hyperplasia (excessive clear epithelial cells, white blood cells, and mucus covering the pink gill tissue).
40X   100X

This caudal fin biopsy sample shows bacterial erosion of the fin margin and inflammation of the fin membrane. The dark colored joints in the two fin rays are normal.

    Gill biopsy samples often reveal parasites within or around the gill filaments. Motile bacteria can also be present in large numbers, indicating a primary or secondary bacterial gill disease. Hyperplasia, or thickening of the cell layers on the gill lamellae, often occurs secondarily to toxins in the water or pathogens on the gills. This results in decreased respiratory efficiency and can even cause death from hypoxia (a too low oxygen concentration). Telangiectasis, or blood clots within the capillaries of the gill lamellae, can also occur due to toxins or infections.

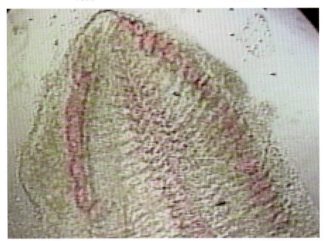

Gill hyperplasia with telangiectasis. White blood cells are abundant in the gill capillaries, and in the epithelium and mucus around the gills.
400X

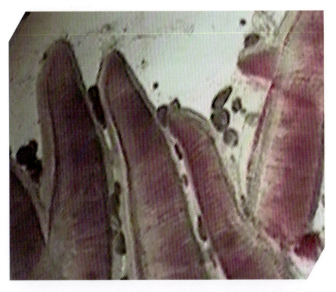

Gill tip biopsy showing numerous *Ichthyophthirius* trophonts (the feeding stage of this protozoan parasite) and hyperplasia of the gill epithelium.   40X

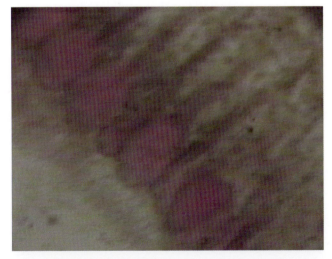

Close-up of dilated capillaries with blood clots (telangiectasis) within the gill lamellae.
1000X

Blood samples can be drawn if needed from the caudal vein below the spine in the caudal peduncle. Use a 1-ml or 3-ml tuberculin syringe with a 22-gauge needle of appropriate length. A butterfly catheter can be attached to the syringe to facilitate handling of the needle separate from the syringe. Fill the hub of the needle with a drop of lithium heparin to prevent the blood from clotting. The needle is inserted at an angle pointing craniodorsally from the ventral midline of the caudal peduncle until it hits the vertebrae. Withdraw the needle slightly and it should be in the caudal vein. Light aspiration on the syringe plunger should be applied to collect the blood.

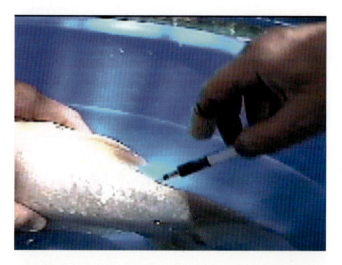

Ventral approach for blood collection from the caudal vein.

In large koi, to facilitate drawing blood without the use of an excessively long needle, the hypodermic needle can be inserted laterally from the middle of the side of the caudal peduncle, ventral to the lateral line. Angle the needle slightly forward and insert it until it touches the spine. Then walk the needle ventrally to the caudal vein below the vertebral column.

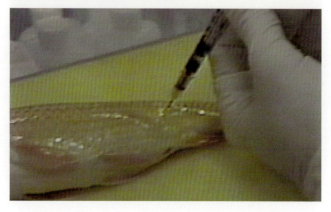

Lateral approach for blood collection from the caudal vein.

Remove the needle from the syringe after blood collection and gently transfer the blood from the syringe into an unstoppered green-top blood vial. This prevents damage to the blood cells and hemolysis that can occur when using vacuum tubes and squirting the blood out through the needle. A hypodermic needle without the syringe can also be used to obtain a blood sample, with microcapillary tubes utilized for collecting blood dripping from the hub of the needle.

Bacterial cultures can be collected from open wounds such as found in "hole in the side" disease. An affected koi is placed on a wet towel, or held in a container of shallow water, and anesthetized if necessary, in order to collect the culture sample. A sterile culturette swab is rolled across the skin lesion, including the margins of the wound, and then replaced into its protective sleeve filled with transport media. Label the tube with the date and the fish that the sample is from, and submit it via overnight mail or courier to the microbiology laboratory.

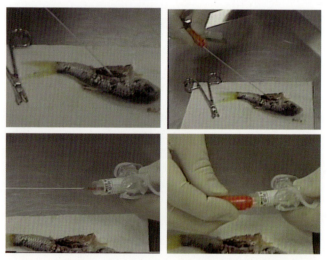

During a necropsy, samples are collected from the liver and kidney for bacterial culture and antibiotic sensitivity testing using a sterile collection swab that is then placed into a sterile tube of media to send to the laboratory.

The bacteria will be grown in culture media, identified, and tested to see what antibiotics are the best for treatment of the fish. This should take about 3-5 days to do. Bacterial cultures taken from fish tissues should be incubated in the laboratory at 68-77°F / 20-25°C. The normal incubation temperature of 98.6°F / 37°C will inhibit the growth of many pathogenic bacteria of fish. Be sure to inform the lab to culture the samples from fish at the lower temperature so that they don't use the higher temperature by mistake.

A fresh fecal sample can be collected with a pipette or syringe from the container of water in which the fish arrived. Place this on a microscope slide and compress it with a coverslip. Examine it for bacteria, protozoa, and helminth ova.

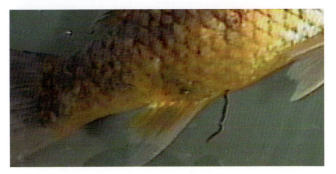

Koi will often defecate when handled or anesthetized.

If the fish is dead upon presentation, obtain the same biopsy (necropsy) samples, but a larger portion of gill tissue should be examined. Remove the operculum to examine the entire gills. Then an internal examination of the abdominal organs is made. Make an incision using sharp dissecting scissors along the ventral midline from the left gill opening to just anterior to the vent. Be careful not to cut the abdominal organs or intestines. Then cut upward to the backbone. Cut anteriorly along the spine through the ribs toward the top of the gill slit. Then elevate the flap of the left body wall, and cut downward to the ventral midline to expose the abdominal organs. Look at the color, size, and position of each of the abdominal organs. Collect tissue samples for bacterial cultures and sensitivities, histopathology, or microscopic squash preparations, as appropriate.

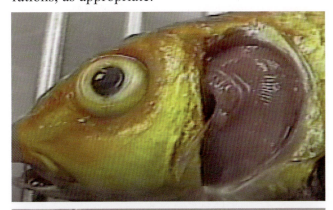

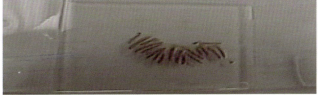

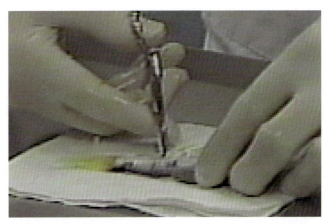

Clean the skin with alcohol prior to opening the abdomen to prevent external bacterial contamination of samples.

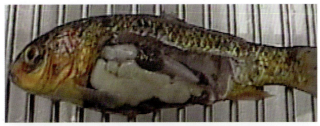

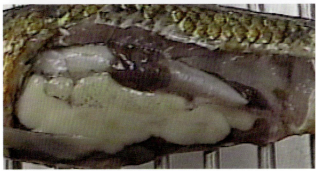

Use sharp scissors to remove the left abdominal body wall. This will allow visualization of all the abdominal organs.

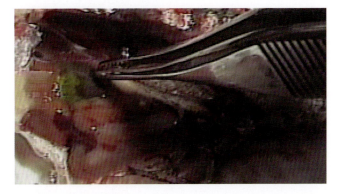

ABOVE: After collecting bacterial culture samples, tissue sections can be removed for a squash-mount microscopic examination or for histopathology preparation.
LEFT: With the operculum removed, the gills can easily be examined and a large section of gill filaments removed for microscopic examination.

Hematology

This branch of clinical pathology studies the blood cells. Koi have blood cells similar to other species of fish. The total volume of blood in koi makes up about 5% of its body weight (50 ml/kg). Up to 20% of the total blood volume can safely be removed in fish that are not excessively ill. This allows for 0.5 ml of blood to be removed from a 50-g fish, or 1 ml from a 100-g fish. Larger blood samples are usually not necessary, even though more blood could be drawn from a large koi. This quantity of blood should be adequate for running the required tests in modern laboratories.

The blood should be collected into a plastic syringe that has been coated with lithium heparin. This is preferable to ammonium heparin or sodium heparin, but they can also be used for hematology testing. The ammonium and sodium heparins will affect those blood values if used in samples for serology or electrolyte testing. A drop of sterile distilled water can be placed into a blood collection tube containing powdered lithium heparin, and then the fluid is withdrawn into the syringe to coat the needle hub and barrel. Depress the syringe plunger to blow out air and excess heparin. Ethylenediamine tetra-acetic acid (EDTA) is not recommended to be used to prevent blood clotting as it may cause erythrocyte lysis.

A drop of blood should be placed on a microscope slide and made into a blood smear sample for microscopic examination. Stain the dried smear with Wright's or Diff-Quik stain. The remaining blood should be kept cool and have the plasma separated into another container as soon as possible. Submit it to the lab immediately for the most accurate test results. Some normal values for koi blood parameters derived from personal clinical experience and from Groff and Zinkl (1999) are listed in the chart below.

KOI COMPLETE BLOOD COUNT (CBC):

Red Blood Cells (Erythrocytes):   Normal Range:

Red Blood Cells (10-13 µm cell length)	1-2 Million/µl
Hematocrit (Packed Cell Volume)	24-35%
Hemoglobin	8-13 g/dl
Methemoglobin	4.8-5.6%
Mean Corpuscular Volume	202 fl
Mean Corpuscular Hemoglobin	49.1 pg/cell
Mean Corpuscular Hemoglobin Concentration	0.24 g/dl

White Blood Cells (Leukocytes):

Total White Blood Cells	5-15 Thousand/µl
Neutrophils/Heterophils (10-15 µm)	750-1500/µl
Neutrophils/Heterophils (% of Total WBC)	12-20%
Band (immature) Neutrophils/Heterophils	0-4%
Small (Mature) Lymphocytes (6.6 µm)	3000-12,000/µl
Small (Mature) Lymphocytes	65-85%
Large (Immature) Lymphocytes (11.8 µm)	0-3%
Monocytes (10-16 µm)	100-600/µl
Monocytes	1-4%
Eosinophils (13.8 µm)	0-150/µl
Eosinophils	0-1%
Basophils (13.8 µm)	0-150/µl
Basophils	0-1%
Thrombocytes (4.6 x 7.7 µm)	50 Thousand/µl

Red Blood Cells (Erythrocytes) – An ellipsoid cell with oval to round central nucleus. These are the most abundant cells in the blood, comprising up to 35% of the total blood volume in koi. These cells transport oxygen and carbon dioxide through the bloodstream. They also transport ammonia to the gills for excretion. Erythropoiesis (red blood cell production) occurs in koi in the anterior kidneys and the spleen. Hemophagocytosis, the removal of worn-out red blood cells, also occurs in the anterior kidneys and the spleen.

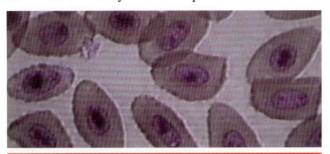

Serum Chemistries (Serology):

ALT(SGPT)	20-50 IU/L
AST (SGOT)	100-300 IU/L
Total Bilirubin	0.1-0.3 mg/dl
Alkaline Phosphatase	10-20 IU/L
GGT	1-3 IU/L
Uric Acid	1-2.5 mg/dl
Blood Urea Nitrogen	5-15 mg/dl
Creatinine	0.2-0.5 mg/dl
BUN/Creat Ratio	10-20
Creatinine Phosphokinase	14.5 IU/ml
Glucose	30-120 mg/dl
Cholesterol	200-400 mg/dl
Triglyceride	50-500 mg/dl
Amylase	25-50 IU/L
Lipase	25-50 IU/L
Total Protein	4-10 g/dl
Albumin	2-6 g/dl
Globulin	2-4 g/dl
A/G Ratio	0.7-1.2
Osmolality	220-420 mOsm/kg
Calcium	8.5-13.5 mg/dl
Phosphorus	10-15 mg/dl
Cal/Phos Ratio	0.6-1.3
Magnesium	3-5 mEq/L
Sodium	100-140 mEq/L
Chloride	90-120 mEq/L
Potassium	4-30 mEq/L
Na/K Ratio	3-30

White Blood Cells (Leukocytes) – There are several types of white blood cells that develop from plasmacytes, which are undifferentiated immature leukocytes. Plasmacytes are only occasionally seen in the blood smears. Each leukocyte has its own structure and function.

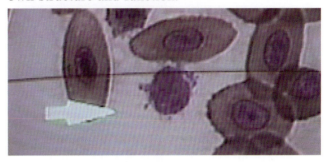

ABOVE: Plasmacyte among red blood cells.
LEFT: Mature nucleated red blood cells.
All these blood smears are stained with Diff-Quik stain.

Neutrophils (Heterophils) - These differ from typical neutrophils (polymorphonucleates) or heterophils from the other vertebrates. They are similar to the other granule-containing cells, the eosinophils and basophils, but are much more numerous. These cells are all referred to as granulocytes. They have an oval to round cell membrane with an eccentric round to lobed nucleus and containing small granules in its cytoplasm. Their function is the phagocytosis of foreign material at sites of inflammation. The number of neutrophils increases in disease conditions. Band neutrophils are immature cells that have a band-shaped nucleus. An increase in band neutrophils indicates new cell formation in response to an ongoing infection or inflammation.

Eosinophils - These granulocyte blood cells are not always present in peripheral blood samples. They are similar to the neutrophils, with a small, eccentric, condensed nucleus. The cytoplasm contains large refractile granules that stain red with eosin stains.

Basophils - These granulocytes have round eccentric nuclei with large refractile granules in their cytoplasm that stain blue. Their function is similar to neutrophils.

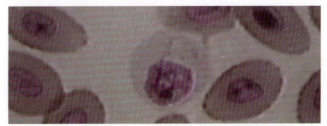

A neutrophil granulocyte among red blood cells.

Lymphocytes - These are small blood cells with irregularly shaped cytoplasmic membranes. The nucleus fills most of the cell, is eccentrically located, and round to oval-shaped. The nucleus stains dark purple and the scant cytoplasm stains blue with blood stains. Lymphocytes are the most abundant white blood cells in the peripheral blood of fish. The large lymphocytes are immature cells and are released in response to inflammation. Lymphocyte counts decrease in conditions of chronic stress or inflammation, as granulocytes increase. One important function of the lymphocytes is antibody production.

Monocytes (Macrophages) - These cells are slightly larger than other white blood cells. They have an eccentric oval nucleus with coarse, granular chromatin. The cytoplasm has abundant vacuoles. The cytoplasm often has pseudopodia along the cell membrane. Their function is the phagocytosis of foreign particles. These cells introduce antigens to lymphocytes to initiate antibody responses.

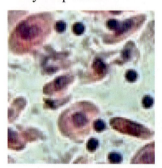 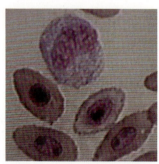

Lymphocytes (left) with dark round nuclei and minimal cytoplasm, and a monocyte (right) among red blood cells.

Platelets (Thrombocytes) – Immature thrombocytes are round, with very little cytoplasm around the nucleus. Mature thrombocytes are more oval or spindle-shaped, with cytoplasm at the poles of the nucleus. Thrombocytes aid in the clotting of the blood.

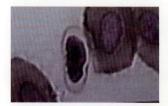 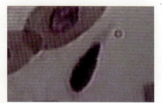

Platelets among red blood cells. The immature platelets appear similar to red blood cells, but are smaller and the cytoplasm is clear. The photograph on the right shows a mature spindle-shaped platelet.

These blood smears are stained with Diff-Quik stain.

Radiology

Standard veterinary radiology equipment can be used to take radiographs of koi. If high-detail films are available, they should be used. Results are often better with the film set on the tabletop, rather than in the bucky tray, but both techniques should be tried to see which is better for each machine. The koi can be anesthetized and removed from the water for taking the radiographs, or it can be restrained in a wet plastic bag held down to the table to keep the fish from jumping. Many times the koi will lie still without jumping even without restraint, but each case must be evaluated individually to determine the amount of restraint needed.

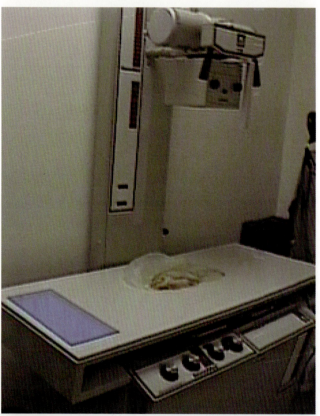

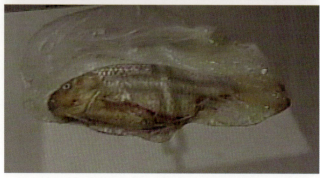

Koi being radiographed in plastic bag with a little water.

Radiographs are good for looking at bone structures and the gas bladder, but individual abdominal organs are often hard to distinguish. Fractures, spinal deformities, and some abdominal tumors can be seen on radiographs. Barium can be administered via a rubber catheter or feeding tube inserted orally passing through the esophagus and into the intestines. This can be used to visualize an intestinal obstruction or displacement of the intestines due to an abdominal mass. Ovaries filled with roe in females can sometimes be visualized on radiographs to help determine the sex of young koi.

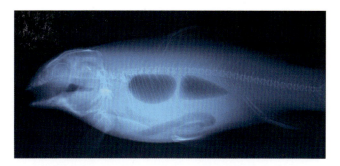

Radiograph of the koi prior to giving it barium. Note the gas visible in the intestines.

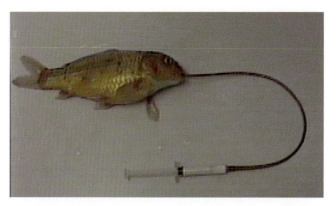

Barium solution is given enterally by placing a rubber French catheter into the mouth and down the esophagus.

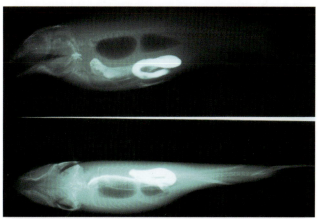

Lateral and DV radiographs taken 15 minutes after giving the barium show the large diameter proximal intestine.

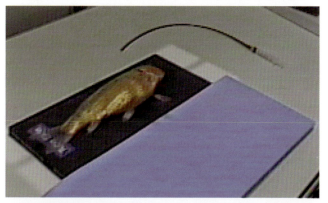

Split plate lateral radiograph of the barium series

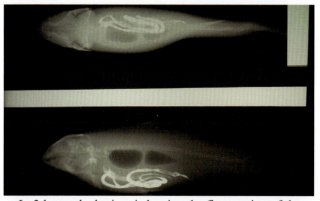

In 3 hours the barium is leaving the first section of the intestines and is filling the thinner distal intestine.

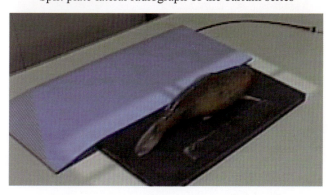

Split plate dorsal-ventral (DV) radiograph of a koi.

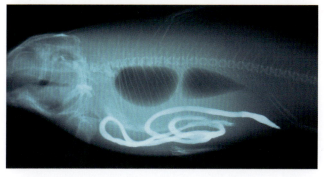

After 6 hours the barium is in the thinner loops of the distal intestines, filling them all the way to the vent.

Sonography

Ultrasound imaging uses high-frequency (3-10 MegaHertz) sound waves to produce a computer-generated cross-section of the body (sonogram). Real-time computer sampling will produce a moving picture that can show the beating of the heart or peristalsis waves of the intestines. Different tissues propagate or reflect sound waves at varying quantities. Sound waves propagate in soft tissues and they will appear in shades of gray, and fluids, which easily transmit sound, appear black. Sound is reflected by bones and air, which send echoes back and appear white.

Ultrasound is a safe, rapid, and noninvasive diagnostic tool that usually does not require sedation of the patient. The koi is kept in the water, which aids in handling the fish and increases sound propagation. The ultrasound transducer (usually 7.5 MHz) is wrapped in a waterproof cover (plastic bag, exam glove, condom) and is placed against the side of the fish while it is still in a shallow container of water. Coupling gel is not necessary for fish in the water and the transducer can be held up to 2 cm away from the skin surface while under water. The transducer is moved until the desired image is obtained. The image can be in motion or frozen into a still picture.

Most units will save the images so they can be replayed or printed. A motion image can be used to guide a biopsy needle into a specific organ or mass for a biopsy sample. Anesthesia may be needed for biopsies, however. Sonography in koi is useful in assessing the swim bladder size and position, monitoring heartbeats during anesthesia and surgery, and can be helpful in diagnosing an abdominal mass, including ovarian tissues.

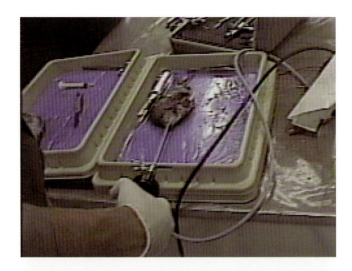

A rigid endoscope probe attached to a video monitor is used to examine with high magnification the oral cavity and pharynx of a fish during a necropsy procedure.

Endoscopy

Rigid endoscopy probes can be used on anesthetized koi to assess the oral cavity and the gills from within the pharynx. Flexible endoscopy probes of small diameter can be passed orally and used to view the esophagus or intestines. There may be some application to surgically sex young koi, as is done with birds, by visualizing the gonads through a small abdominal laproscopic incision.

Having a video monitor attached to the endoscopic probe makes its use easier than having to look down the optical eyepiece on the probe. Images can also be recorded on videotape.

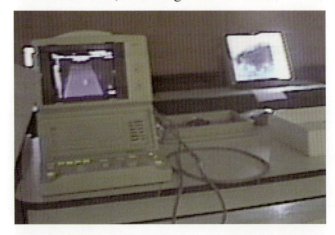

While ultrasound units are still rather expensive, the cost is coming down and the units are getting smaller. Portable units are available that can be used pond-side.

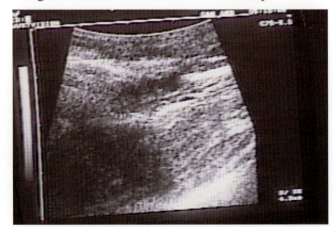

With practice, sonograms are as easy to read as radiographs. Fluid filled organs appear black, and bones and the swim bladder appear white.

Anesthesia

When handling koi for examination or disease treatment, it is often desirable to use an anesthetic agent to calm the fish in order to reduce stress and trauma. Surgery can also be performed on anesthetized koi to repair wounds, remove skin and fin tumors, or to remove abdominal masses. Many chemicals have been used to induce anesthesia in fish. All have some element of risk, but when used carefully they have successfully induced sedation or anesthesia.

Each of the following anesthetics is added to clean well-oxygenated water in a suitable glass or plastic container. The water is thoroughly mixed to ensure all of the chemical is dissolved and dispersed evenly. The water containing the anesthetic solution should be the same temperature and pH as the pond water. Use a thermometer to monitor the water temperature during surgery, and also monitor the dissolved oxygen concentration.

After the procedure is accomplished, the fish is placed into clean, aerated fresh water without any anesthetic in order to recover safely, before being returned to the pond. Never leave a fish unattended while it is under anesthesia. Monitor the respiration rate (opercular movements) to assess the depth of anesthesia. The fish will lie on its side and the respiratory rate will slow as the chemical induces anesthesia. Introduce fresh water into the container with anesthetic if the level of anesthesia becomes too deep.

Anesthetic Doses

Benzocaine (ethyl p-aminobenzoate) –
Dose at 50–500 mg (may need to dissolve in ethanol first) / liter of water.
Induction time is 1 minute, recovery in fresh water occurs in 3-15 minutes.

Carbon dioxide (CO_2) –
A dose of 100–400 mg/L will cause unconsciousness, excessive exposure will cause death. Adding one Alka-Seltzer tablet per liter water will produce adequate levels of carbon dioxide for short term sedation. Use with caution, under constant observation to prevent death! Carbon dioxide is approved by the AVMA for euthanasia.
Induction is in 1-2 minutes and recovery in 5-10 minutes in fresh water.

Diazepam (Valium) –
A sedative and muscle relaxant, that is used as a preanesthetic agent.
Can be injected intramuscularly at 0.1-0.5 mg/kg, or mixed in food.

Ethanol (ethyl alcohol) –
1% added to the water will produce sedation, 3% or more will result in euthanasia. Using 20 ml of 100-proof (50%) grain alcohol in 1 liter of water will produce a 1% solution.

Ether (dimethyl ether) –
Dose at 10-15 ml/L water.
Induction occurs in 2-3 minutes, recovery in clean water in 2-3 minutes.
HIGHLY EXPLOSIVE! Do not use near flames or sparks! Keep tightly sealed, store in a cool area.

Eugenol (clove oil) –
Use 40-80 mg/L (1-2 drops/liter of water).
Mix in the water vigorously to evenly disperse.
Induction occurs in 2-3 minutes and recovery in 5 minutes in fresh water.

Isofluorane (1-chloro-2,2,2-trifluoroethyl difluoromethyl ether) –
Dose at 0.5-1 ml/L water. Spray the required dose through a 25-gauge needle under the water while mixing.
Induction in 2-8 minutes, recovery in clean water in 3-30 minutes. The longer the time under anesthesia, the longer it takes to regain consciousness.

Ketamine hydrochloride –
Dose at 1 g/L added to the water, or 66-100 mg/kg injected intramuscularly.
Provides sedation and immobilization for handling or transportation. Does not produce analgesia.

Quinaldine sulfate (2-methylquinolinesulfate) –
Dose at 25-200 mg/L.
Induction in 2-6 minutes, recovery in fresh water in 5-20 minutes.
Acidifies low alkaline water, use buffer in water as necessary.

Tricaine methane sulfonate, MS-222 (3-aminobenzoic acid ethyl ester) –
Dose at 10-40 mg/L for sedation (handling/shipping).
Dose at 50-100 mg/L for anesthesia.
Induction in 1-5 minutes, recovery in 3-15 minutes in clean water.
Acidifies water – use buffered or hard water.

After the koi is anesthetized in the anesthetic bath, it can be removed from the water for short-term examination or diagnostic procedures. If the koi is removed for longer procedures, anesthesia can be dripped across the gills through an IV bag and drip line, by hand with a syringe, or with a recirculating water pump or aquarium filter powerhead. Have oxygenated fresh water on hand to syringe across the gills if the plane of anesthesia becomes too deep.

Recuperation after anesthesia is accomplished by transferring the koi into a container of fresh well-aerated water. Moving the fish gently in a forward direction will aid the flow of fresh water across the gills, hastening anesthesia release from the gills. Do not slosh the fish back and forth in the water. Once there are steady opercular movements let the koi rest and gradually recover in a quiet, dim environment. Monitor it until it is swimming normally and can be transferred back into the pond.

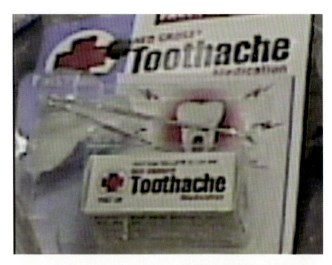

Over-the-counter toothache remedy containing eugenol from a pharmacy makes an effective emergency anesthetic.

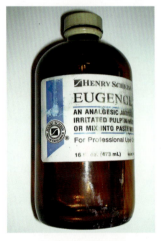

Eugenol anesthetic from a dental supply company is easy to use and inexpensive.

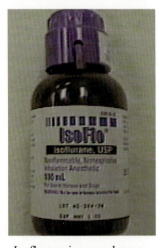

Isoflurane is a good anesthetic choice for abdominal surgical procedures.

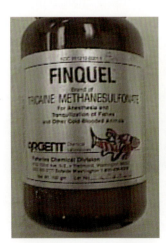

MS-222 must be ordered from aquaculture suppliers and is more expensive than other veterinary anesthetics.

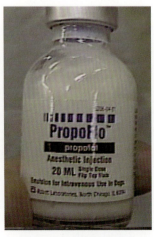

Propofol is an intravenous anesthetic that can be injected into the caudal vein in fish.

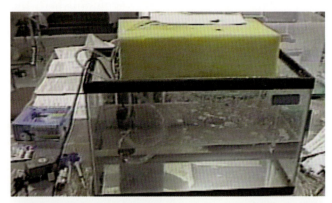

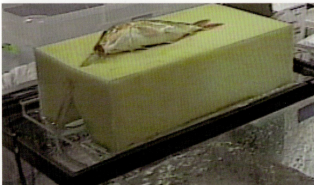

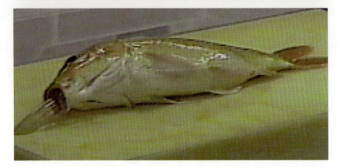

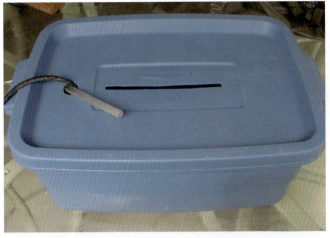
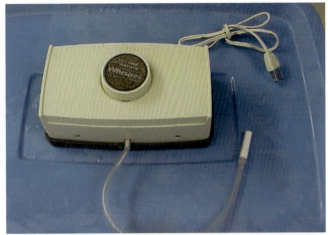
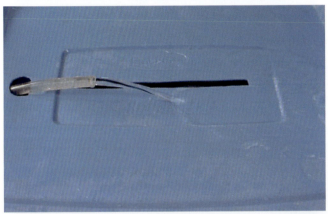
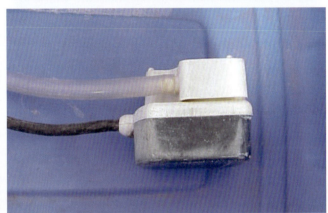
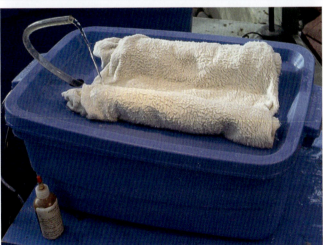
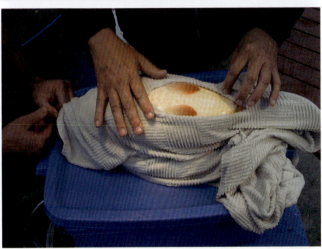

LEFT: Anesthesia chamber designed by veterinarians Dr. Craig Harms and Dr. Gregory Lewbart uses a 10-gallon aquarium with a recirculationg water pump that squirts water through a hose placed in the fish's mouth. An open-cell foam pad to hold the fish is placed on top of a perforated plastic cover over the tank. The foam pad is flat on one side to lay the fish in lateral recumbancy, and notched on the opposite side so that the koi can be held in a dorsally recumbant position for abdominal surgery. The water pumped through the mouth goes out the gill slit and drips back into the anesthetic tank for reuse.

ABOVE: The author's portable, light-weight, unbreakable and inexpensive anesthesia induction chamber and field surgery table. A slit and a hole are cut into the recessed lid of a plastic tub. A small water pump or an aquarium powerhead is used to recirculate the water. An aquarium air pump has an attached air stone that is placed into the solution to provide aeration. Pure oxygen can also be bubbled through tubing into the water to increase the dissolved oxygen level. A wet towel is rolled on each end to support the dorsally recumbant koi, then it is covered with another wet towel with a slit in it to expose the surgery field; finally a sterile surgical drape covers the whole unit and the koi.

Surgery

A number of surgical procedures have been performed on koi, primarily for external skin and fin tumor excisions, and abdominal exploratory surgeries to remove abdominal masses. Other surgical procedures have been performed for repair of lacerations from traumatic injuries, resection of prolapsed cloacal tissues, and orthopedic procedures on koi with spinal fractures. General surgical knowledge and experience will facilitate successful koi surgery, as will familiarity with normal koi anatomy. Aseptic surgical technique should be maintained as best as possible.

After the fish is in an adequate plane of anesthesia, it is placed on wet chamois cloth, towel or foam in the appropriate position for surgery. Rolled up cloth can be placed on either side of the body to maintain the koi in dorsal recumbency (belly up). Exposed tissues not in the surgical field are covered with wet gauze to prevent desiccation. Ophthalmic ointment should be placed on the eyes to keep them moist. The surgical site is gently cleaned with a 1:10 diluted solution of 1% povidone-iodine (Betadine) in 0.9% physiological saline. A clear plastic surgical drape can be placed over the surgery site; small dabs of Vaseline will help it adhere to the skin.

The aerated anesthetic solution is dripped over the gills to maintain anesthesia, or plastic tubing can be placed in the fish's mouth and the solution slowly pumped in and across the gills. The anesthetic solution flow can be maintained via a motorized pump such as an aquarium powerhead, by gravity using an IV bag and drip set filled with anesthetic solution, or by hand with a syringe attached to IV tubing or aquarium air line. A raised drainboard or grate under the fish will allow the excess solution to run out from under the fish and into a catch basin.

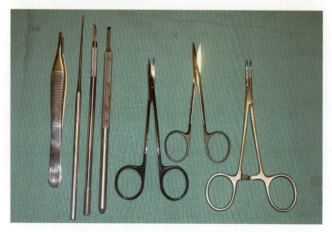

Assorted microsurgical instruments useful in koi surgery.

The best surgical instruments for fish surgery are ophthalmic or microsurgery instruments because of their small size; but many surgeries can be performed with a scalpel with a #11 or #15 blade, iris scissors, Metzenbaum scissors, mosquito hemostats, and a pair of fine forceps. A jeweler's loupe or other magnifying lens is very helpful.

Abdominal surgery is performed in koi through a ventral midline incision. Start the incision cranial to the vent and continue forward to the pectoral fin bones, as needed. Scales along the incision may be cut through, or removed with forceps prior to making the incision. The pelvic girdle may be separated with Mayo scissors or bone cutters if necessary. Use gentle blunt dissection with the hemostats, Metzenbaum scissors, or gloved fingers to isolate the desired tissues. Ligate blood vessels as needed with 3-0 or smaller absorbable suture material such as Vicryl or Maxon. Stainless steel Hemoclips may also be used for ligation. Bipolar cautery units are useful for small vessel hemostasis.

Successful abdominal surgeries have been performed on koi to remove both testicular and ovarian gonadal tumors. These appear as large (as much as 10% of the total body weight in size), irregular, fibrous masses in the caudal abdomen. They often cause the abdomen to appear quite distended (called "choman" by the Japanese). These can be bluntly dissected free from fibrous attachments, using appropriate hemostasis. After removal, survey the abdominal organs to assess any damage from pressure necrosis or obstruction. The contralateral gonad should also be assessed.

Occasionally the gas bladder will become traumatized and distended, creating an appearance similar to an abdominal tumor. A radiograph or ultrasound examination will distinguish between an enlarged gas bladder and a tumor. The gas bladder in koi consists of two compartments joined by an isthmus. The caudal compartment is connected to the esophagus by the pneumatic duct. The damaged compartment of the gas bladder can be isolated and ligated for removal. The cranial compartment when removed is ligated at the isthmus. The caudal compartment is ligated distal to the pneumatic duct, leaving it attached to a remnant of the caudal compartment near the isthmus. The fish will gradually stabilize its buoyancy with the remaining portion of the gas bladder.

Muscle layers can be closed with absorbable suture material in a simple continuous suture pattern. Trapped air in the abdomen should be removed by suction after closing the muscles and before closing the skin. In smaller fish, the muscle layer and skin may be closed in one layer. For skin closure use small monofilament nylon suture material with a swaged-on reverse cutting needle. Simple continuous or simple interrupted suture patterns are most often used to oppose the margins of the skin incision. The incision may be covered with cyanoacrylate tissue glue (Nexaband) to ensure a waterproof closure. Remove the skin sutures in 2-3 weeks, or when the skin appears adequately healed.

Skin and fin wounds can be sutured using fine (3-0) monofilament nylon sutures. To repair split fin membranes, gently scrape the apposing edges with a scalpel blade to remove scar tissue, and then tightly appose the fin edges with a series of simple interrupted sutures. Start at the base of the tear, and work outward toward the edge of the fin. Incorporate one or more fin rays in each side to keep the suture from tearing through the fin membrane. Apply Betadine solution topically to the fin before and after suturing. Remove the sutures in 3 weeks. Hyperplasia of the epidermis will grow over the suture sites, but will regress after the sutures are removed, and it can be trimmed back at the time of suture removal.

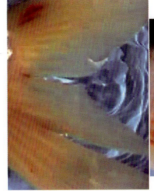
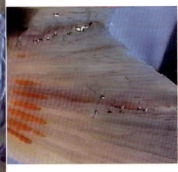

Tears in the center and in the lower half of the caudal fin in a Shusui koi.

The two tears were sutured with monofilament nylon in a continuous pattern. Sutures were removed at 3 weeks.

The fin is completely healed at 8 weeks.

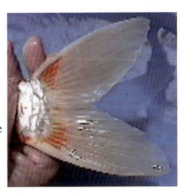

Scale injuries from netting or handling can also be repaired if the sloughed scale still contains adequate attached epidermis, and is immediately replaced in its normal position. Hold the scale in place with a few small simple interrupted sutures through the surrounding tissue. Clean the skin with topical iodine solution (Betadine). Remove the sutures in 7 days, or when the tissue has reattached.

On certain color varieties of koi a stray black sumi mark (called a shimi) in the wrong section of color will detract from its appearance. These small pigmented areas can be surgically excised, although pigment cells (melanophores) occur both in the epidermis and in the dermis, so sometimes the pigment is below the scale. A microscalpel with a #67 Beaver mini-blade, or even a #11 standard scalpel blade is used to incise around the shimi and elevate it from the skin. Deep pigmentation may need a cone-shaped excision of tissue to get through the scale (without removing the whole scale) into the dermis layer.

Afterwards apply topical antibiotic ointment. The wound is allowed to heal by epithelial migration. White and orange skin usually heals with normal color, although scarring can occur or the pigmentation shade may vary from the surrounding tissue. The ethical aspect of cosmetic modifications must be considered.

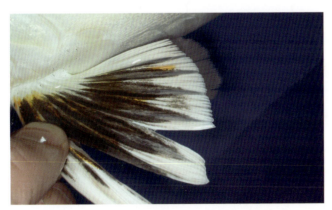

The left pelvic fin was torn on this Doitsu koi during transportation.

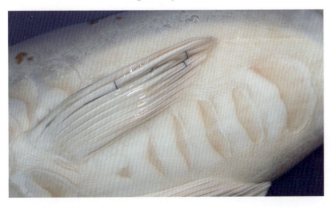

Ventral view of the same left pelvic fin after suturing the fin rays together along the two tears in the fin.

Abdominal Surgery to Remove a Testicular Tumor from a Koi (Choman Belly)

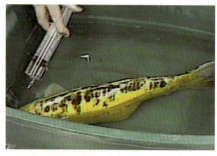

Isoflurane anesthetic is injected into fresh, dechlorinated water at 1ml/L to anesthetize the koi for exploratory abdominal surgery.

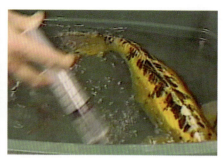

Rapid stirring motion while injecting the Isoflurane into the water through a 25-gauge needle will increase its dispersion in the water.

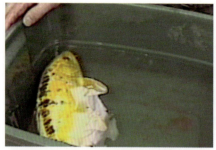

After one minute, the koi is beginning to show the effects of the Isofluorane. It begins to list to one side and slows its opercle motions (respiration).

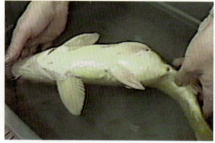

After only three minutes the koi is anesthetized and unable to right itself. The caudal abdomen is distended from the abdominal mass.

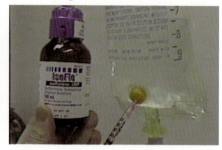

Isofluorane for anesthesia maintenance while in surgery is injected at a dose of 0.5 ml/L into an IV bag filled with sterile water and oxygen.

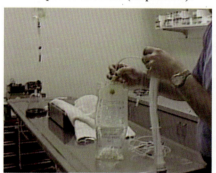

Prior preparation of the interoperative anesthesia delivery system by filling an empty IV bag with sterile water.

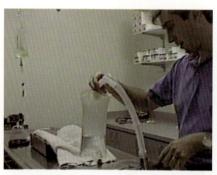

Then the bag is filled with oxygen and an IV drip line is attached to keep the oxygen from escaping.

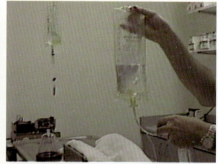

The IV drip line is placed in the koi's mouth to provide the anesthesia. Flow of the solution is by gravity.

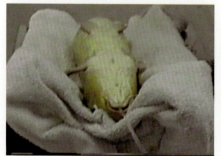

The koi is positioned on a wet towel placed over a V-tray. The IV tubing is adjusted so the oxygenated water with the anesthetic flows out the gills. The gravity flow is controlled by a valve.

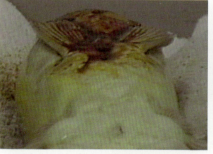

The koi is placed in a dorsal recumbant position on the V-tray. Betadine solution is sprayed onto the abdomen where the incision will be made.

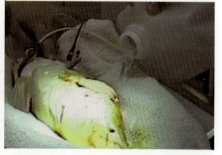

Sterile water is added to the towel as needed to keep the koi wet. The ECG leads are clipped onto hyodermic needles inserted into the muscles on either side of the pectoral fins.

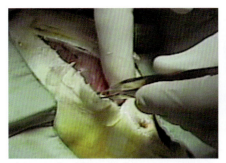
A ventral midline incision is made 1-2 cm anterior to the vent, and carefully extended to the pelvic girdle as necessary for exposure.

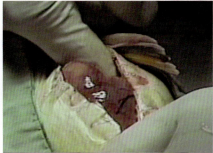
A gloved finger is used to bluntly dissect the tumor from the body wall and the abdominal organs. The tumor is isolated and exposed.

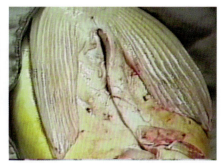
The blood supply to the tumor was ligated with Hemoclips and then it was removed. The abdomen was flushed with saline solution.

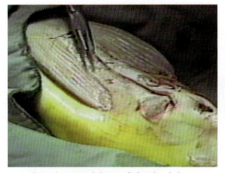
Good apposition of the incision edges should occur when closing the incision.

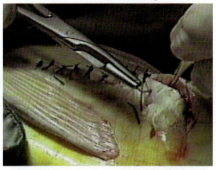
A reverse cutting needle facilitates penetration of the skin and body wall when suturing the incision.

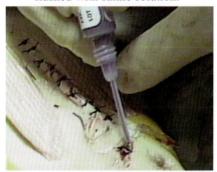
Tissue glue can be applied over the sutured incision to form a temporary water-tight seal.

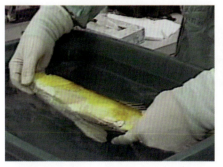
Fresh water is flushed across the gills to lessen the anesthesia, and then the koi is placed in clean water to awaken.

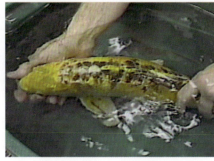
Gentle forward motion is used to help water flow through the mouth and across the gills.

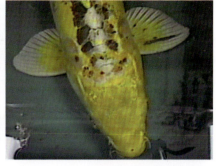
Surgery time length will affect how long it takes the koi to awaken from anesthesia.

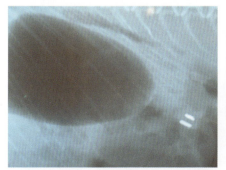
Post-operative radiograph showing two Hemaclips to the right of the caudal chamber of the swim bladder used to ligate the blood supply to the tumor.

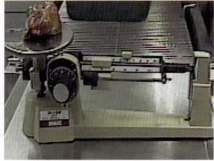
The testicular tumor weighed 161 grams and was 8 cm in diameter. It was sectioned, placed in 10% formalin, and submitted for histopathology.

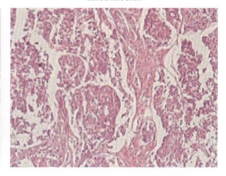
Microscopic photograph of the histopathology slide of the testicular tumor, which was diagnosed as a gonadal sarcoma.

Electrocardiogram

During a surgical procedure, an electrocardiogram (ECG) reading can be taken to monitor the heart rate and rhythm. Three ECG lead clips can each be attached to the metal part of 22-gauge hypodermic needles. These needles then are placed through the skin and just into the muscle tissue at the base of the right pectoral fin (RA lead), the left pectoral fin (LA lead), and cranial to the vent opening (LL lead). The P-QRS-T waves produced are of low amplitude (1 mV QRS complex), but similar to those in other animals. Heart rates are temperature dependant, as well as being affected by anesthesia. Normal heart rates are 30-40 beats per minute, but can range from 15 to 100 beats per minute.

Pulse Oximeter

Anytime a koi is anesthetized a pulse oximeter can be attached to a thin area of the caudal fin, or other fin. The pulse oximeter measures the oxygen saturation (in percent) of the blood flowing through the capillaries, and also records the pulse rate. This is helpful information to know to determine if more aeration of the water is needed, including using pure oxygen from a canister to bubble through the water to increase the dissolved oxygen content. The pulse rate will decrease as the koi is more anesthetized, so the pulse rate can be used to judge the depth of anesthesia. Increase fresh water flow across the gills to lessen the anesthesia and cause the pulse to increase if it slows too much.

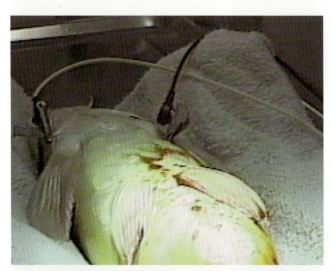

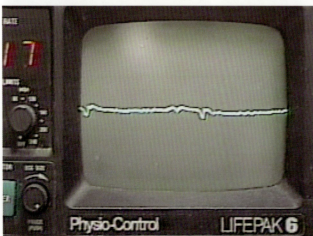

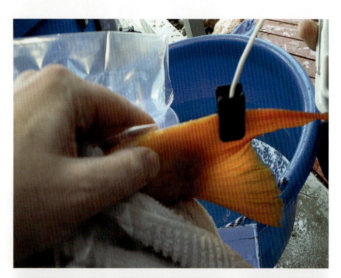

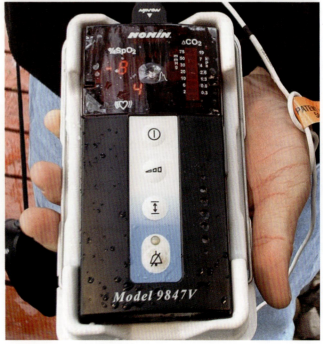

ABOVE: The ECG leads are clipped to the metal hypodermic needle inserted into the muscles of the anesthetized koi. The ECG monitor shows an inverted p-wave followed by an inverted QRS complex. The heart rate is 17 beats/min. RIGHT: The Pulse oximeter is clamped onto the caudal fin. The display shows oxygen saturation percent and pulse rate.

Injections

Koi can be anesthetized briefly for injections if warranted, or can be gently restrained with wet hands, or wrapped in a wet chamois cloth, towel or wet plastic bag. Using a butterfly catheter between the syringe and needle can increase the ease of giving injections, and reduce the risk of injury to the koi, especially when it is not anesthetized for the injection.

Intramuscular (IM) injections are given to koi in the epaxial muscles along the back. A 22 or 25-gauge hypodermic needle is most often used, and it is inserted along either side of the dorsal fin between scales, angling the tip toward the head. As fish skin is not very elastic, the medication will leak out the hole made by the needle if the needle is not inserted far enough forward from the hole when depositing the medicine. Hold a finger over the scales when removing the needle to keep from pulling out an impaled scale, and also to help seal the skin hole so medication doesn't leak back out.

The IM injection can also be given into the epaxial muscles by inserting the hypodermic needle on the dorsal midline behind the dorsal fin, and angling it forward and to either side into the muscles. This area of the skin does not have scales, so it is easier to insert the needle and there is no danger of accidentally removing a scale impaled on the needle. It also produces less skin reaction at the injection site. Small volume IM injections can also be given into the muscle at the fleshy base of the pectoral fin.

Intraperitoneal (IP), or intracoelomic, injections are given on the belly of the koi, lateral to the ventral midline and caudal to one of the pelvic fins, passing the needle through the body wall and just into the peritoneal cavity. Angle the needle toward the head so it penetrates the body wall obliquely. Be careful to insert the needle only through the body wall and not into abdominal organs, or into the ovarian egg mass in females, which are in this area.

Intravenous (IV) injections can be given through the caudal peduncle into the caudal vein ventral to the vertebrae.

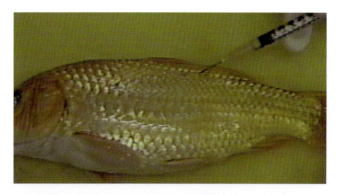

IM injection in the epaxial muscle lateral to the dorsal fin.

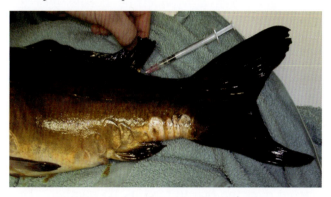

IM injection given behind the dorsal fin.

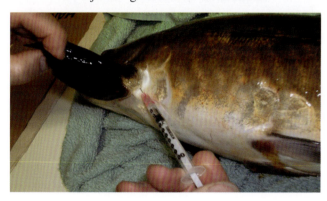

IM injection given in muscle at base of pectoral fin.

BELOW: Intraperitoneal injection being given through the abdominal body wall into the coelomic cavity.
LEFT: Care must be taken in giving IP injections as organs (such as an egg-filled ovary) lie just beneath the body wall.

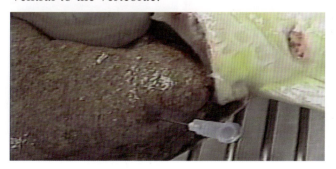

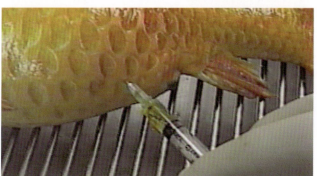

Microchip Identification

The insertion of a tiny (2 x 12 mm) passive radio-frequency transponder into koi provides a permanent method of identification. The transponder consists of a glass-encased electromagnetic coil, tuning capacitor, and a microchip. Each microchip contains a unique identification number that cannot be altered. The transponder is activated by a hand-held scanner emitting a low-frequency 125 kHz radio signal, and transmits its unique ID code to the scanner. The transponder is injected through a hypodermic needle into the epaxial muscle, or intraperitoneally, where it remains permanently. Although the transponder is very small, the 12-gauge hypodermic needle used to implant it can be traumatic to small fish. Koi of 6 inches (15 cm) or more will do best for implanting. Anesthesia can be used when inserting the transponder.

A central registry is kept to record which microchip number is given to each animal. The registry can be contacted to locate the owner of a lost animal. A hand-held electronic scanner is passed over the fish to read its ID number. This permanent invisible ID system makes is possible to prove ownership of koi at shows, or when recovering stolen koi. It is an excellent way of identifying breeder koi for keeping accurate breeding records each year. Many koi change color as they mature, and this ID would show it is the same koi. A certificate of ownership is provided with each transponder that can be used to transfer the ID number from the previous owner to the new owner, providing proof of sale.

This is an enlarged image of the passive microchip transponder that can be implanted in koi for permanent positive identification.

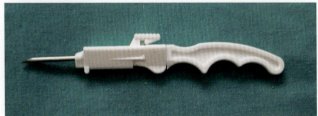
The hypodermic applicator for implanting the microchip transponder has a 12-gauge needle that is preloaded with the sterile microchip. After inserting the needle into the koi, the thumb tab is pushed forward to inject the microchip transponder into the fish.

Euthanasia

Sometimes severely sick or injured koi may need to be humanely euthanized. One commonly used technique is to place the fish in a plastic container of 1% salt water (10 teaspoons/gallon) to supposedly calm it, and then place the whole container in the freezer, slowly lowering its metabolic rate until it dies. However, freezing is not an acceptable method of euthanasia by the American Veterinary Medical Association (AVMA) standards. It is preferable and more humane to use an overdose of anesthesia, which will render the fish unconscious quickly, and cause its respiration to cease. Use up to 10 times the recommended anesthetic dose, and leave the fish in the solution for an hour after it has stopped opercular movements.

In some cases appropriate anesthesia is not available for humane euthanasia. In this case, sodium bicarbonate (baking soda) can be used as an alternative. Baking soda added to the water produces narcosis (unconsciousness) by increasing carbon dioxide. It is effective in water with pH 6.5-8.5. The fish will lose consciousness and then the opercular movements (respiration) will stop. Waiting up to an hour after the opercular movement ceases should ensure the fish has expired. Using carbon dioxide for euthanasia is approved by the AVMA.

To make the euthanasia solution, add 1-2 ounces (30-60 grams) of baking soda to each quart (or liter) of water and mix well, until all the powder is dissolved. Add the fish to be euthanized to the solution and wait until the fish has expired before removing it.

Alka-Seltzer can also be used to produce carbon dioxide in the water for euthanasia of small fish. Use 2 or more tablets per liter of water, then add the fish to be euthanized to the solution and wait until the fish has expired before removing it.

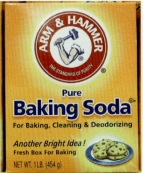 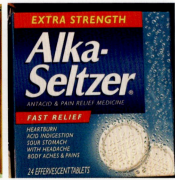
Baking Soda, as well as Alka-Seltzer tablets, can be used to produce carbon dioxide in the water for fish euthanasia.

REFERENCES:

Bond, Carl E. 1979. *Biology of Fishes,* W.B. Saunders, Philadelphia.

Campbell, Terry W. and Frank Murru. 1990. "An Introduction to Fish Hematology" in *Practical Exotic Animal Medicine,* Veterinary Learning Systems, Trenton, NJ.

Francis-Floyd, Ruth. 1995. *Incorporating Pet Fish Into Your Small Animal Practice,* University of Florida, Gainesville, FL.

Francis-Floyd, Ruth. 1999. "Clinical Examination of Fish in Private Collections" in *The Veterinary Clinics of North America – Exotic Animal Practice,* vol. 2, no. 2, W.B. Saunders, Philadelphia.

Groff, Joseph M. and Joseph G. Zinkl. 1999. "Hematology and Clinical Chemistry of Cyprinid Fish" in *The Veterinary Clinics of North America – Exotic Animal Practice,* vol. 2, no. 3, W.B. Saunders, Philadelphia.

Harms, Craig A. 1999. "Anesthesia in Fish" in *Zoo & Wild Animal Medicine* 4, W.B. Saunders, Philadelphia.

Harms, Craig and Gregory Lewbart. 2000. "Surgery in Fish" in *The Veterinary Clinics of North America – Exotic Animal Practice,* vol. 3, no. 3, W.B. Saunders, Philadelphia.

Johnson, Erik L. 1997. *Koi Health and Disease,* Reade Printers, Athens, GA.

Lewbart, Gregory A. 1998. *Self-Assessment Color Review of Ornamental Fish,* Iowa State University Press, Ames, IA.

Lewbart, Gregory A. et al. 1998. "Surgical removal of an undifferentiated abdominal sarcoma from a koi carp (*Cyprinus carpio*)," in *The Veterinary Record* 143, p. 556-558, UK.

Noga, Edward J. 1996. *Fish Disease: Diagnosis and Treatment,* Mosby, St. Louis, MO.

Ranson, Stan (editor). 1997. *Practical Koi Keeping*, vol. 3, Koi USA, Midway City, CA

Stetter, Mark. 1999. *Ultrasonography of Nondomestic Species,* North American Veterinary Conference Fish Wetlab, Orlando, FL.

Stoskopf, Michael K. (editor). 1988. "Tropical Fish Medicine" in *The Veterinary Clinics of North America – Small Animal Practice*, vol. 18, no. 2, W.B. Saunders, Philadelphia.

Stoskopf, Michael K. (editor). 1993. *Fish Medicine,* W.B. Saunders, Philadelphia.

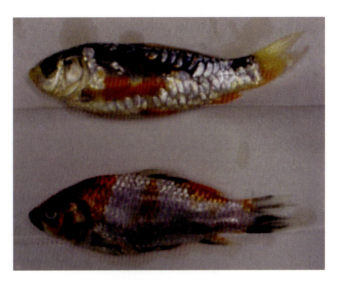

Deceased koi brought into the clinic for diagnostic testing and necropsy examination. Note the Doitsu "mirror" (kagami) scales on the upper koi, and the normal scales (wagoi) on the bottom koi.

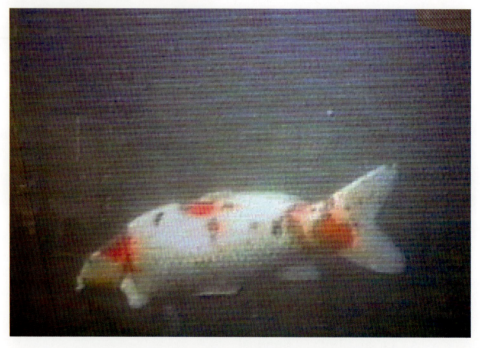
Having an underwater video camera is one way of monitoring the health of the koi without needing to catch them!

CHAPTER 3: INFECTIOUS DISEASES

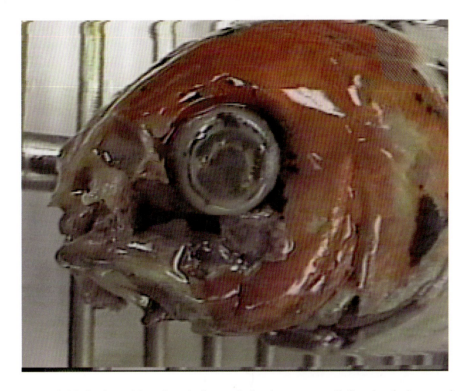

Bacterial infections (above) and viruses (below) can cause disfiguring lesions, and ultimately death if not diagnosed properly and treated appropriately in a timely manner.

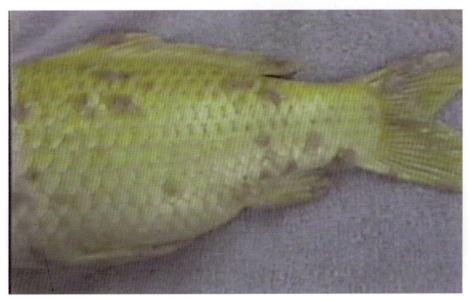

VIRAL DISEASES

Carp Pox

This disease is not caused by a poxvirus but by *Herpesvirus cyprini* (Cyprinid Herpesvirus 1). It produces epidermal hyperplasia, presenting as superficial milky white to pink-colored plaques on the skin and fins. They extend 1-2 mm above the surface of the skin, and are usually smooth. Adjacent plaques may merge into larger raised areas. The lesions are benign and eventually slough. The disease is not fatal but can produce scarring. In severe cases large areas of the body and fins can be covered with plaques. The fish swim and eat normally in most instances.

The virus is transmitted by direct contact of an infected fish with healthy fish. Overcrowding in the pond will increase the prevalence of the disease. Inbred fish also appear more susceptible. It may be seasonal in occurrence and is more prevalent in cold or cool water temperatures. Isolation of affected koi is suggested. No treatments are completely effective against viruses, but a cleaning the lesions with a disinfectant solution and surgical removal, followed by topical application of Acyclovir ointment may be helpful.

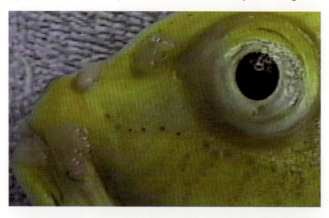

The pink masses are typical carp pox lesions, but this koi has a greater number than is usually seen on a koi.

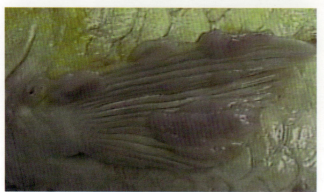

Herpes-Associated Gill Disease (Koi Herpesvirus)

In the spring of 1998, severe common carp and koi mortalities occurred at fish farms in Israel. In the summer of 1999 a similar disease occurred in koi that had been entered into a Japanese-style koi show in New York. Since then veterinary researchers have isolated a herpesvirus believed to be the cause of this disease. Electron microscopy of the Israeli fish revealed intranuclear inclusions in the cells of the hematopoietic (anterior) kidney and the gill epithelium. The virus' envelope was 140-172 nanometers (nm) diameter, with a 94-nm nucleocapsid. The New York koi were examined at the University of California – Davis and had viral inclusions with a loose envelope of 230-250 nm diameter, and a central hexagonal nucleocapsid of 108 nm diameter.

Fish affected with Koi Herpesvirus (KHV) became anorectic, lethargic, floated at angles or swam erratically, and had erythema of the skin and increased mucus production. On examination, the gills were pale and had severe necrosis. There was rapid mortality once signs occurred after exposure, with incubation time dependant on temperature, approximately 30 days at 50°F / 10°C and 3 days at 75°F / 23.8°C. The larger fish were affected earliest. Mortality rates of 80-90% are typical for affected koi ponds. In ponds with other fish present, no species other than common carp or koi appeared to be infected.

The KHV appears most virulent at temperatures between 68-85°F / 20-29°C. The pathogen is highly contagious, transmitted even with brief contact, and can be spread via equipment such as nets and hoses. It causes a decreased immune response (immunosuppression) thereby allowing myriad secondary bacterial infections to occur, confusing the diagnostic process.

The KHV destroys epithelial cells of the gills, and on the skin causes excess mucus production. Death occurs from hypoxia due to gill damage. As yet there is no treatment for the herpesvirus, but perfect water quality, high oxygen concentration, and treatment of secondary infections are all important. Raising the water temperature above 86°F / 30°C may help infected koi. ALWAYS QUARANTINE FISH BEFORE PUTTING THEM INTO AN ESTABLISHED POND! This would limit the spread of the disease to other fish.

A Polymerase Chain Reaction (PCR) test has been developed to identify the KHV DNA, but only detects it in infected fish, not the carriers.

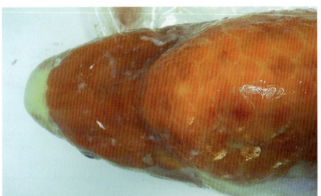
This extremely overfed Kohaku koi is infected with KHV. The skin and fin capillaries are congested, with excess mucus production covering the body.

The head is covered with lumps of mucus. These are not attached to the epidermis as with Carp Pox Herpesvirus.

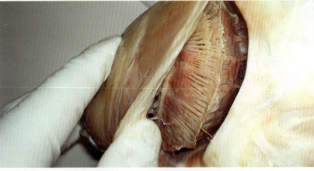
KHV causes the gill epithelium to slough off, leaving the cartilage of the filament exposed with no tissue over it.

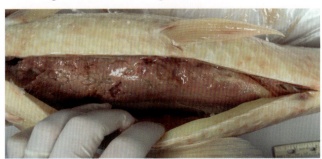
In addition to the external lesions, KHV caused hepatic inflammation and hemorrhage in this koi, although the amount of fat tissue indicates possible hepatic lipidosis.

Carp Gill Necrosis Iridovirus

This is a disease of common carp in Russia, caused by nonenveloped iridovirus particles that measure 190-210 nm diameter. The virus is found as cytoplasmic and intranuclear inclusions. The virus causes gill edema and necrosis, with discoloration and increased mucus production. There is no known treatment as yet, and affected fish should be isolated as soon as diagnosed.

Spring Viremia of Carp (Infectious Dropsy)

This fish disease is caused by *Rhabdovirus carpio* (120 x 60-90 nm). It occurs in Europe and Asia, each area having its own strain of virus. It has now been introduced into North America; the European strain was found in Wisconsin in 1989, and the Asian strain in North Carolina in 2002. It produces a wide variety of signs, including a distended ascitic abdomen (dropsy), exophthalmia (popeye), inflamed and protruding vent, uncoordinated swimming, weak respiration, and gill and skin hemorrhages. The virus is shed in the feces, and the gills are the site of virus entry and primary replication. Virus will spread in the blood to the internal organs. Internal visceral hemorrhages and serosanguinous ascitic fluid are seen on necropsy. Eggs can be infected at breeding. Fish lice and leeches can also carry the virus between fish.

The disease is more severe in cool water temperatures, hence the prevalence of signs in spring, as the water temperature warms above 48°F / 8°C. Warming the pond water up to 68°F / 20°C will protect the fish from the virus. Ultraviolet irradiation of the pond water will inactivate the virus and help prevent its spread. Formalin added to the pond (25 mg/L) will also inactivate the virus in the water. An autogenous vaccine can be made from formalin-inactivated virus and administered by intraperitoneal injection. This will not help already infected fish, but will prevent infection in exposed healthy fish. They should be vaccinated in the summer or fall to prevent disease outbreak in the spring.

Confirmed cases of this virus were diagnosed in koi farms in the United States in April of 2002. World-wide shipping of koi as the koi keeping hobby expands will inevitably spread disease and parasites with the fish. Proper diagnostic examinations, prophylactic treatments and quarantine of new fish are imperative to prevent further transmission of exotic diseases.

BACTERIAL DISEASES

Bacterial Hemorrhagic Septicemia

This serious disease is caused by a number of species of bacteria from the *Aeromonas* genus. Most often identified are *Aeromonas hydrophila* (= *A. liquefaciens*, = *A. punctata*) and *A. sobria*, but other species of *Aeromonas* may also be found. The organisms are motile, Gram-negative, rod-shaped bacteria about 1 x 2.0-4.5 µm in size. They have a single polar flagellum.

Aeromonas bacteria are almost always present in pond water, and even on the fish itself. It is an opportunistic pathogen that proliferates when the fish is weakened or injured. Signs of infection include hemorrhages of the gills, skin and base of fins, loss of scales, and skin ulcers. Eye swelling (exophthalmia) and abdominal swelling (dropsy) may also occur, secondary to circulatory disturbances and fluid accumulation. Parasites such as fish lice cause skin wounds that can become infected with *Aeromonas*.

Treatment consists of antibiotic injections, antibiotics in the food or water, and topical applications of antimicrobial solutions such as povidone-iodine directly on the skin ulcers. The bacteria have become resistant to many commonly used antibiotics (especially ampicillin and tetracycline), so culture and sensitivity testing is necessary prior to choosing an antibiotic. Water quality improvement is indicated for all disease conditions.

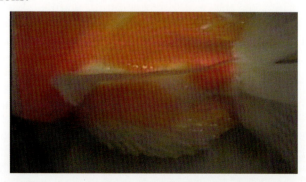

Dropsy (ascites) in this oranda goldfish, causing the scales to protrude, and vent inflammation are signs of septicemia.

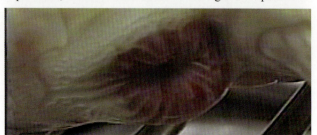

Carp Erythrodermatitis (Furunculosis, Ulcer Disease)

Severe epizootics of this disease occur most frequently in the spring when the water temperature is rising (increased bacterial growth) and the fish are stressed from over-wintering (decreased fish resistance). The signs are erythema (redness) on the skin and base of fins. Raised skin lesions (furuncles) may form, which then ulcerate exposing the underlying muscles. Congestion and hemorrhage of the internal organs also occurs.

The causative organism is atypical *Aeromonas salmonicida achromogenes*, a Gram-negative, nonmotile, short rod (0.5 x 1.5 µm) bacterium. It occurs singly, in pairs, chains, or clumps. It is inactive in water temperatures below 40°F / 4.4°C or above 68°F / 20°C. Disease outbreaks occur when water temperatures rise into this range in the spring. It is contagious and infected koi should be isolated if possible.

Treat with antibiotic injections (Azactam, Baytril, Fortaz, or NuFlor have been effective) and topical disinfection (Betadine) of the lesions. Tube-feeding a mixture of antibiotics and soaked, mashed koi pellets can be used on koi in treatment tanks. Keep the water temperature in the treatment tank above 68°F / 20°C, preferably 73°F / 23°C or higher to increase the fish's immune response and aid healing. Prevent osmotic stress due to skin lesions by adding salt to the water (0.1-0.3% solution). Raising the water temperature in the spring may prevent outbreaks.

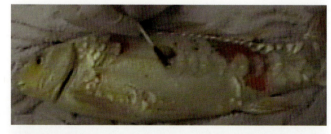

Primary ulcer treatment includes swabbing the lesions with Betadine solution and using topical and injectible antibiotics.

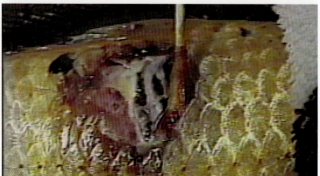

SEQUENTIAL STAGES OF ULCER DISEASE

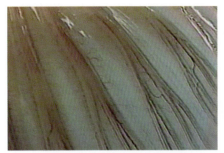

Early signs include redness (congestion) of the fins and skin.

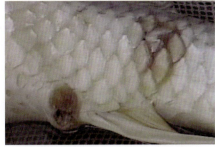

Skin inflammation and a red, protruding vent indicate septicemia.

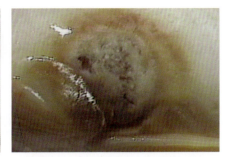

Raised red furuncles may occur, or the skin can ulcerate without them.

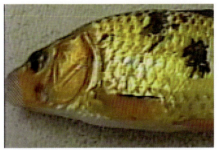

There is a small erosion on the cheek exposing the bone of this koi.

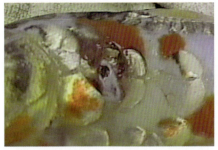

A single ulcer penetrates a scale in the center of the inflamed tissue.

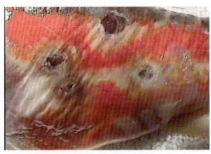

Multiple small ulcers affect the skin on both sides of this Shusui koi.

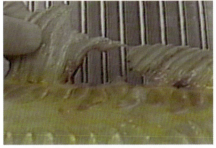

This dorsal fin has been eroded through and is missing fin rays.

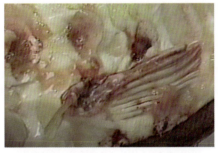

Multiple ulcerations around the pectoral fin, exposing the pectoral bones.

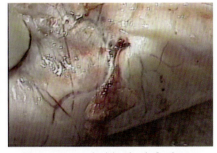

Necropsy on koi in the left photo, lesion goes through the body wall.

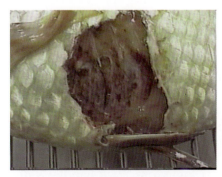

This large ulceration over the pelvic fin extends completely through the body wall, exposing muscle, rib bones, and ovarian tissue within the abdomen. With aggressive treatment, even koi with an exposed abdomen may survive.

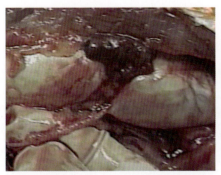

Hemorrhage and congestion in the kidney, swim bladder, and the pneumatic duct. This can lead to buoyancy disorders if the koi cannot properly regulate the air pressure in the swim bladder through the inflamed pneumatic duct.

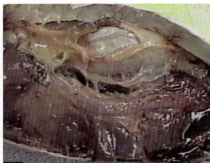

Fibrin adhesions on the abdominal organs indicate septicemia and peritonitis (coelomic inflammation). Organ dysfunction and failure can occur, causing ascites (dropsy), organ necrosis, and death.

Currently there is a vaccination against *Aeromonas salmonicida* available commercially (Furogen from Aqua Health Products). It is given every 6 months by immersion or injection to build resistance in the koi to this bacterium. Another commercially available product to help reduce *Aeromonas* infections is KoiZyme from Koi Care Kennel. This product contains probiotic bacteria that competitively inhibit the *Aeromonas* bacteria. While it does lower the concentration of *Aeromonas* bacteria from the water column, they may be still present in the sediment and debris on the pond bottom.

Bacterial Fin and Gill Rot

This is usually caused by the Gram-negative, short (0.5-1 x 1.5-4 µm), motile rod bacteria *Pseudomonas fluorescens*, *P. putida*, or *P. putrefaciens,* but *Aeromonas* or other species of bacteria can also be involved. Fin and tail erosions are the usual signs, but hemorrhages and skin ulcers sometimes occur, similar to furunculosis. Some suspected cases of furunculosis have been found to be *Pseudomonas* when cultured. A wet mount of infected organs or tissue may reveal motile bacilli that would quickly differentiate these bacteria from the nonmotile *Aeromonas salmonicida*. Traumatic injuries to the fins often result in this secondary bacterial infection.

Treat with antibiotics in food or water, antibiotic injections, and topical wound disinfection. Chloramine-T is often helpful in treating bacterial gill disease. Severely damaged fin margins can be trimmed off with a scalpel or sharp scissors, and the fin topically disinfected. This may hasten healing and fin regeneration. Fin rot is commonly associated with poor water quality.

Columnaris (Cotton Mouth) Disease

Flexibacter (Cytophaga, Flavobacterium) columnaris bacteria is an opportunistic pathogen that causes reddened areas on the skin with cottony white growths, often mistaken for fungi. The lesions occur mostly on the lips and fins, and across the top of the caudal peduncle. The bacterium is a long (10-12 µm), thin, flexingly motile rod.

It will grow in water from 39-95°F / 4-35°C, but is more pathogenic in water above 64°F / 18°C. On the surface of the fish large masses of this bacteria will align themselves into "haystack" formations. It occurs on previously injured tissues. Most healthy fish are resistant to this infection.

Treat with antibiotics in the food and with copper sulfate baths. The disease is worse at higher water temperatures so lower the temperature if possible to slow bacterial growth. Other stresses (poor water quality, other diseases) make this organism more virulent (pathogenic).

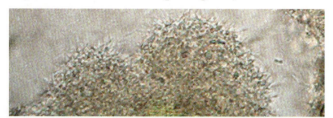

Flexibacter columnaris is one of the few bacteria that can be identified microscopically, due to its long, thin rods creating a haystack appearance.

Mycobacteria (Fish Tuberculosis)

The Mycobacteria are the smallest organisms that are capable of self-replication. Unlike other bacteria, they lack a cell wall. Three species can be found in koi – *Mycobacterium marinum, M. fortuitum,* and *M. smegmatus*. They are Gram-positive, nonmotile coccobacilli measuring 1 µm in length by 0.2-0.6 µm wide. They can live in both fresh and salt water, and can survive in the pond environment for 2-4 days outside of the host, but only for approximately 5 hours out of water.

The infection causes an acute, necrotizing peritonitis to a chronic granulomatous peritoneal response. Occasional giant cells are found in the granulomata. Signs in the fish include lethargy, anorexia, skin lesions, exophthalmia, and ascites. Diagnosis is made by culturing the bacteria at 86-89.6°F / 30-32°C, and by acid-fast staining of affected tissues and examining them microscopically for the bacteria. Treatment is usually unrewarding, but a combination of enrofloxacin (10-14 mg/kg) and rifampin (10-20 mg/kg) can be tried. Minocycline (2 mg/kg) also shows promise for *Mycobacterium* treatment.

A zoonotic potential exists with mycobacteria, and people handling infected fish can get lesions on their hands from contamination of cuts or scrapes. This is known as "fish handler's disease." It is especially of concern in persons with immune deficiencies, who may develop respiratory disease in addition to the localized skin infection. Wear examination gloves when handling fish suspected of having this or any other disease.

Swim Bladder Disease (Submarine Koi)

Abnormalities of the swim bladder can occasionally be caused by bacterial infections, especially *Aeromonas*. An infection that alters the pneumatic duct can allow water to enter the swim bladder, affecting the buoyancy of the koi. These fish lose their positive buoyancy as the air is replaced by water. They have difficulty swimming, and often sit on the bottom of the pond. They will even "hop" on the bottom rather than swim. There may be lesions on the abdomen and ventral fins from rubbing on the pond bottom. The abdomen may also appear bulging due to abnormal distension of the swim bladder. A radiograph will help identify water in the swim bladder and differentiate it from an abdominal mass.

Treat affected koi by percutaneous aspiration of the fluid in the swim bladder while under anesthesia. Use a 22-gauge, 1 ½ inch long needle and place it through the body wall 1-2 cm below the lateral line at the caudal end of the abdominal cavity, which is at about the end of the pelvic fin but before the vent. Angle the needle acutely forward so it passes obliquely through the body muscle and then into the caudal chamber of the gas bladder. Hold the koi out of the water with its head higher than the tail and aspirate all the fluid out of the swim bladder.

Then inject enrofloxacin (10-14 mg/kg) into the gas bladder by switching syringes on the inserted needle. Follow this with enough air injected into the bladder to produce slightly positive buoyancy. Hold a finger over the hole as the needle is withdrawn to prevent pulling out any scales, and also to keep the air from leaking out the hole. Treat any abdominal skin lesions with topical antibacterial solution. This process may need to be repeated weekly until no more fluid can be aspirated from the swim bladder.

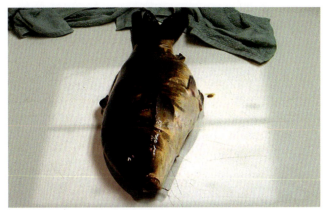

Radiographing a Karasu koi with a swim bladder lesion that prevents it from swimming off the bottom of the pond.

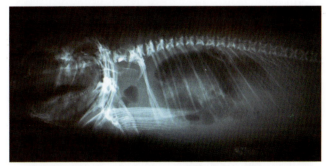

ABOVE: Radograph of the Karasu koi showing minimal air in the gas bladders, but some free air in the abdomen.
BELOW: The ventral lesions by the pelvic fins, and the smaller ones by the pectoral fins are from rubbing on the pond bottom, and are not from a bacterial infection, although they could become secondarily infected.

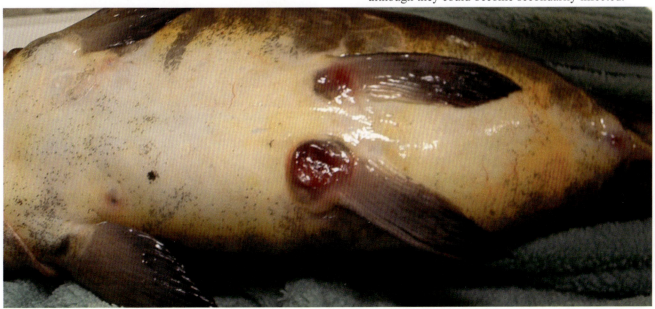

FUNGAL DISEASES

Saprolegnia, Achlya

These aquatic Oomycetes occur as external fungal infections on koi fish. They appear as white cottony tufts on the skin or gills, and also on fish eggs. These fungi can grow in water with up to 0.7% salinity, and in temperatures ranging from 32-96.8°F / 0-36°C, and in the pH range of 4-8.3.

Microscopic examination shows transparent nonseptate branching hyphae, about 20 μm in diameter. The hyphae develop zoosporangia at their tips, which asexually produce by mitosis spherical zoospores. Motile biflagellate primary zoospores (5μm diameter) are released from the zoosporangium (100 μm long) on the tip of *Saprolegnia* mycelium. Each primary zoospore may encyst and divide internally to produce many secondary zoospores. Encysted nonmotile primary zoospores of *Achlya* cluster around the exit papilla of the zoosporangium while dividing. The zoospores attach to damaged tissue or other decaying organic matter and germinate to produce hyphae. They can also reproduce sexually (by meiosis) to produce diploid oospores that also germinate to produce hyphae.

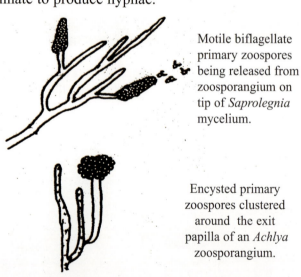

Motile biflagellate primary zoospores being released from zoosporangium on tip of *Saprolegnia* mycelium.

Encysted primary zoospores clustered around the exit papilla of an *Achlya* zoosporangium.

Fungal growth occurs on tissue that has been previously damaged by trauma or other disease conditions. The hyphae produce proteolytic enzymes that cause destruction of adjacent healthy tissue. The fungus also attacks unfertilized fish eggs, but once established will spread to the viable eggs, causing their death by obstructing oxygen absorption with hyphae. Remove any white opaque eggs from the spawning mats, if possible, to prevent their decay and fungus proliferation.

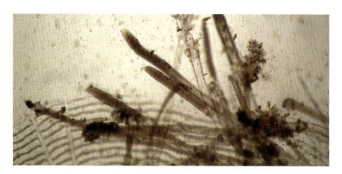

Saprolegnia fungal mycelia, with zoosporangia at the tips.

Treatment consists of adding formalin/malachite solution to the water, and using topical antifungal disinfectants (e.g., Betadine) on the affected skin. Fungus proliferates in ponds with large amounts of organic debris (dead plants and leaves, dead fish, uneaten food), so detritus removal and water changes are helpful. Prevent fungal growth on egg masses with methylene blue (4 mg per gallon of pond water daily for 3 days), malachite green (0.38 mg per gallon daily for 3 days), or hydrogen peroxide 3% (1 ml per gallon of water).

Fungal Gill Rot

Branchiomyces sanguinis and *B. demigrans* fungi invade the blood vessels of the gills, obstructing the flow of blood. Infected gill filaments become brownish with white or gray streaks and raised patches. The gill filaments fuse together and have areas of avascular necrosis due to the

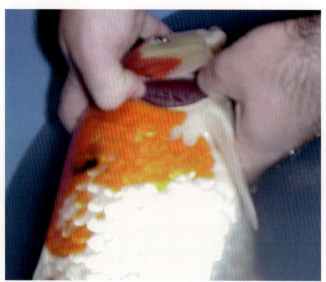

Sanke koi infected with *Branchiomyces demigrans* on its gills. There are raised white fluffy masses of fungal hyphae on the gills that can be removed by scraping.

fungal hyphae blocking the blood vessels of the gill. Gill biopsy of affected tissues will reveal telangiectasis and hyperplasia of gill lamellae. Affected fish become lethargic and appear to be gasping.

Zoosporangia on the fungal hyphae asexually produce nonmotile spores (5-9 µm diameter), which are released into the water and will attach to the gill surface. The spores then germinate branched nonseptate hyphae (8-30 µm diameter) that penetrate into the gill tissue. *Branchiomyces sanguinis* only grows within the gill capillaries, while *B. demigrans* will grow throughout the gill tissue and form masses of hyphae on the surface of the gills. This fungus grows in water temperatures of 57-95°F / 14-35°C.

High levels of un-ionized ammonia in the water increase the incidence of fungal gill rot due to gill epithelial hyperplasia. Accumulation of organic debris in the pond, and suspended particulate matter, may also predispose fish to this infection. Death due to hypoxia can occur rapidly in affected fish, in as little as 2 days after infection. Mortality rates in affected ponds can be high.

Treat daily with methylene blue or malachite green, and add salt to the pond (0.3-0.5%) until gill tissue is healthy. Prevent by keeping the water cool and clean, reducing overcrowded conditions, and avoiding accumulations of decomposing organic matter.

Dermocystidium koi

As the name implies, this fungus causes cysts in the dermis of koi. The spore-filled hyphae infiltrate the skin and gills and cause 1-cm raised nodules to form. These may be surgically removed to improve the koi's appearance. Microscopic examination of a removed cyst will show many spores (3-6 µm x 6-12 µm). Each spore has an eccentric nucleus, a large vacuole, and an inclusion body.

Treat the skin with topical antifungal solutions such as Betadine or chlorhexidine, and treat the water with antifungal dyes such as malachite green or methylene blue.

REFERENCES:

Ariav, Ra'anan. 1999. *Proceedings of the 9th International Conference,* European Association of Fish Pathologists.

Bullock, Graham L., et al. 1971. *Diseases of Fishes,* Book 2: *Bacterial Diseases of Fishes,* T.F.H. Publications, Neptune, NJ.

Dawson, Verdal K., et al. 1994. *Hydrogen Peroxide is Fungicidal on Trout Eggs,* National Fisheries Research Center, La Crosse, WI.

Dixon, Beverly. 1991. "Fungus Among Us" in *Aquarium Fish Magazine,* vol. 3, no. 8, Fancy Publications, Irvine, CA.

Dixon, Beverly A. and Gerard Issvoran. 1993. "Antibacterial Drug Resistance in *Aeromonas* spp. Isolated from Domestic Goldfish and Koi from California" in *Journal of the World Aquaculture Society,* vol. 24, no. 1, Baton Rouge, LA.

Kebus, Myron. 1999. *Koi Mortalities Associated with Koi Viral Agent,* Wisconsin Aquatic Veterinary Service, Madison, WI.

Lansdell, W., et al. 1993. "Isolation of Several *Mycobacterium* Species from Fish," in *Journal of Aquatic Animal Health,* 5:73-76, American Fisheries Society, Bethesda, MD.

Lewbart, Gregory A. 1998. *Self-Assessment Color Review of Ornamental Fish,* Iowa State University Press, Ames, IA.

Neish, Gordon A. and Gilbert C. Hughes. 1980. *Diseases of Fishes,* Book 6: *Fungal Diseases of Fishes,* T.F.H. Publications, Neptune, NJ.

Plumb, John A. 1999. *Health Maintenance and Principal Microbial Diseases of Cultured Fishes,* Iowa State University Press, Ames, IA.

Roberts, Ronald J. 1989. *Fish Pathology,* 2nd ed., Bailliere Tindall, London.

Stoskopf, Michael K. 1993. *Fish Medicine,* W.B. Saunders, Philadelphia.

Talaat, A.M. et al. 1997. "Pathogenesis of Experimental Mycobacterial Infection in Fish" in *Proceedings of the 28th Annual IAAAM Conference,* International Association for Aquatic Animal Medicine, Hardowijh, Netherlands.

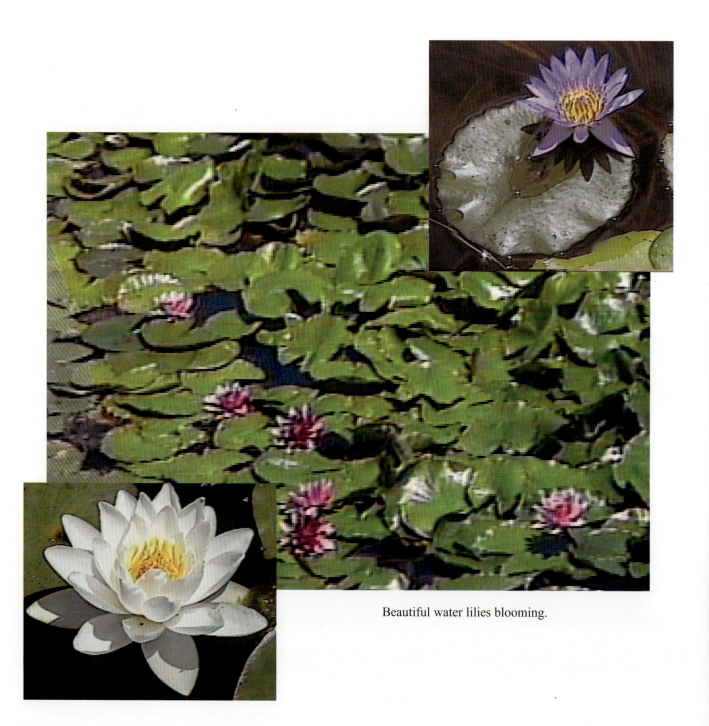

Beautiful water lilies blooming.

CHAPTER 4: PARASITIC DISEASES

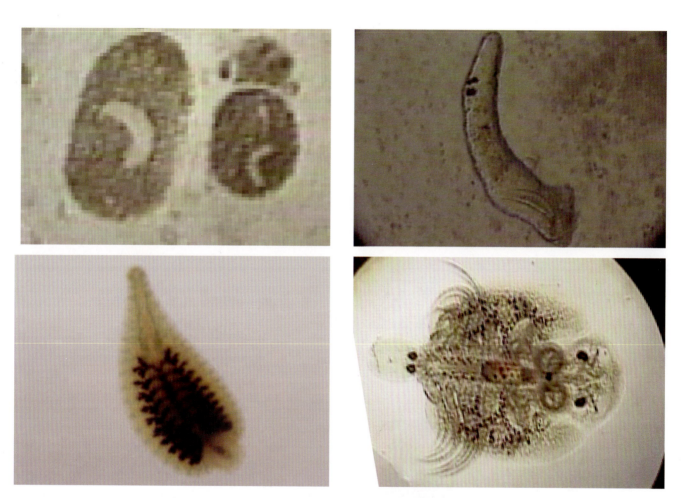

Many types of parasites can infest koi. Pictured are commonly encountered ones from four taxonomic groups: (top) protozoan parasites, *Ichthyophthirius;* a flatworm, *Dactylogyrus;* (bottom) an annelid leech; and a crustacean, *Argulus*.

PROTOZOAL PARASITES

Diagnosis of protozoal infestation is best done by examination of a live fish, or a freshly dead refrigerated fish. Frozen specimens or fish dead for very long will not yield accurate samples of protozoa. The soft-bodied protozoa will disappear rapidly from delayed specimens. Samples taken and examined microscopically right at the pond location, or having the live fish brought to the clinic for examination, are better than taking samples at the pond and then bringing them into the laboratory for examination.

Affected fish should have a small area of skin scraped and the mucus examined under a microscope. A small section of a fin and of a gill filament should also be clipped off for examination. Fresh wet mounted samples must be microscopically examined quickly to visualize the motility of many protozoa species. A blood sample can be drawn and checked for blood parasites. Feces should be examined for intestinal protozoa.

SPORE-FORMING PROTOZOA (SPOROZOA)

Eimeria, Goussia (Coccidiosis)

These are intracellular protozoal parasites that cause inflammation of the intestines. Affected fish are thin and depressed. The feces are often yellowish. Microscopic examination of the feces will reveal the coccidioid oocysts (20-40 μm). Each oocyst contains four sporocysts, each of which contains two sporozoites. Treat with tetracycline antibiotic in the food.

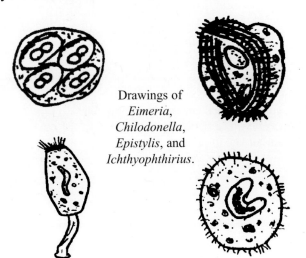

Drawings of *Eimeria*, *Chilodonella*, *Epistylis*, and *Ichthyophthirius*.

CILIATED PROTOZOA (CILIATA)

Chilodonella cyprini

This motile ciliated protozoan attaches to the skin and gills causing respiratory distress, depression, fins clamped to sides, and excessive mucus production that makes the skin look white or bluish. The gills may appear pale and covered with mucus. A smear taken from the mucus will contain many of the organisms. The organism is notched at the posterior pole, giving it a heart-shaped appearance. It is 20-40 x 30-80 μm in size. The cilia are in parallel rows forming a band around the body.

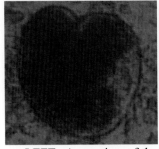 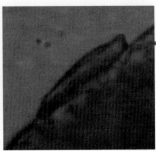

LEFT: A top view of the heart-shaped *Chilodonella*.
RIGHT: A side view of *Chilodonella* gliding across the hyperplastic surface of a gill filament.

It is an especially important parasite during the winter, when the fish are dormant. *Chilodonella* can reproduce in cold water and prefers temperatures as low as 41-50°F / 5-10°C. They reproduce by simple division (binary fission) and their life cycle is direct. Their numbers can increase when the fish is in a weakened state from the cold water. Fission ceases at 68°F / 20°C, and the parasite dies in warm water.

Treating the pond with formalin/malachite solution is effective against most protozoan parasites. The standard solution uses 14 grams of zinc-free malachite green granules added to one gallon of formalin (37% formaldehyde solution). Use this at a dose of 1 ounce (30 ml) per 300 gallons of pond water every 2-3 days for 1-2 weeks. This gives a dosage level of 25 mg/L of formalin and 0.10 mg/L of malachite green. Be sure to monitor the pond water quality when using this medication. Copper sulfate can also be used for treatment, or a 2% salt solution for a 10-20 minute bath. Keeping a 0.2-0.3% salt concentration in the pond will help prevent outbreaks. Also, avoid overcrowding, overfeeding, and accumulation of organic debris.

Epistylis, Heteropolaria (Red Sore Disease)

These sessile, colonial, ciliated parasites attach to the body, fins, and gills of fish by a long retractable stalk (50 μm wide). They have a direct life cycle and reproduce asexually by binary fission. They are filter feeders that ingest organic debris and do not feed on the fish itself, but use it as a substrate for attachment. This can lead to secondary *Aeromonas* or *Saprolegnia* infections at the attachment sites. Heavy infestation causes light-colored cottonlike patches on the skin. Fish may scrape their sides on rocks (flashing) because of irritation. They may also attach on fish eggs, causing them to appear fuzzy. Standard doses of Formalin/malachite solution will reduce the growth of these parasites, as will adding salt to the pond. Decreasing the organic load in the pond is also important.

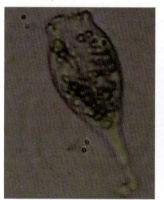 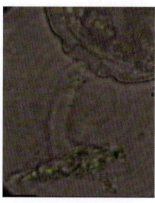

LEFT: A single *Epistylis* organism showing its body attached to the stalk. The mouth is at the top of the body.
RIGHT: The hold-fast at the end of the stalk can cause damage to the epithelium of the host to which it attaches.
BELOW: A typical colonial group of the organisms.

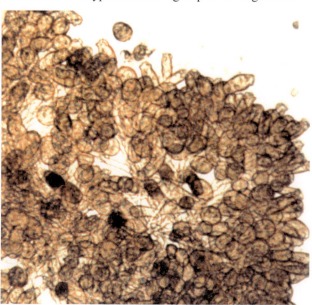

Ichthyophthirius multifiliis (Ich)

These holotrichously ciliated parasites embed in the epithelium of the gills, fins and skin. They appear as small white spots on the fish, but many times affected koi will have Ich on the gill filaments, and no visible signs on the skin. Hyperplasia of the gill epithelium makes the gills look pale and results in hypoxia. Flashing is very frequently seen.

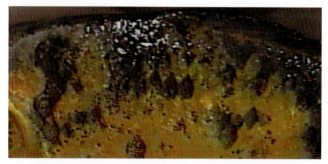

The white specks on this koi's skin are embedded *Ichthyophthirius* trophonts. In many koi with Ich, they will be seen on gill biopsy microscopic examination, but there will be no visible lesions on the skin.

The embedded feeding stage (trophozoite, or trophont) grows in the epidermis for 3-30 days, depending on temperature. After feeding, the trophont (up to 1 mm in size) breaks out of the epidermis leaving epithelial destruction. It drops from the fish to the bottom of the pond where it encysts (tomont stage) and divides by binary fission within the cyst. Hundreds of free-swimming tomites (20 x 50 μm) are released from the cyst after 8-24 hours. These then search out a host fish on which to feed. They must attach to a host within 24-48 hours or they will die. The tomites secrete hyaluronidase to allow penetration of the fish's epithelium. There it matures into the trophozoite feeding stage, completing the cycle.

The optimum water temperature for the Ich parasite is 70-77°F / 21-25°C, at which it will complete a full life cycle in 3-7 days. At cooler water temperatures it takes longer; 15 days at 59°F / 15°C, and as long as 5-6 weeks at 50°F / 10°C.

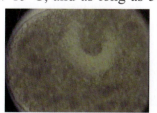 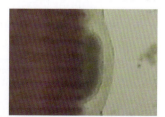

LEFT: Microscopic photograph showing the characteristic horseshoe-shaped macronucleus of an Ich trophont.
RIGHT: Side view of a trophont embedded in the gills.

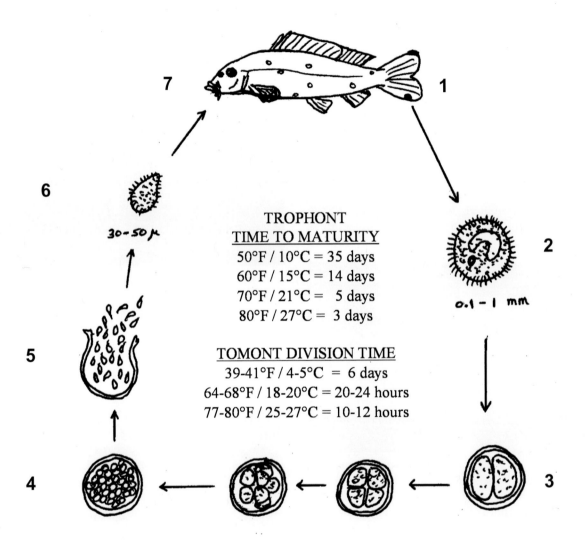

1) Koi infested with *Ichthyophthirius* trophonts.
2) Trophonts (trophozoites) - embedded feeding stage: spherical cell completely covered in cilia with a U-shaped macronucleus. Grows up to 1 mm diameter in epidermis of fish until mature. Feeds by absorption of tissue fluid.
3) Trophont leaves the host when mature and attaches to plant, gravel, or other substrate. There it forms a cystic capsule (tomont stage) and begins mitotic cell division.
4) Mitotic division continues for up to 10 times (2^{10} = 1024 cells) producing hundreds and up to a thousand new protozoa.
5) The tomont's cystic capsule ruptures and the free-swimming ciliated tomites (theronts) are released. This is the only stage of *Ichthyophthirius* that is susceptible to treatments.
6) Free swimming tomite will die if it does not find a host within 24-48 hours.
7) Tomite penetrates and embeds in the epidermis of the skin or gill epithelium, where it matures as a trophont. The cycle repeats -- length of time depends on water temperature.

The free-swimming tomites will not survive in water warmer than about 84-86°F / 29-30°C. This can be useful in treating for this parasite. Ultraviolet light will also kill the tomites.

Standard dosages of formalin/malachite solution or copper sulfate will kill the free-swimming tomite stage, but the trophont and tomont stages are resistant to treatments. This is why treatment must continue long enough for all the trophonts to develop into tomonts and then into new tomites, when they are susceptible to treatments. Salt in the pond at 0.3% (3 g NaCl/liter water) will inhibit Ich infestations.

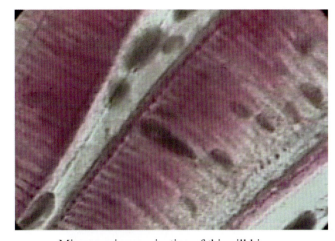

Photographs below (not to scale) are of the Ich lifecycle stages depicted in the chart to the left.

Microscopic examination of this gill biopsy reveals many *Ichthyopthirius* trophonts.

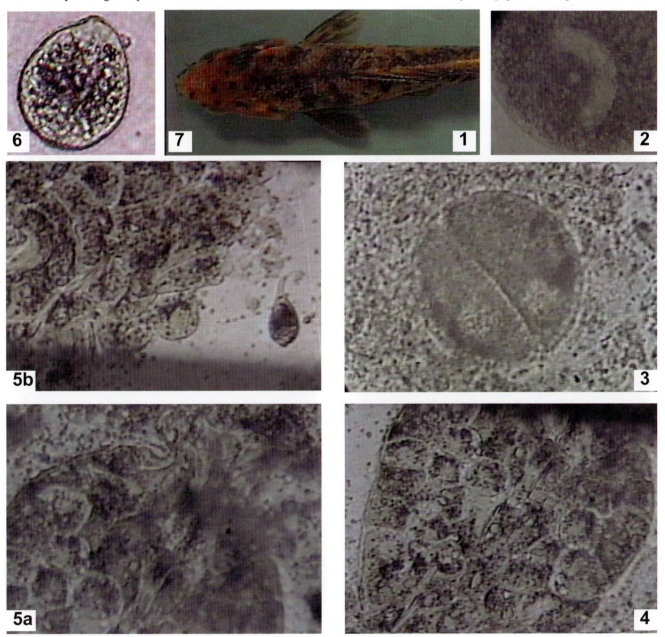

Trichodina Complex

Several genera (*Trichodina, Trichodonella, Tripartiella*) of similar protozoa cause this disease. They are peritrichously ciliated, circular parasites (40-100 μm diameter) that are flattened ventrally. They reproduce by binary fission and have a direct life cycle. They are freely motile on the surface of the fish and can swim through the water. They live on the skin and gills where they damage tissue with their rotating denticular (toothed) ring. Affected fish may produce excessive mucus and develop a white cast to the skin. Small hemorrhages may appear on the skin and fins.

Formalin/malachite solution is effective in killing these parasites. Individually infested fish may be bathed in a 2% salt solution (20 g NaCl/liter water) for 10-20 minutes to remove these parasites. Add up to 0.3% salt in the pond when infestations occur. Decreasing organic debris and stocking densities will reduce risk of infestation.

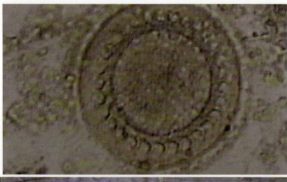

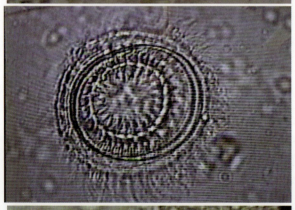

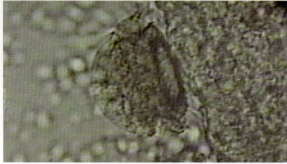

FLAGELLATED PROTOZOA (MASTIGOPHORA)

Hexamita (= *Octomitus*), *Spironucleus*

These similar organisms infest the intestines of fish. In many cases they do not cause disease, but in large numbers they can cause anorexia, weight loss, and even death. Stress from shipping, overcrowding, poor water quality, or malnutrition allows rapid reproduction of these protozoa in the intestinal tract, leading to disease. Microscopic examination of feces will show highly motile pyriform (*Hexamita*) or elongate (*Spironucleus*) protozoa with six anterior flagella and two posterior somatic flagella. They are 4-8 x 10-12 μm in size.

Improved nutrition, fresh vitamin C (ascorbic acid) supplementation, and metronidazole in the food or in the water can be used for treatment.

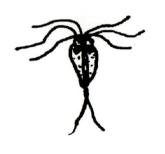   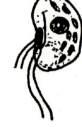

Hexamita   *Ichthyobodo*

Ichthyobodo necator (= *Costia necatrix*)

This small (10 x 20 μm) flagellated protozoan attaches to the skin and gills by a hold-fast organelle. The hold-fast is on the narrow end of the pyriform body. The parasite feeds on the epithelial cells of the fish, resulting in sloughing of the epidermis. A bluish white film may develop on the skin from excessive mucus production. The fish will have respiratory difficulty and be depressed. Death occurs by asphyxiation due to damage of the gill epithelium. Large numbers of koi may be affected in a short period and die suddenly.

> TOP LEFT: Dorsal-ventral view of a *Trichodina*. The small clear pyriform cells around it are *Ichthyobodo necator* protozoa.
> CENTER: Oblique view with peritrichous cilia clearly visible. Note the denticular ring.
> BOTTOM: Side view of a *Trichodina* crawling along a koi gill filament.

It has two long flagella that project posteriorly from the body and cause the parasite to swim in a jerky spiral, which can be seen microscopically on gill or skin biopsy. It reproduces by binary fission and four flagella, two long and two short, may be seen prior to cell division. It spreads from fish to fish by swimming and it will encyst when conditions become unfavorable. It will survive in temperatures from 36-86°F / 2-30°C, but its optimum temperature for reproduction is 75-77°F / 24-25°C.

Treat with standard formalin/malachite solution, 1 ounce per 300 gallons of pond water, or 2% salt bath for 10-20 minutes. This will kill the trophic (feeding) stage, but the encysted stage may survive, so treatment should be repeated on a weekly basis as long as necessary. Adding salt to the pond to the 0.3% level is helpful when outbreaks occur.

Trypanosoma, Trypanoplasma, Cryptobia

These flagellated blood parasites (40-100 µm long) live within the circulatory system of fish and can be found in the gills. They can cause obstructions in the blood vessels of the gills. Signs include lethargy, weight loss, anemia, and ascites. They are spread between fish by leeches. Diagnosis is made by examining blood smears and gill biopsies under a microscope. The organisms appear as undulating flagellated cells moving rapidly among the red blood cells. Collect the blood from the gill biopsy or from the caudal vein ventral to the spine in the caudal peduncle. Prevent the disease by controlling leeches.

MYXOSPORIDIA

Myxobolus (= Henneguya) koi

Protozoa from the family Myxobolidae are parasites of poikilotherms (cold-blooded vertebrates), primarily fish, with an intermediate host of an invertebrate, usually an annelid worm such as a *Tubifex* worm. They are obligate parasites that are very specific to the species of host and the tissue they invade. Their life cycle will not be completed if both intermediate and primary hosts are not present in the pond environment.

The spores *of Myxobolus koi* are found in the connective tissue (cartilage) of the gill filaments of koi and may be found on microscopic examination of gill biopsies. The spores can obstruct blood flow in the gill filaments, causing damage resembling bacterial gill disease. The mature spore (10-16 µm) consists of an oval or pyriform bivalvulid shell around a binucleate sporoplasm and two polar capsules. Each polar capsule contains a coiled polar filament that is extended from the spore and used for locomotion when the mature spore is released from the fish. The spores are released when the fish dies, and remain stable in the pond environment for a year, or possibly longer. Eventually the spores are ingested by an intermediate host (an annelid worm). Eliminating live worms in the pond would prevent completion of the parasites life cycle and its spread to the other koi fish.

Once ingested by the intermediate host, the valves of the spore open, releasing the sporoplasm. The sporoplasm then transforms into the infective

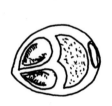
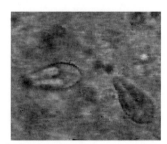

ABOVE: *Myxobolus koi* spores

BELOW: *Hoferellus carassii (= Mitraspora cyprini)*

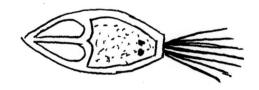

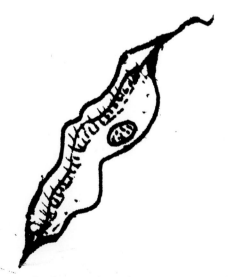

An undulating membrane runs along the *Trypanosoma* cell.

actinosporean stage in the worm. These wait to enter the fish host by ingestion of the intermediate host (the worm). Once inside the fish host, the actinosporean develops into a plasmodium that migrates to its specific tissue site in the fish (the cartilage of the gill filament). In the gill cartilage the plasmodium grows in size and produces many spores that are released into the fish's tissue. In some cases the plasmodium and the spores do not cause much tissue damage and the fish acts normally. In severe infestations there can be damage to the gill filaments causing noticeable lesions and gill necrosis.

In natural ponds, where infected fish that die remain in the water to decay, and annelid worms inhabit the substrate, the life cycle of this parasite can progress to spread to other fish. In most koi ponds, however, dead fish are removed so that the spores would less likely be able to spread in the pond. The cement, fiberglass, or plastic pond liners on the bottom of the koi pond – as opposed to natural soil – would reduce the likelihood of the annelid worm living in the pond as well. The risk of the parasite spreading in a hobbyist's koi pond is much less than in a natural pond or a mud bottomed breeding pond. As a precaution, affected koi should be removed and isolated to avoid spreading the parasite to other fish. Also, don't use live annelid worms such as *Tubifex* worms to feed the fish. Treat affected koi with Fumagillin added to the diet (0.1%).

Hoferellus carassii (= *Mitraspora cyprini*)

Another myxosporidian protozoa, this causes "kidney bloater disease" in goldfish and can infect common carp. The fish are infested by ingesting spores in the water, and the sporoplasm leaves the spore, penetrates through the intestinal mucosa, and circulates through the blood system. When passing through the kidney blood vessels, it penetrates into the epithelial cells of the renal tubules. There it reproduces asexually before releasing spores that pass into the water with the fish urine. The spores are shed in the urine on a seasonal basis, with their release usually occurring in late winter. The protozoa's multiplication causes kidney enlargement and ultimate kidney failure. Grossly, the fish will look bloated, and on necropsy one or both kidneys will be greatly enlarged. Histopathology of affected kidney tissue reveals papillary cystic hyperplasia and protozoal trophozoites visible in the kidney tubules. The spores are long ovals, similar to those of other Myxosporea.

HELMINTH PARASITES

MONOGENEAN TREMATODES (FLATWORMS)

These parasitic flatworms in the phylum Platyhelminthes have a complete life cycle that involves only a single host. There are two types that infest koi, *Dactylogyrus* and *Gyrodactylus*.

Dactylogyrus (Gill Flukes)

These monogenean trematodes live on the tips of the gills and occasionally on the skin of fish. They grow up to 1 mm in length. They cause gill filament hyperplasia resulting in hypoxia. Signs include rapid respiratory movements, clamped fins, and flashing. Gill tip biopsy will reveal the flukes upon microscopic examination. They have a four-pointed anterior end with four dark eyespots and a sucker disc. The posterior end (opisthohaptor) has one or two large pairs of hooks and 12, 14, or 16 smaller peripheral hooklets.

Each fluke is hermaphroditic, having both a testes and an ovary, and releases a single large egg (40 μm) after mating with another fluke. The oval egg has a hooked projection that may keep it attached to the fish or to aquatic plants. The eggs hatch in 1-4 days, depending on temperature. Newly hatched flukes (oncomiracidia) are ciliated and swim to find a new host. Their photosensitive eyespots are used to detect shadows of fish as the fish swim by and obstruct the light. They attach to the fish's gills or onto the body where they will then crawl to the gills. On the gills, the larvae will mature in 3-6 days. The adult parasites often die in cold water in winter, but the eggs are capable of surviving the winter on the bottom of the pond, as low temperature will arrest their development.

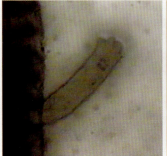 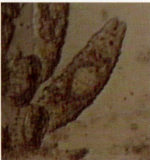

Comparison of *Dactylogyrus* (left) with *Gyrodactylus* (right). Note the four pronged anterior end with four eyespots, versus the two pronged end and no eyes.

Gyrodactylus (Skin Flukes)

These monogenean flukes occur mainly on the skin and fins, but occasionally are found on the gills. They are hermaphroditic and give birth to live young, one at a time. An embryo with hooks is often visible microscopically within the adult. The young are parasitic immediately after birth.

They have two points on the anterior end and an anterior sucker, but no eyespots. The opisthohaptor has one pair of median hooks and 16 marginal hooklets. The attachment of the hooks causes localized hemorrhaging of the skin and excessive mucus production. Secondary bacterial infections can also occur at the site of attachment.

Treat flukes with formalin/malachite solution, potassium permanganate, trichlorfon, Chloramine-T, or praziquantel. Dosages for medications are in the Formulary chapter.

Gyrodactylus rearing its ugly head! Note the hooks attaching to the epithelium.

DACTYLOGYRUS   GYRODACTYLUS

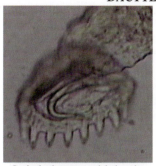
Opisthohaptor with hooks

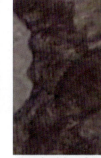
Egg inside of *Dactylogyrus*

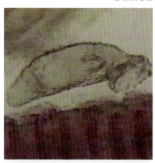
Gyrodactylus on a gill

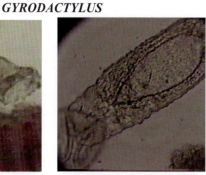
Opisthohaptor and uterus

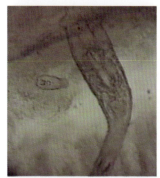
Oncomiracidia and adult

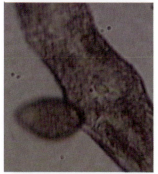
Dactylogyrus laying egg

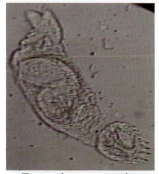
Two points on anterior end are visible

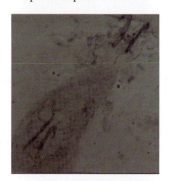
Embryo and adult's hooks both visible

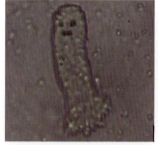
Dactylogyrus oncomiracidia

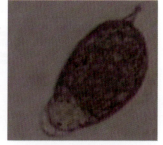
Egg with hooklet

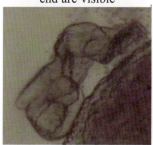
Gyrodactylus flukes mating

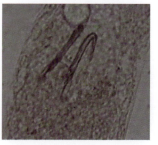
Embryo's hooks in adult

DIGENEAN TREMATODES

Digenean trematodes require multiple hosts to complete their life cycle. Fish serve as secondary intermediate hosts for these (snails fish birds). The immature trematode is encysted in the tissue of the fish, and matures to adult when the fish is eaten by another animal. The encysted Digenean trematode is a 1 to 4-mm black (*Neascus*), white or yellow (*Clinostomum*) "grub" seen in the muscles, internal organs, or in the eyes (*Diplostomum*) of the fish.

Eliminating snails from the pond will prevent transmission of the immature stage (cercaria) to the fish. Surgical excision of the cysts is possible if they are near the surface of the fish's body. Intramuscular praziquantel injections (25 mg/kg body weight [BW], one time) may eliminate the encysted metacercariae.

Sanguinicola inermis (Blood Flukes)

This digenean trematode uses fish as its final host. It lives in the blood vessels, heart, and the gills. Its triangular-shaped eggs can cause blockages of the circulatory system. The eggs hatch releasing miricidia that penetrate through the gills and enter the water in search of their intermediate host, a mollusc. After developing to the cercarial stage in the mollusc, they return to the fish and re-enter the gills. There they reach sexual maturity and deposit eggs. Digeneans are hermaphroditic, so each individual reproduces after mating with another one.

Gill damage occurs from the larval penetrations and from blood vessel blockages. Secondary bacterial infections can occur on the necrotic tissues.

Eliminating snails from the pond will prevent the spread of this parasite. Affected fish can be treated with a praziquantel injection (25 mg/kg BW, intramuscularly).

CESTODES (TAPEWORMS)

Fish serve as definitive hosts for some species of tapeworms that live in their intestinal tracts. The adults of the tapeworms *Bothriocephalus acheilognathi* and *Caryophyllaeus fimbriceps* can be found in koi intestines. Koi also are secondary intermediate hosts for larval stages (plerocercoids) of tapeworms such as *Ligula intestinalis*, which encyst in their muscles and abdomen.

Bothriocephalus acheilognathi

The Asian tapeworm has been imported into the United States in the grass carp, and can be found in many fish species. It is large (up to 20 cm) and has a prominent head end (scolex) that has a groove (bothria) on each side. The segments (proglottids) are rectangular. The adult tapeworm can damage or even obstruct the anterior intestines. Signs include swollen abdomen, lethargy, and muscle loss. Koi become infested with this tapeworm by ingesting copepod crustacea (the intermediate host) that contain plerocercoids. Treat with praziquantel injection (25 mg/kg) or with praziquantel 0.50% medicated food; prevent by not feeding live copepods to the fish. Treat the pond with antiparasitic medications used for other crustacean parasites (e.g., trichlorfon) to eliminate copepods in the pond.

Caryophyllaeus fimbriceps

This nonsegmented tapeworm is parasitic in the intestines of koi. Its intermediate hosts are oligochaete annelids of the genera *Tubifex* and *Limnodrilus*. Eating the annelid worm host infests the koi. Large numbers of tapeworms can cause intestinal inflammation and weight loss.

Treat with praziquantel 0.50% added to the food. Avoid feeding live annelid worms to koi.

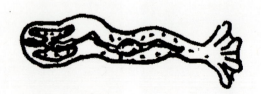

Caryophyllaeus fimbriceps is a tapeworm that can occasionally be found in the intestines of fish, which are its primary host.

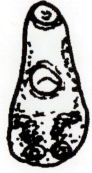 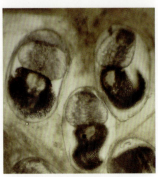

Adult stage of a digenean trematode.   Digenean metacercariae encysted in muscle.

NEMATODES (ROUNDWORMS)

Capillaria

This long thin worm from the phylum Nematoda is found within the fish's intestines. Its attachment to the wall of the intestines can lead to areas of necrosis and secondary bacterial infections. It may reduce growth rate and reproductive ability of the fish. Feces of affected fish may contain excessive mucus.

Diagnosis can be made from microscopic examination of a fecal sample. Ova with bipolar caps will be seen in infested koi. Treat with fenbendazole 0.25% in the food for 2 days, then repeat treatment in 2 weeks. Recheck fecal sample to evaluate treatment success. Repeat treatment as necessary.

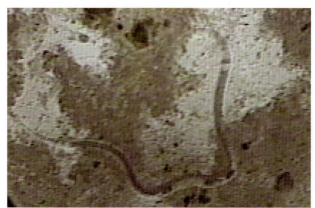
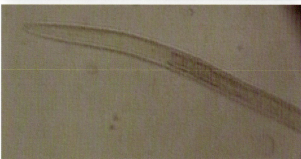
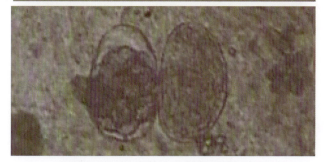

TOP: Nematode in a biopsy sample.
CENTER: Close-up of its anterior end.
BOTTOM: Two nematode ova; the left is in early development and the right is more developed.

ANNELIDS (SEGMENTED WORMS)

Leeches (*Piscicola geometra*)

Leeches are in the phylum Annelida, class Hirudinea. While some leeches are blood-sucking parasites, many species feed on the debris at the bottom of a pond, and are not parasitic. Leeches can be introduced into the pond with plants, rocks, snails, or on fish. Parasitic leeches can cause anemia and can spread protozoal blood parasites between fish. After feeding they leave the host fish to breed. The hermaphroditic adults mate and lay egg sacs in the pond substrate.

Leeches have a mouth within an anterior sucking disc (oral sucker) and an anus within the posterior sucker. They move along a surface using the two sucker discs, similar in motion to an inchworm. They can also swim freely through the water, using undulating motion of their body for propulsion.

Leeches should be picked off fish when seen and the skin swabbed with a disinfectant. Soaking affected fish in a 2% salt solution for 10-20 minutes will cause the leeches to drop from the host. Trichlorfon at 0.25-0.50 mg/L added to the water will kill leeches in the pond.

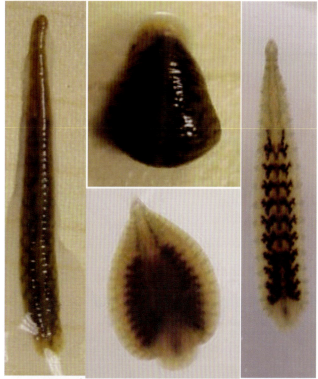

Dorsal (left and top center photographs) and ventral views of a leech elongated and contracted, using its anterior (pointed end) and posterior (wider end) suckers to walk along the surface.

CRUSTACEAN PARASITES

Lernaea cyprinacea (Anchor Worms)

These copepod crustacea have free-swimming larval stages. Once mature, the adult male (170 x 780 µm) will mate with a female and then die. The fertilized female (10-40 mm long) develops an anchor-shaped head, which it embeds into the skin of the host fish. This causes a reddened sore, which may become secondarily infected with bacteria. The female anchor worm develops two large egg sacs on its external end, containing several hundred eggs each. The egg sacs are shed when the eggs are ready to hatch. The nauplii hatch from the eggs and break out of the egg sac. The female will then develop new egg sacs. The mature female may be up to 4 cm long.

At the optimal temperature of 77°F / 25°C, egg sacs are produced every 2 weeks. Temperatures below 57°F / 14°C inhibit their reproduction. In winter, anchor worms can hibernate in the pond and cause an epidemic in early spring as the temperature warms.

Treat by gently extracting the parasite with forceps, being careful not to leave any of the anterior anchor behind. Treat the wound with topical disinfectant. Trichlorfon organophosphate (0.25 mg/L) or Dimilin (0.06 mg/L) can be used to kill the free-living juvenile stage. *Lernaea* are also inhibited by 2% salt solutions for short-duration (10-20 minutes) baths.

Ergasilus (Gill Maggots)

These parasitic copepods attach to fish's gill filaments with specialized claws formed from the second pair of antennae. They feed on blood and body tissues. Only the gravid female (1-2 mm long) is parasitic. After they mate, the male dies and the female finds a host on which to feed while developing eggs. The two large white egg sacs that develop on the female's posterior resemble maggots. The eggs are retained in the female's egg sacs until they hatch. After hatching, the juveniles are free-living in the pond until they mature and mate. Treat with trichlorfon (0.25 mg/L) or Dimilin (0.06 mg/L) once weekly for 3 doses.

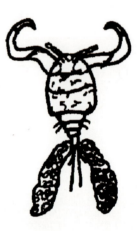

Female *Ergasilus* carrying two egg sacs ("maggots")

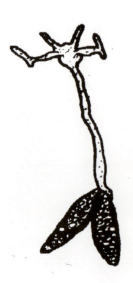 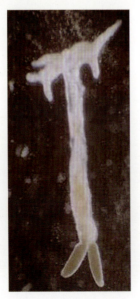

Female *Lernaea cyprinacea*

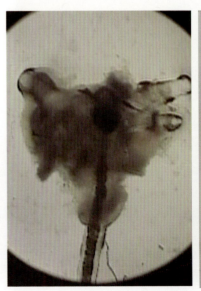 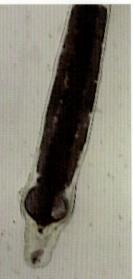

Close-up microscopic photographs of the anterior end (anchor) and the posterior end of a female *Lernaea*. Note the flesh from the koi still attached to the anchor.

Argulus foliaceus (Fish Lice)

These are oval, flattened Branchiurans with two prominent eyes, two sucking discs, and a stylet mouthpart. This stylet repeatedly pierces the skin of the fish and releases toxic secretions. They feed on the tissue fluids released by this trauma. They are freely moving on the host and swim well. Affected fish flash frequently. Skin ulcers from secondary bacterial or fungal infections are common on koi affected with *Argulus*.

The adult female fish louse lays a thin strip of eggs on submerged objects near the banks of the pond. The eggs hatch in 2-8 weeks, depending on temperature. The larvae must attach onto a fish to feed within the first 3 days, but can swim between fish after feeding. They are mature in 3-6 weeks. Adults can grow to 1 cm long. Reproduction ceases in temperatures below 57°F / 14°C.

Mosquito fish (*Gambusia affinis*) and bitterlings (*Rhodeus sericeus*) may eat immature forms of the parasite. For best control, treat the pond with trichlorfon (0.25 mg/L) on a weekly basis for 4-8 weeks. Dimilin (0.06 mg/L) and lufenuron (409.8 mg tablet/1000 gallons) have also been used for control of fish lice.

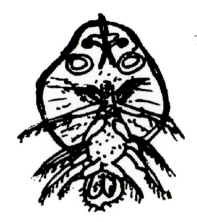

The fish louse, *Argulus*

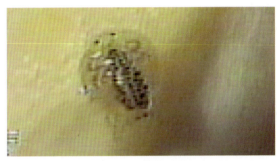

Argulus on the operculum of a koi.

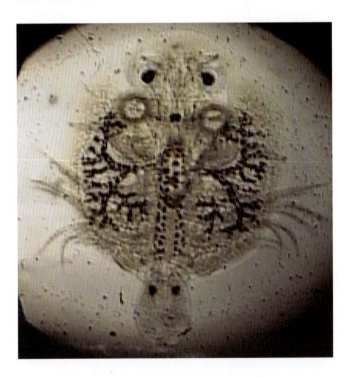

Dorsal-ventral view of an *Argulus*. There are two clear sucking discs below the eyes which it uses to hold onto the skin of a fish while it feeds. It swims well to find a new host fish, using its 10 legs and its rudderlike tail.

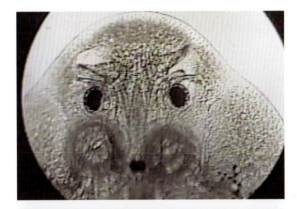
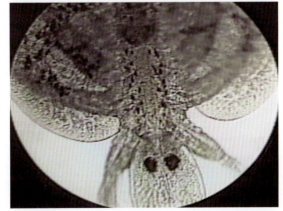

Close-up microscopic photographs of the anterior end and the posterior end of an *Argulus*.

MOLLUSC PARASITES

Freshwater Clams

The larvae (glochidia) of freshwater bivalve molluscs of the families Unionidae and Mutelidae attach to the fins and gills of fish. There they feed by osmotic absorption from the surrounding tissue. After a feeding period of several months, they drop off and mature to filter-feeding adults.

In most cases the glochidia does little harm to the host fish However, in very young koi, or if there are a large number of glochidia per fish, there could be significant damage. Also, there is a chance of secondary bacterial or fungal infection occurring at the site of attachment. Not placing freshwater clams into the pond will prevent possible infestation from this temporary parasite. Organophospates such as trichlorfon, and copper sulfate may also be used to eliminate molluscs (including snails) from the pond.

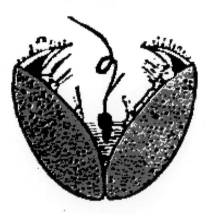

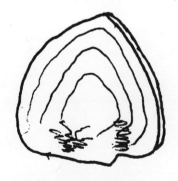

Illustrations of glochidia from Unionidae family of clams.
TOP: Side view of open shell.
BOTTOM: Top view of closed shell.

REFERENCES:

Amlacher, Erwin. 1970. *Textbook of Fish Diseases,* T.F.H. Publications, Neptune, NJ, English translation.

Anderson, Douglas P. 1974. *Diseases of Fishes, Book 4: Fish Immunology,* T.F.H. Publications, Neptune, NJ.

Andrews, Chris, Adrian Excell, and Neville Carrington. 1988. *The Manual of Fish Health,* Tetra Press, Blacksburg, VA.

Axelrod, Herbert R., Albert Spalding Benoist, and Dennis Kelsey-Wood. 1992. *The Atlas of Garden Ponds,* T.F.H. Publications, Neptune, NJ.

Baer, J.G. 1971. *Animal Parasites,* World University Library, New York.

Butcher, Ray L. 1992. *Manual of Ornamental Fish,* British Small Animal Veterinary Association, Gloucestershire, UK.

Brown, E. Evan and John B. Gratzek. 1980. *Fish Farming Handbook,* AVI Publishing, Westport, CT.

Dogiel, V.A. 1958. *Parasitology of Fishes,* T.F.H. Publications, Neptune, NJ, English translation 1970.

Dulin, Mark. 1979. *Fish Diseases,* T.F.H. Publications, Neptune, NJ.

Francis-Floyd, Ruth. 1993. *The Use of Salt in Aquaculture,* Fact Sheet VM 86, University of Florida, Gainesville, FL.

Gratzek, John B. (editor). 1992. *Aquariology: The Science of Fish Health Management,* Tetra Press, Morris Plains, NJ.

Grzimek, Bernhard. 1968. *Animal Life Encyclopedia,* Van Nostrand Reinhold, New York, English translation 1984.

Herwig, Nelson. 1979. *Handbook of Drugs and Chemicals Used in the Treatment of Fish Diseases,* Charles C. Thomas, Springfield, IL.

Hoffman, Glenn L. and Fred P. Meyer. 1974. *Parasites of Freshwater Fishes,* T.F.H. Publications, Neptune, NJ.

Hoffman, Glenn L. 1981. *Two Fish Pathogens, Parvicapsula sp. and Mitraspora cyprini (Myxosporea), New to North America,* U.S. Fish and Wildlife Service, Fish Farming Experimental Station, Stuttgart, AR.

Kabata, Z. 1970. *Diseases of Fishes,* Book 1: *Crustacea as Enemies of Fishes,* T.F.H. Publications, Neptune, NJ.

McDowall, Anne (editor). 1989. *The Tetra Encyclopedia of Koi,* Tetra Press, Morris Plains, NJ.

Noga, Edward J. 1996. *Fish Disease: Diagnosis and Treatment,* Mosby, St. Louis, MO.

Post, George. 1987. *Textbook of Fish Health,* T.F.H. Publications, Neptune, NJ, Revised edition.

Reichenbach-Klinke, Heinz-Hermann. 1965. *Fish Pathology,* T.F.H. Publications, Neptune, NJ, English translation.

Roberts, Ronald J. 1989. *Fish Pathology,* 2nd ed., Balliere Tindall, London.

Saint-Erne, Nicholas. 1984. *A Veterinarian's Guide to the Diseases of Freshwater Aquarium Fishes,* Kansas State University College of Veterinary Medicine, Manhattan, KS.

Sarig, S. 1971. *Diseases of Fishes,* Book 3: *Diseases of Warmwater Fishes,* T.F.H. Publications, Neptune, NJ.

Stoskopf, Michael K. 1993. *Fish Medicine,* W.B. Saunders, Philadelphia.

Untergasser, Dieter. 1989. *Handbook of Fish Diseases,* T.F.H. Publications, Neptune, NJ, English translation.

Waddington, Peter. 1995. *Koi Kichi,* Infiltration, Cheshire, UK.

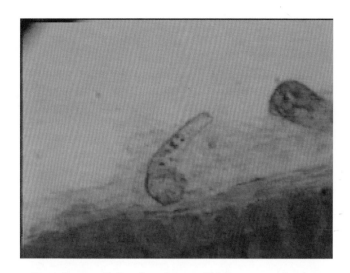

Dactylogyrus flukes found on a gill biopsy examination.

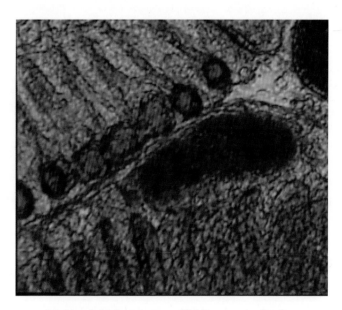

Ichthyophthirius seen on gill biopsy examination. It is embedded in the gill epithelium, and the gill capillaries are showing telangiectasis.

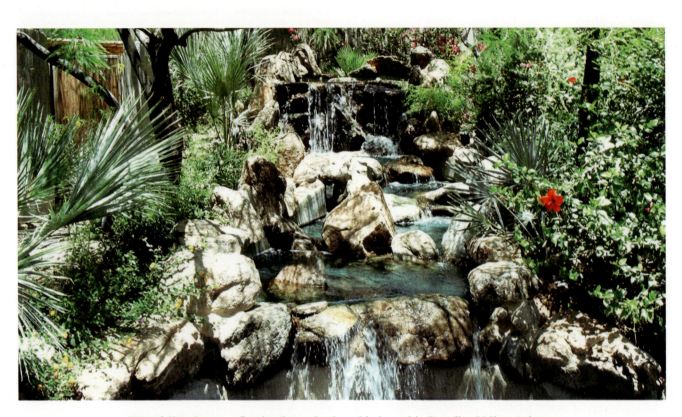
Waterfall and stream flowing into a backyard koi pond in Paradise Valley, Arizona.

CHAPTER 5:
ENVIRONMENTAL MANAGEMENT

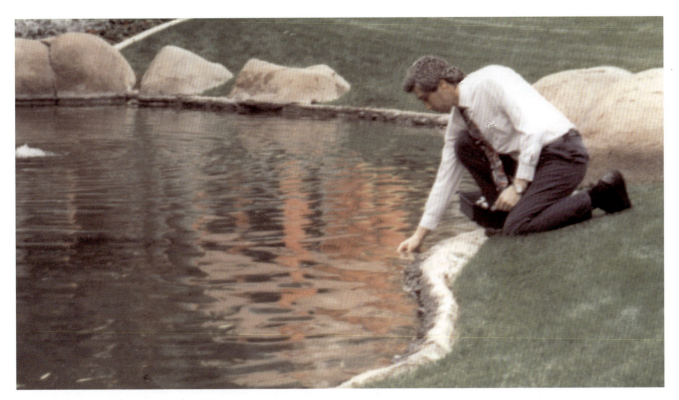

The author testing the water quality in the koi pond at the Tropicana Resort and Casino in Las Vegas, Nevada

KOI NUTRITION

Fish are poikilothermic (cold-blooded), therefore their rate of metabolism depends on the temperature of the surrounding water. Food consumption and nutritional requirements vary with their metabolic rates. The warmer the water temperature, the greater will be their nutritional requirements. Feed koi more frequently during warm weather, and decrease feeding when the water temperature cools. In cold climates, reduce the quantity and frequency of feeding when the temperature drops below 50°F / 10°C and discontinue feeding when water temperature remains below 45°F / 7.2°C.

Like the higher vertebrates, fish require proteins, fats, carbohydrates, vitamins, minerals, and water from their diet. The last of these is readily acquired by fish from their aquatic environment. In the wild, carp will eat insects, worms, fish eggs, algae, aquatic plants, and decaying organic matter. Since koi are omnivores – eating almost anything – a wide variety of foods are available to meet their nutritional needs.

Feeding koi a floating pelleted food makes it easier to see if the fish are eating, and to tell how much to feed them. An adequate amount of food is the quantity they will consume in about 5 minutes. If all the food is gone in less time, they probably should be given more. If there is food remaining after 5 minutes, they have been given too much. Carp are grazers and, as they have no stomach to store large meals, eat small amounts frequently. Young koi should eat 3-5 times daily. Older koi can be fed once or twice daily. Overfeeding is as much a health risk as is starvation. Older healthy koi can go for days or even weeks without being fed. However, overfeeding will cause obesity, fatty liver syndrome, and foul the water producing toxic ammonia.

Overfeeding is especially a risk when neighbors take care of the pond while the owner is on vacation! In this situation, place the proper amount of food for each feeding in individual plastic zip-lock bags, and label the bags with the time and date they are to be used for feeding the koi. Secure all remaining food so it is unavailable for the temporary caregivers to prevent additional feedings. The owner should leave an emergency telephone number where they or the veterinarian can be reached.

Besides commercially prepared diets, fresh foods should be fed to koi as well. Cooked vegetables such as peas and corn are relished by koi, as are leafy vegetables. Koi can be trained to come to a certain spot when being fed, and will even eat out of one's hand. In general, feed adult koi 1-3% of their body weight per day, and young koi 2-6% of their body weight per day.

PROTEINS

Proteins make up the major portion of a fish's diet on a dry matter basis. Young growing koi require 40-47% protein in their diet, while mature koi need 30-38% protein diets. The proteins in the diet are broken down into 20 different amino acids by enzymes in the digestive tract. These amino acids are then absorbed and resynthesized into new protein in the fish's tissues. There are 10 essential amino acids which must be supplied by the fish's protein consumption: arginine, histidine, isoleucine, leucine, lysine, methionine, phenylalanine, threonine, tryptophan, and valine. Deficiency of any of these essential amino acids, or an insufficient quantity of total protein will result in reduced growth and reproduction rates, and increased mortalities.

In nature, ingested protein is in the form of phytoplankton, zooplankton, algae, higher plants, bacteria, protozoa, crustacea, worms, insects, and sometimes other fish. In a koi pond, the fish's nutritional needs are usually met by feeding a processed commercial flake or pelleted food. Prepared foods decrease in nutritional value over time, especially if exposed to air, sunlight, moisture, or high temperatures. Be sure to keep fish foods in closed airtight containers stored at refrigerated or room temperatures. All stored food should be used up within a 3-month period to ensure freshness.

A good homemade protein supplement for feeding koi can be made from eggs. Hen's eggs are 100% nutritious, contain all 10 essential amino acids, and are high in lecithin and linoleic acid as well. They also contain 22 important minerals. Spinach or other dark green leafy vegetables can be added to the eggs as a source of vitamin A and other nutrients. The mixture is blended until it is homogenous and is then cooked until firm using a stove or microwave oven. Once cooked, it can be crumbled into bite-sized pieces and stored in airtight containers in the refrigerator or freezer.

Excess proteins not needed for growth or reproduction are utilized as an energy source instead of fats or carbohydrates. However, because proteins average 16% nitrogen, the breakdown products of protein metabolism are ammonia (NH_3) and a small amount, less than 2%, of urea [$2(NH_2)CO$]. The ammonia is passively released into the water through the fish's gills and can lead to toxicity if levels increase. Nonprotein energy metabolism does not cause ammonia production. Fats and simple carbohydrates added to the diet have a protein-sparing effect in that they can be used for energy instead of protein, without increasing ammonia production.

FATS

Fats (lipids) are another nutrient necessary in the fish's diet. Only low melting point unsaturated fats (oils) are readily digested and used by koi. Saturated (solid) fats are poorly digested, and at water temperatures below 68°F / 20°C can solidify and cause intestinal blockages. Rapidly growing fish utilize oils over carbohydrates or proteins as their primary source of energy. That is why young fish need higher fat in the diet than do mature fish. Fat metabolism produces CO_2 and H_2O as its byproducts, which are nontoxic. Fats are an efficient energy source because they contain 9 kilocalories (kcal or Cal.) per gram, while proteins and carbohydrates only produce 4 kcal/gram.

In koi foods, 10% fat in the diet is optimal for young, rapidly growing fish, and 7-8% fat for mature koi. Excess of fats can lead to hepatic lipidosis (fatty degeneration of the liver). High fat levels can also discolor the white color of the koi's skin. Deficiency of fats, including the essential fatty acids, causes fin erosions, slow growth, and neuromuscular shock. The fat-soluble vitamins (A, D, E, and K) will not be absorbed without adequate fat in the diet.

Fats are used in formation of cell structures and membranes, and in the formation of some steroids and other hormones. Two polyunsaturated fatty acids, linolenic acid (18:3 ω-3) [= 18 carbons, 3 double bonds, first double bond is on the 3rd carbon away from the end omega (ω) carbon] and linoleic acid (18:2 ω-6), are essential for koi growth. They should be provided at 1% of the total diet on a dry matter basis for each of the omega-3 (ω-3) and omega-6 (ω-6) fatty acids.

Unsaturated fatty acids oxidize readily and will go rancid if exposed to oxygen, light, and heat. The oxidation metabolites can be toxic to fish. Sekoke disease in koi occurs when oxidized (rancid) fats destroy α-tocopherol in the food, resulting in vitamin E deficiency. Keep fish food in closed containers away from sunlight or heat. Do not use food that is moldy or has a rancid odor.

CARBOHYDRATES

Carbohydrates are not a major nutrient source in fishes. Most fish cannot utilize complex starches (polysaccharides). Simple sugars (monosaccharides) are a readily digestible energy source, but they are not available in most of the natural diet of fish. Adding small amounts of monosaccharides or disaccharides to koi food will have a protein-sparing effect for energy production. Microflora (beneficial bacteria) in the intestines of koi will break down some complex carbohydrates from plants, but it is the least digestible nutrient for fish. Carbohydrates are only about 34% digestible by fish, compared to 85-95% digestibility of proteins and fats. Carbohydrate digestion produces carbon dioxide, water, and energy.

Total carbohydrates in the diet should be 25-40%, which includes indigestible fiber at no more than half the total amount of carbohydrates. Fiber consists of indigestible plant polysaccharides such as cellulose, hemicellulose, and lignin. Excess carbohydrates are stored in the liver as glycogen or converted into stored fat. Diets too high in carbohydrates can produce liver cell degeneration (hepatic lipidosis).

VITAMINS

Both water-soluble and fat-soluble vitamins are necessary in the diet of fishes. Most water-soluble vitamins (B complex and C) are coenzymes used in cellular metabolism. A constant supply of these vitamins is required in the diet as they are not stored in the body tissues. Fat-soluble vitamins (A, D, E, K) may be stored in the liver or other tissues after ingestion.

One of the first signs of any vitamin deficiency is a decreased appetite, resulting in poor growth. More specific signs of a particular vitamin deficiency will develop after several weeks of feeding a vitamin-deficient diet. See chart for specific vitamin deficiency signs.

Vitamin C deficiency is a common problem of koi fish. Vitamin C (L-ascorbic acid) is necessary for the metabolism of collagen for bones and joints. A deficiency causes poor bone and cartilage formation resulting in scoliosis, or curvature of the spine. It is usually due to decay of vitamin C in processed fish food. Vitamin C can decay in food in as short a period as 3-6 months after processing. Excess heat and exposure to the air hastens the process. A newer form of stabilized Vitamin C (L-Ascorbyl-2-polyphosphate) is available, and increases the shelf life of prepared foods to as long as two years. It is advisable, however, to use as fresh of a supply of fish food as possible.

Always keep fish food in airtight containers and in dry, cool storage areas. Additional vitamin C can be given to koi by floating orange slices in the pond, which koi will nibble on, and by soaking pelleted foods briefly in orange juice before feeding on an occasional basis.

In Japan, koi fed a vitamin E (α-tocopherol) deficient diet of oxidized silkworm pupae developed a condition called Sekoke disease, which is characterized by a marked loss of muscling on the back of the fish. It was treated by adding DL-α-tocopheryl acetate (50 mg/100g food) to the diet. This form of vitamin E is stable during food storage.

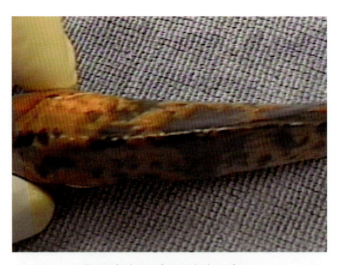

Dorsal view of muscle loss from Sekoke disease in a koi, which is due to Vitamin E deficiency.

Essential vitamin dosages and deficiency signs:

VITAMIN	DAILY REQUIREMENT	DEFICIENCY SIGNS
WATER-SOLUBLE VITAMINS:		
Thiamin (B1)	0.15-0.20 mg/kg Body Weight	Fin congestion, fading color, neurologic signs
Riboflavin (B2)	0.5-1.0 mg/kg	Skin & fin hemorrhages, poor growth, death
Niacin (B3, nicotinic acid)	3-7 mg/kg	Skin hemorrhages, death
Pantothenic acid (B5)	1.0-1.5 mg/kg	Skin hemorrhages, anemia, exophthalmia, gill hyperplasia
Pyridoxine (B6)	0.2-0.4 mg/kg	Nervous disorders, ascites
Cyanocobalamin (B12)	0.0005-0.0007 mg/kg	Hematological disorders
Biotin	0.03-0.07 mg/kg	Poor growth, anemia
Choline	50-60 mg/kg	Fatty liver
Folacin (folic acid)	0.15-0.20 mg/kg	Poor growth, anemia
Inositol	18-20 mg/kg	Skin lesions, poor digestion
L-Ascorbic acid (C)	3-5 mg/kg	Spinal deformities, hemorrhages, deformed gill opercula
FAT-SOLUBLE VITAMINS:		
Vitamin A (retinol)	100 International Units/kg BW	Hemorrhages, paleness, poor vision, exophthalmia, abnormal gill opercle
Vitamin D_3 (cholecalciferol)	72 IU/kg	Poor growth, bone deformities
Vitamin E (α-tocopherol)	1.0 IU/kg	Muscular dystrophy, death
Vitamin K (methyl-naphtho-quinones)	0.1 IU/kg	Skin hemorrhages

MINERALS

Fish have mineral requirements similar to the other vertebrates. There are 7 minerals that are needed in large amounts (calcium, chloride, magnesium, phosphorus, potassium, sodium, and sulfur) and 14 that are needed in only trace amounts (chromium, cobalt, copper, fluorine, iodine, iron, manganese, molybdenum, nickel, selenium, silicon, tin, vanadium, and zinc). Most minerals are obtained directly from the food, although some essential and nonessential compounds are absorbed from the water through the gill membranes. Mineral ions capable of being diffused through the gill membranes include calcium, chloride, cobalt, iodine, iron, magnesium, phosphorus, potassium, sodium, and zinc. The rest must be provided in the food.

Deficiencies of minerals cause a multitude of signs, including stunted growth, anorexia, anemia, cataracts, and increased mortalities, depending on the mineral lacking. Placing fish in deionized or distilled water would result in mineral imbalances, as a result of mineral losses from the fish into the water by osmosis.

WATER

Most prepared commercial fish foods contain about 9-10% moisture when packaged. Foods higher in water content will spoil more rapidly and may need to be kept refrigerated or even frozen. Freshwater fish do not drink water, as they are constantly trying to eliminate excess water from their bodies. Their kidneys' primary function is water excretion, and waste excretion occurs through the gills.

ADDITIVES

Pigments are non-nutrient food additives used to enhance colors. The Japanese call the practice of enhancing koi colors through dietary pigments "iroage." Carotenoid pigments (found in *Spirulina* algae, carrots, corn, alfalfa, peppers, broccoli, and many other plants, and in shrimp and bee pollen) such as β-carotene and xanthophylls produce yellow to orange colors. Paprika contains capxanthin, which produces a red-orange color. Crustacea such as krill, shrimp, and crab contain astaxanthin.

Some foods available commercially contain antibiotics such as Romet (sulfadimethoxine-ormetoprim), Terramycin (oxytetracycline), or tetracycline. These are useful to feed fish with internal bacterial infections, or septicemia. The problem of bacterial resistance can occur if the antibiotics are used indiscriminately. Also, many sick fish will refuse to eat, making the feeding of medicated foods futile, unless tube-fed.

New food additives include products such as Aquagen, which is an immunostimulating agent developed by Aqua Health, Ltd. to protect koi from *Aeromonas* infections. It is added to a pelleted food that helps to build the fish's immunity against the bacterial infection.

INGREDIENTS

Always check the ingredients list on a koi food to be sure it is made from quality ingredients. They are listed in descending order. The Guaranteed Analysis panel gives the percentages of the nutrients in the food, and is useful for comparing quality between different brands of food.

The following diet's Guaranteed Analysis is an ideal nutrient blend for a koi food to produce rapid growth. It has a high protein level for growth and high fat for energy. The vitamin and mineral components would be at or above the required amounts.

For mature koi, decrease the protein to 35%, and the fat to 8%, and increase the digestible carbohydrate to 27%. The growth rate will be less, but so will the ammonia production and the cost of the food. The total energy will be only slightly lower as both protein and carbohydrates produce 4 kcal/gram, so changing protein for digestible carbohydrate does not affect the energy level, but fat produces 9 kcal/gram, so decreasing the fat percentage will lower the total energy.

High Growth Diet - Guaranteed Analysis:

Protein	45%
Fat (should be polyunsaturated fat plus 1% ω-3 and 1% ω-6 fatty acids)	10%
NFE (nitrogen-free extract, the digestible carbohydrates)	15%
Fiber (the indigestible carbohydrates)	10%
Ash (minerals)	9%
Vitamins	1%
Moisture (maximum)	10%
TOTAL	100%

Total energy = 330 kcal/100 g of food

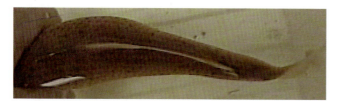

Spinal curvature from collapsed vertebrae due to Vitamin C deficiency in the diet.

REFERENCES:

Blazer, Vicki. 1983. *General Fish Nutrition,* College of Veterinary Medicine, University of Georgia, Athens, GA.

Gratzek, John B. (editor). 1992. *Aquariology: Fish Anatomy, Physiology, and Nutrition,* Tetra Press, Morris Plains, NJ.

Horne, Mike. 1997. "New Approaches in Koi Health" in *Koi Health Quarterly,* Autumn 1997, Koi Health Group, UK.

National Academy of Sciences. 1981. *Nutrient Requirements of Coldwater Fishes,* National Academy Press, Washington, DC.

National Academy of Sciences. 1983. *Nutrient Requirements of Warmwater Fishes and Shellfishes,* Revised Edition, National Academy Press, Washington, DC.

Pannevis, Marinus C. 1993. "Nutrition of Ornamental Fish," *Waltham International Focus,* vol. 3, no. 3, Waltham Centre for Pet Nutrition, Leicestershire, UK.

Post, George. 1987. *Textbook of Fish Health,* 2nd ed., T.F.H. Publications, Neptune, NJ.

Saint-Erne, Nicholas. 1982. *Nutritional Requirements of Tropical Aquarium Fishes,* Kansas State University College of Veterinary Medicine, Manhattan, KS.

Stoskopf, Michael K. 1993. *Fish Medicine,* W.B. Saunders, Philadelphia.

Wilson, Robert P. 1991. *Handbook of Nutrient Requirements of Finfish,* CRC Press, Boca Raton, FL.

Yanong, Roy P. E. 1999. "Nutrition of Ornamental Fish," in *The Veterinary Clinics of North America - Exotic Animal Practice,* vol. 2, no. 1, W.B. Saunders, Philadelphia.

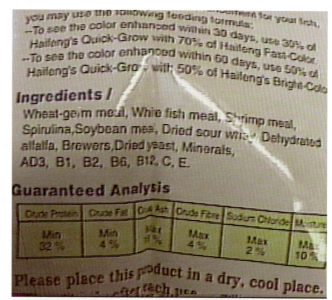

The Nutrition Panel on a bag of koi food lists the ingredients in descending order and the Guaranteed Analysis lists the percentages of nutrients.

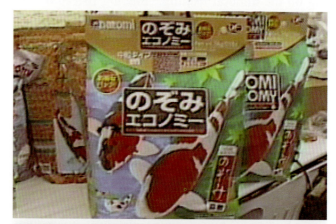

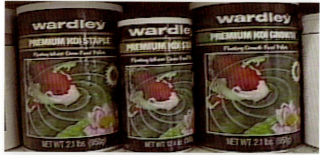

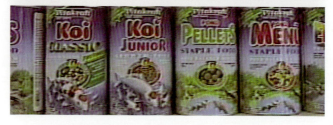

Koi foods come in a variety of styles and qualities. Compare nutrients to select an appropriate diet.

WATER QUALITY IN THE KOI POND

It is difficult to control or prevent infectious and parasitic diseases of koi fish without considering the quality of the pond water in which they live. Many diseases are fatal to fish populations only when the water quality is less than optimum. By improving water quality, stress on the fish is reduced and its immune system can keep many other diseases in check.

Water quality can be measured with test kits available through pet stores or pond supply companies. The most important parameters to measure are temperature, pH, ammonia, nitrite, nitrate, and dissolved oxygen. Other elements that can be tested are hardness, alkalinity, carbon dioxide, chloride, chlorine, salinity, and other compounds dissolved in the water such as heavy metals (e.g., copper, iron).

The following are general guidelines for the safe ranges and optimal levels of these parameters in koi ponds.

Temperature

Koi will survive in water temperatures from 35-95°F / 2-35°C, although they prefer cool water temperatures of 65-77°F / 18-25°C. Gradual changes in water temperature within a fish's optimum range seldom cause health problems. Ideally, water temperature differences should be no more than 5°F / 3°C change per day. Temperature shock can occur with rapid changes, especially from warmer water to cooler water.

Increasing the water temperature will lower the saturation point of dissolved oxygen (warmer water holds less oxygen than cooler water). It will also increase the toxicity of dissolved substances such as ammonia, chlorine, and heavy metals. Most pathogens' activity will increase as the water warms as well.

To convert from degrees Fahrenheit to degrees Celsius: (°F - 32) x 0.555 = °C.

To convert from degrees Celsius to degrees Fahrenheit: (°C x 1.8) + 32 = °F.

Celsius and Fahrenheit temperature equivalents:

Celsius	=	Fahrenheit	Celsius	=	Fahrenheit
-5	=	23	23	=	73.4
-4	=	24.8	24	=	75.2
-3	=	26.6	25	=	77
-2	=	28.4	26	=	78.8
-1	=	30.2	27	=	80.6
0	=	32	28	=	82.4
1	=	33.8	29	=	84.2
2	=	35.6	30	=	86
3	=	37.4	31	=	87.8
4	=	39.2	32	=	89.6
5	=	41	33	=	91.4
6	=	42.8	34	=	93.2
7	=	44.6	35	=	95
8	=	46.4	36	=	96.8
9	=	48.2	37	=	98.6
10	=	50	38	=	100.4
11	=	51.8	39	=	102.2
12	=	53.6	40	=	104
13	=	55.4	41	=	105.8
14	=	57.2	42	=	107.6
15	=	59	43	=	109.4
16	=	60.8	44	=	111.2
17	=	62.6	45	=	113
18	=	64.4	46	=	114.8
19	=	66.2	47	=	116.6
20	=	68	48	=	118.4
21	=	69.8	49	=	120.2
22	=	71.6	50	=	122

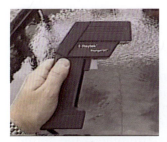 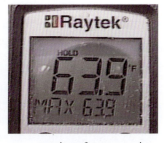

Infrared digital thermometers are convenient for measuring water temperature from a distance, and in multiple areas.

Water pH (Acid/Base Balance)

The symbol pH stands for *potentia Hydrogenii*, which is Latin for "power of Hydrogen." It is an indication of whether a solution is acidic or basic. The pH number is the reciprocal (or negative) logarithm to the base ten of the hydrogen ion molarity (in moles/liter).

$$pH = \log_{10} 1/[H^+] \quad \text{or} \quad pH = -\log_{10} [H^+]$$

In a neutral solution, the number of hydrogen cations (H^+) equals the number of hydroxyl anions (OH^-). If there are more hydrogen ions, the solution becomes acidic and if there are more of the hydroxyl ions the solution is basic.

$$H_2O \text{ (water)} = H^+ + OH^-$$

The pH of a neutral solution is 7. Neutral water has 0.0000001 moles of hydrogen per liter. That equals 10^{-7} m/L, or $\log_{10} -7$, or $-\log_{10} 7$. Therefore the pH = 7. An acidic solution has a pH less than 7, and a basic solution has a pH above 7 up to 14. Because the pH is logarithmic, a change of 0.3 units approximately doubles the Hydrogen or hydroxyl activity. A change of 1 unit has 10 times the acid/base activity! This is why pH changes should be made slowly in a pond or aquarium.

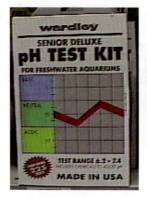
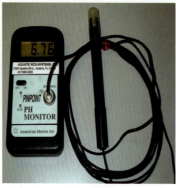

The pH can be tested using chemical test kits or by digital electronic instruments.

Koi are relatively tolerant of pH changes as long as they are gradual. They will survive in pH ranges from 6 to 10, although the optimum is about 7-7.5. The use of chemicals to adjust pH is not recommended because the resulting pH changes are usually temporary, so the koi become subjected to frequent fluctuations of the pH. It is safer for a koi to adjust to a pH of the local water of 8.2, for example, than to be constantly stressed from the pond owner's changing of the pH with chemical treatments to get it to the 7-7.5 range.

Be aware that the higher the pH, the more toxic any ammonia in the water becomes. Hard water tends to be more basic and resists changes in pH, whereas soft water is usually acidic and the pH will fluctuate more easily.

Signs of low pH toxicity include increased mucus production, hyperactivity and erratic swimming, and chronic stress. Treat by doing a partial water change with water of the appropriate pH, and removing organic debris from the pond that can lower the pH as it decays. Buffers (calcium carbonate) can be added to soft water to prevent pH changes. Do not raise the pH in water with elevated ammonia nitrogen levels, as increasing the pH will convert ionized ammonium into toxic ammonia. Any changes in pH should be made slowly if possible, not more than about 0.3-0.5 units per day.

Ammonia

This is the end product of microbial decomposition of nitrogenous organic material (amino acids) in decaying plant and animal tissues, or uneaten fish food. Ammonia is also excreted by fish via kidney waste and through the gills.

Increased ammonia in the water irritates the gill tissues causing hyperplasia, which reduces the oxygen absorption and waste excretion ability. Depending on water pH and temperature, some ammonia (NH_3) is ionized into ammonium (NH_4^+), which is nontoxic. Low pH and low temperature, as well as increases in salinity, will increase the ionization to ammonium.

$$NH_3 + H_2O = NH_4OH = NH_4^+ + OH^-$$

Measure the total ammonia dissolved in the water, as well as the pH and temperature. If the water test kit measures ammonia-nitrogen, rather than total ammonia, multiply the ammonia-nitrogen reading (in mg/L or PPM) by 1.3 to get the total ammonia level. Then, using the chart, approximate the percentage of un-ionized ammonia that would be present. Multiply that percentage by the measured dissolved total ammonia, and the product will be the actual toxic ammonia present. The optimum level for toxic ammonia in the water is less than 0.02 milligrams NH_3 per liter of water (mg/L).

For example, if the measured total ammonia was 2.0 mg/L with a pH of 7.5 and temperature around 68°F / 20°C, then the toxic ammonia would be 1.25% x 2.0 = 0.025. This is slightly higher than the preferred maximum level, so the fish could become stressed. If the pH was 6.5 and the temperature at 77°F / 25°C, then 0.18% x 2.0 = 0.0036 mg/L, well below the toxic level. Use the next higher temperature value for temperature readings that are between the given values. This will give a higher percentage reading, which will act as a safety factor in determining if the ammonia level is in the toxic range.

Percentages of total dissolved ammonia as toxic un-ionized ammonia (NH_3):						
Water pH:	**Temperature:**					
	41°F / 5°C	**50°F / 10°C**	**59°F / 15°C**	**68°F / 20°C**	**77°F / 25°C**	**86°F / 30°C**
6.0	0.01 %	0.02 %	0.03 %	0.04 %	0.06 %	0.08 %
6.5	0.04	0.06	0.09	0.13	0.18	0.25
7.0	0.13	0.19	0.27	0.40	0.57	0.80
7.2	0.20	0.29	0.43	0.62	0.90	1.26
7.4	0.32	0.46	0.68	0.98	1.41	1.98
7.5	0.40	0.59	0.86	1.25	1.73	2.48
7.6	0.49	0.73	1.08	1.55	2.21	3.10
7.8	0.76	1.16	1.68	2.44	3.46	4.82
8.0	1.23	1.83	2.65	3.83	5.28	7.46
8.2	1.95	2.86	4.15	5.90	8.26	11.3
8.4	3.04	4.45	6.43	9.04	12.5	16.8
8.5	3.89	5.56	7.98	11.2	15.3	20.3
8.6	4.74	6.88	9.81	13.6	18.4	24.2
8.8	7.30	10.5	14.7	20.0	26.4	33.6
9.0	11.1	15.7	21.5	28.5	36.3	44.6
9.2	16.5	22.7	30.2	38.6	47.3	56.0
9.4	23.9	31.8	40.7	49.9	58.7	66.9
9.5	28.5	37.1	46.4	55.7	64.3	71.8
9.6	33.2	42.5	52.1	61.2	69.3	76.2
9.8	44.0	53.9	63.2	71.4	78.1	83.5
10.0	55.5	65.1	73.3	79.9	85.1	89.0

When toxic levels of un-ionized ammonia are encountered, rapid measures must be taken to lower the ammonia level. Make water changes of 20-50% on a daily basis until levels are normal. Add salt to the water at the rate of 1 pound per 100 gallons (0.1%) to increase ionization of ammonia. Slowly decrease the water temperature and pH if possible, also. Increasing biological filtration will gradually lower the ammonia, but this may not be rapid enough without other measures. Decrease feeding to reduce added proteins and fish waste. Remove any decaying organic material in the pond. Ensure adequate oxygenation of the water is present because ammonia irritates the gill epithelium causing hyperplasia that reduces oxygen absorption, and it also reduces the hemoglobin's oxygen-carrying capacity in the blood. The breakdown of ammonia by bacteria also requires oxygen. There are also commercial water treatments available (e.g., AmQuel, AmmoLock2) that can be added to the pond water and will bind ammonia into a nontoxic form.

Chlorine, chloramine, formalin and certain other medications such as the ammonia binders that are added to the pond can interfere with accurate ammonia testing when using the Nessler method ammonia test. In these cases, use the salicylate method ammonia test; however nitrite, nitrate, phosphate, and sulfate at high levels will interfere with the accuracy of this test method. Check the nitrite and nitrate levels first, then the ammonia level. In ponds with low levels of nitrite and nitrate, the salicylate method ammonia test will be accurate.

Nitrite

The aerobic oxidation of ammonia (NH_3) in the water by chemoautotrophic bacteria produces nitrite (NO_2^-).

$$2NH_3 + 3O_2 = 2H^+ + 2NO_2^- + 2H_2O$$

High levels of nitrite in the water will be absorbed by the fish's gills. In the blood, it oxidizes the iron in hemoglobin producing methemoglobin that prevents the red blood cells from carrying oxygen. Methemoglobinemia causes the blood and gills to turn brown. Death in the fish occurs from hypoxia. Toxic conditions occur when the nitrite level is above 0.10 mg/L in soft water or 0.20 mg/L in hard water.

Some kits used for water analysis test for nitrite-nitrogen, rather than total nitrite. With these test kits, multiply the nitrite-nitrogen value

THE NITROGEN CYCLE IN A POND:

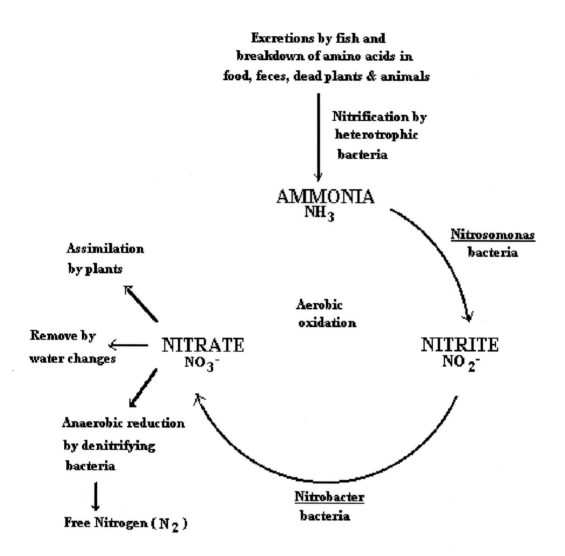

The nitrogen cycle is most rapid at pH 7.1-7.8 and temperatures of 77-95°F / 25-35°C, with saturation levels of dissolved oxygen. Decreased oxygen levels, and pH or temperatures above or below optimum levels will reduce the rate of nitrification.

(in mg/L or PPM) by 3.3 to get the total value of nitrite present.

Treat nitrite toxicity by partial water changes, increasing the oxygen concentration in the water, increasing the aerobic biological filtration, and by adding salt to the water. The chloride ions (Cl⁻) from sodium chloride (NaCl) compete with nitrite ions for absorption by the gills, reducing the toxicity. There should be 6 mg/L of chloride ion present for every 1 mg/L of nitrite ion to prevent toxicity. Add salt at a rate of one teaspoon per gallon of water, or one pound per hundred gallons, to achieve 0.12% salinity (1200 mg/L). This dose is very safe for the koi and enough to reduce nitrite toxicity. Salinity tests are available to monitor salt levels in the pond water. Chloride test kits can also be used, with 1 mg/L of chloride ion equivalent to 1.67 mg/L of sodium chloride.

Nitrate

Nitrate (NO_3^-) is produced by aerobic oxidation of nitrite by chemoautotrophic bacteria. The nitrifying bacteria oxidize the nitrite to nitrate to produce energy, and unlike photosynthesis, this can occur even in the dark, as long as oxygen is present.

$$2HNO_2 + O_2 = 2HNO_3 = 2H^+ + 2NO_3^-$$

Nitrate is relatively nontoxic, and koi can survive at levels up to 200 mg/L, but do best if nitrate is kept below 20 mg/L. The accumulation of nitrate will reduce the buffering capacity (alkalinity) of the water over time, which will allow the pH to decrease (become acidic). Nitrate acts as fertilizer for algae, and high levels will stimulate algal blooms. Also high nitrate levels will interfere with salicylate method ammonia testing. Keep the level low by periodic water changes and removal of dead plant material from the pond.

Some water test kits give the results of nitrate tests as nitrate-nitrogen, which is the measure of only the nitrogen component of the nitrate molecule. To obtain the total nitrate level with these test kits, multiply the value of nitrate-nitrogen (in mg/L, or PPM) by 4.4 to equal the total nitrate level.

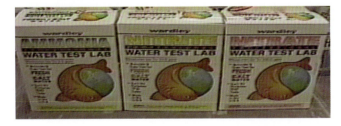

Chemical test kits for ammonia, nitrite, and nitrate.

Dissolved Oxygen

The amount of oxygen dissolved in water is dependent on multiple factors such as temperature, turbulence, and salinity. High population densities (overcrowding) in fish ponds, decreased water circulation (aeration), plant respiration in absence of sunlight for photosynthesis, addition of certain chemicals like formalin, and bacterial decomposition of decaying organic matter all lower the oxygen level in the water. Higher water temperatures will increase the biochemical oxygen demand by fish and other organisms in the water. Koi utilize 7.2 mg of oxygen per kilogram of body weight per hour at 36°F / 2°C, but 300 mg oxygen per kg BW per hour at 86°F / 30°C. Higher water temperatures will also decrease the amount of oxygen that can be dissolved in the water.

Saturation levels of dissolved oxygen in fresh water at sea level (760 mmHg):

Water temperature	Mg oxygen/liter water
32°F / 0°C	14.6 mg/L
41 / 5	12.8
50 / 10	11.3
59 / 15	10.1
68 / 20	9.1
77 / 25	8.3
86 / 30	7.6
95 / 35	7.0
104 / 40	6.5
113 / 45	6.0

At higher elevations the dissolved oxygen levels will be slightly lower than listed on this chart. Increases in salinity will also decrease the amount of oxygen dissolved in the water. Seawater at 3.5% salinity holds 18% less oxygen than distilled water.

Dissolved oxygen is depleted at lower depths first so measurements should be made at least 2 feet down from the surface of the pond. While koi will survive in water with oxygen levels as low as 5 mg/L, they do best at 9 mg/L or more. Because both animals and plants consume oxygen for respiration at night, the dissolved oxygen level will be lowest at dawn. Turning off waterfalls or fountains at night ("because no one is there to see it") can cause significant reduction in dissolved oxygen when it is required most.

Respiration:

O_2 (oxygen) + $C_6H_{12}O_6$ (glucose)
=> CO_2 + H_2O + Energy

Photosynthesis:

CO_2 (carbon dioxide) + H_2O + Sunlight
=> O_2 + $C_6H_{12}O_6$

Fish suffering from hypoxia will "gasp" at the surface of the pond, especially near water inlets. They will die with their opercula flared and mouths open, with a pale gill color. Do not feed fish in conditions of low oxygen as this will increase the biochemical oxygen demand.

Remove organic debris and algae, and reduce overcrowding to prevent low oxygen levels. A partial water change will also increase the dissolved oxygen in the pond and dilute chemicals that lower available oxygen. In an emergency, 3% hydrogen peroxide can be added to the pond at 0.25 ml/L (1 ml/gallon) to instantly increase the oxygen concentration.

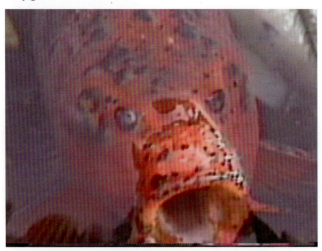

A koi gulping air (piping) at the surface of a pond due to low disslolved oxygen level.

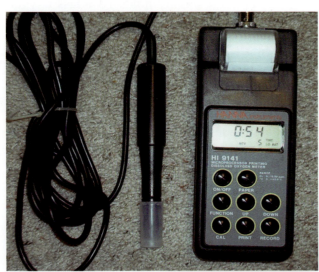

ABOVE: Electronic digital dissolved oxygen meter makes monitoring oxygen levels in different parts of the pond easy.

RIGHT: Test kit for measuring water hardness.

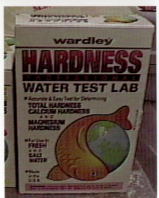

Hardness

This term is used to describe the characteristic of water that represents the total concentration of polyvalent metal cations, expressed as their calcium carbonate ($CaCO_3$) equivalent. Calcium (Ca^{++}) and magnesium (Mg^{++}) are the main ions that contribute to hardness, along with aluminum, barium, copper, iron, lead, strontium, and zinc to a lesser extent. The greater the concentration of metals cations in the water, the higher its hardness.

Terms used to describe calcium carbonate concentration in water (mg $CaCO_3$ / L H_2O):

VERY SOFT WATER	0 - 25
SOFT	25 - 75
MODERATELY HARD	75 - 150
HARD	150 - 250
VERY HARD	Over 250

Hardness, alkalinity, and pH are very closely related water properties. Soft water is usually acidic, while hard water usually has a basic pH. Highly alkaline waters also have a basic pH. Alkalinity measures the mineral anions and hardness measures the metal cations, but since calcium carbonate is the single largest source of these ions in natural waters, the alkalinity and hardness values expressed as mg $CaCO_3$/L water will be similar.

Another term for measuring hardness is DH or dH, which stands for Deutsche Hartgrad or "German degrees of hardness." This is often called degrees hardness, and 1 DH is 1 part CaO in 100,000 parts of water, which equals 17.9 mg $CaCO_3$/L H_2O. Thus, very soft water would have a DH of approximately 1-1.5.

Hard water reduces osmotic work required for fish to replace blood electrolytes (sodium, potassium, calcium, chloride, phosphorus, bicarbonate) lost in urine. Koi will do well in water with hardness of 100 mg/L or more, but very hard water, with higher pH, will make ammonia toxic and so increases in ammonia levels must be avoided in water with high hardness. The hardness of water will increase with time as water evaporates, leaving behind and concentrating the dissolved minerals. Removing water from the pond (partial water change) will take out the old hard water, and replacing it with fresh water will lower the total hardness. In ponds with too soft water, calcium carbonate (limestone, crushed oyster shells, or commercial pond blocks) or calcium hydroxide (slaked lime) can be added to raise the hardness.

Alkalinity

Buffers help to reduce abrupt or radical changes in water chemistry that could be harmful to the fish. Water's buffering capacity is measured as alkalinity, which is the ability of the water to resist changes in the pH. The greater the alkalinity, the more stable the pH of the water will be. However, increasing alkalinity will cause an increase in the pH value (making it more basic).

Alkalinity is due to dissolved mineral anions: mainly carbonate (CO_3^{--}), bicarbonate (HCO_3^-), and hydroxide (OH^-), and in lesser amounts borate, chloride, phosphate, silicate, and sulphate. Total alkalinity measures all of the mineral anions, but is expressed in terms of calcium carbonate (mg $CaCO_3$/L H_2O). The optimum alkalinity is 100 mg/L, but koi will do well in water with 20-300 mg/L alkalinity.

Add calcium carbonate ($CaCO_3$), calcium hydroxide [$Ca(OH)_2$], or sodium bicarbonate ($NaHCO_3$) to soft water to increase its alkalinity. Sodium bicarbonate is common baking soda, and can be added safely to the water at 1 teaspoonful/10 gallons whenever the alkalinity is too low in order to buffer the water and raise the pH.

Calcium Carbonate

As mentioned in the Hardness and Alkalinity sections, calcium carbonate ($CaCO_3$) is the most common mineral in fresh water. It comes from dissolved limestone, mollusc shells, and other sources. It dissolves readily in water containing carbon dioxide, forming carbonic acid. This will then form the highly soluble calcium bicarbonate [$Ca(HCO_3)_2$] which exists only in solution.

$$CaCO_3 + CO_2 + H_2O = Ca^{++} + 2HCO_3^- = Ca(HCO_3)_2$$

The presence of calcium carbonate and calcium bicarbonate buffers the water to prevent pH changes upon additions of acid or basic solutions. Acids react with bicarbonates to form the weaker carbonic acid and carbon dioxide, only slightly lowering the pH. Basic solutions react with the bicarbonates to form the carbonate ion (CO_3^{--}) which only slightly raises the pH, and is easily neutralized. Without the buffers the pH changes would be more extreme and could be detrimental, or even fatal, to the fish.

Acid: $2H^+ + Ca(HCO_3)_2 = H_2CO_3 + CO_2 + H_2O + Ca^{++}$
Base: $2OH^- + Ca(HCO_3)_2 = 2CO_3^{--} + 2H_2O + Ca^{++}$

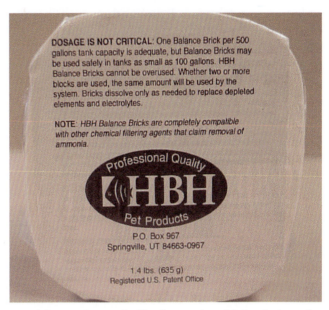

A calcium carbonate buffer that can be added to koi ponds.

Carbon Dioxide

Respiration from fish and other aquatic animals, and plants in the absence of sunlight, produces carbon dioxide (CO_2). In solution, CO_2 acts as an acid by combining with water (H_2O) to form carbonic acid (H_2CO_3) and then dissociating to release hydrogen ions (H^+) and bicarbonate (HCO_3^-).

$$CO_2 + H_2O = H_2CO_3 = HCO_3^- + H^+$$

As dissolved CO_2 increases, pH value decreases (becomes more acidic). Pure water saturated with CO_2 will have a pH of 4.5-5.6, depending on temperature. This is why the pH drops in ponds and aquariums with soft water. Since this change is gradual, the fish are seldom affected, but new fish introduced into the water will go into pH shock. Agitation of the water will allow the dissolved CO_2 to be released from the water, preventing acidification. Ideal range of CO_2 in the water is 1.5-5.0 mg/L. Levels of CO_2 over 10 mg/L are harmful to fish.

In hard water with high levels of metal cations, the dissolved CO_2 combines with the calcium carbonate to form calcium bicarbonate. This prevents the pH from dropping as it does in softer water.

$$CO_2 + H_2O + CaCO_3 = Ca(HCO_3)_2$$

Calcium bicarbonate is 30 times more soluble in water than is calcium carbonate. The rate of calcium carbonate dissolution is dependent on the availability of carbon dioxide. If plants use up CO_2, the equation goes backward and the calcium bicarbonate is broken down to release CO_2. If excess CO_2 is present from respiration, the equation moves to form calcium bicarbonate. This reaction can cause the pH of the water to fluctuate between day and night as plants change from photosynthesis to respiration.

These diurnal changes, especially in low-alkalinity water (unbuffered), can result in fish deaths from either the wide pH fluctuations or from oxygen depletion by dawn. Preventing large algal blooms in the pond will reduce the major plant impact on carbon dioxide in the water. Adding carbonates or bicarbonates to the water will also raise the alkalinity to buffer pH changes. Maintaining adequate water circulation, especially at night, will release dissolved carbon dioxide and increase oxygen.

Chlorine

Most municipal water departments add chlorine or chloramine to the water supplies for sanitation purposes. The usual amount is 0.5-1.5 parts per million (PPM = mg/L) of chlorine, but some locales may add more. The chlorine gas dissolves in water and forms hypochlorous acid and dissociated hydrochloric acid.

$$Cl_2 + H_2O \Rightarrow HOCl + H^+ + Cl^-$$

Chlorine levels of 0.2 mg/L or higher will kill fish fairly quickly. Lower doses can cause extensive gill damage and gradual deaths. Signs include trembling, flashing, discoloration, listlessness, and death due to hypoxia because of gill damage. Secondary bacterial or fungal gill infections frequently occur in chlorine-damaged gills.

Chlorine will dissipate from water over time, and agitation, aeration, and ultraviolet light will increase the rate of chlorine evaporation. Allowing chlorinated water to sit exposed to the atmosphere will take 15 days to completely dissipate the chlorine, 7 days are required if it is aerated. Activated carbon will remove chlorine from the water, and dechlorinators such as sodium thiosulfate ($Na_2S_2O_3$) bind it to make it nontoxic.

$$Cl_2 + 2(Na_2S_2O_3 \cdot 5H_2O) =$$
$$Na_2S_4O_6 + 2NaCl + 10H_2O$$

Whenever adding tap water into a pond or an aquarium, appropriate measures must be taken to prevent chlorine toxicity. There should never be any detectable chlorine in a koi pond!

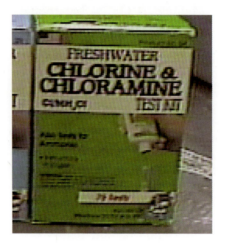

Chlorine and Chloramine test kits are available with liquid reagents, and also as dip test strips.

Chloramine

Some municipal water supplies contain high levels of organic matter or "humic acids." Organic matter in water will react with chlorine to produce chloroform, dichlorobromine, and other trihalomethanes. These compounds are considered to be carcinogenic, so many municipalities use chloramine ($ClNH_2$) for water purification, which is more stable. But chloramine eventually can be broken down into chlorine and ammonia, both of which are toxic to fish, so it's more of a concern than chlorine alone! Also chloramine is a weaker disinfectant than chlorine, so water treatment facilities may use 1.0–4.0 mg/L residual chloramine.

$$Cl_2 + NH_3 \Rightarrow Cl^+ + Cl^- + NH_2^-$$
$$+ H^+ \Rightarrow ClNH_2 + HCl$$

$$HOCl + NH_3 \Rightarrow OH^- + Cl^+$$
$$+ NH_2^- + H^+ \Rightarrow ClNH_2 + H_2O$$

Tap water for use in ponds or aquaria should be chemically dechloraminated. Sodium thiosulfate ($Na_2S_2O_3$) will break the chlorine-ammonia bond and remove the chlorine, but leaves the ammonia. Fresh activated carbon will also adsorb the chlorine component, leaving the ammonia free in the water. Zeolite clay will remove the ammonia, but must be recharged regularly and is not effective in pond water with salt added to it. Biological filtration will convert ammonia to nitrite and then to nitrate, but the rate of this oxidation by the aerobic bacteria may not be fast enough to prevent ammonia and nitrite toxicity to the fish from the added tap water.

A practical alternative treatment is to add sodium hydroxymethanesulfonate ($HOCH_2SO_3^-Na^+$) to the water. This "ambidextrous" chemical breaks the chlorine-ammonia bond, and the sulfonate end reacts with chlorine (Cl_2) and hypochlorite (OCl^-) to produce nontoxic chloride ions (Cl^-). The hydroxymethane end of the molecule will bind with ammonia to produce a stable, nontoxic water-soluble compound, aminomethanesulfonate, which will not release the ammonia back into the water, and is ultimately removed by biological filtration. This chloramine eliminator is available in commercial aquarium and pond products (AmmoLock2, AmQuel, AquaSafe, and A.C.E.).

$$ClNH_2 + HCl + HOCH_2SO_3^-Na^+ => H_2NCH_2SO_3Cl + Na^+ + Cl^- + H_2O$$

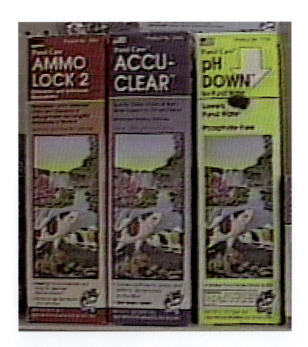

Commercially available products to remove ammonia, remove particulates, and to control elevated pH levels.

Sodium Chloride

Sodium chloride (NaCl) is the chemical name for table salt, or *halite*. Natural fresh waters contain about 0.02% sodium chloride. Seawater contains about 3.1% sodium chloride (and 0.4% other salts), the Great Salt Lake in Utah varies between 15-28% sodium chloride, and the Dead Sea in Israel contains 9.7% sodium chloride and 17.3% magnesium chloride ($MgCl_2$). A measure of 1% salt is often expressed as 10 parts per thousand (PPT = mg/ml) or 10,000 parts per million (PPM = mg/L).

Dissolved salt in fresh water is important in the osmoregulation of the fish's body fluids, which contain about 0.9% sodium chloride. It also increases the production of the slime coat, protecting the skin and helping the fish to glide through the water with less resistance. The dissociated chloride ion from dissolved salt also prevents nitrite toxicity by competing for absorption with the nitrite ion by the fish's gills. A useful level of salt in a koi pond would be from 0.1% to 0.3% (1000-3000 PPM or mg/L).

Salt solutions in the pond may be toxic to aquatic plants at concentrations above 0.3%. Delicate pond plants such as water hyacinth, water lettuce, and water cress are especially sensitive to salt levels, and may be affected by even 0.1% salt concentrations. Also, if you are using Zeolite (clinoptilolite clay) in your pond for ammonia removal, the addition of salt will cause the Zeolite to release some ammonia back into the water in exchange for adsorbing the salt. Be sure to remove the Zeolite, or monitor the ammonia level carefully, when adding salt to the koi pond.

Salinity

Many people assume that salinity is the sodium chloride concentration of water, but it is actually the concentration of ALL dissolved salts (mineral ions) in a solution. In seawater, sodium chloride is the main component of dissolved salt, but in dilute fresh water, calcium bicarbonate and calcium carbonate are the most common salts. The dissolved salts dissociate into their positive cation and negative anion components. The predominant mineral ions in natural waters are sodium (Na^+), potassium (K^+), calcium (Ca^{++}), magnesium (Mg^{++}), chloride (Cl^-), bicarbonate (HCO_3^-), carbonate (CO_3^{--}), and sulfate (SO_4^{--}).

Increases in salinity occur in koi ponds when water is added to replace only what has evaporated, without actually removing some pond water first. Over time the dissolved salt concentration increases, raising the water's pH, hardness, alkalinity, and total dissolved solids (TDS) content. High salinity also reduces the amount of oxygen soluble in the water. By performing periodic partial water changes (20-30%) rather than just topping-off the pond water, increased salinity is avoided.

Salinity is measured with hydrometers and refractometers as specific gravity, a measure of density relative to pure water, or with salinometers that measure electrical conductivity. Temperature must be taken into account to get accurate readings.

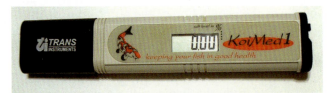

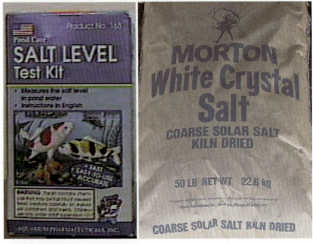

TOP: Digital salinity meter simplifies salt testing
LEFT: Liquid salt test kit is inexpensive way to test pond
RIGHT: Pure salt (sodium chloride) is used for ponds
BELOW: Salt is a standard at fish breeding facilities.

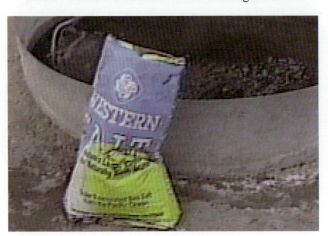

Conductivity

Electrolytic conductivity is the capacity of dissolved mineral ions in a solution to carry electrical current. The current is carried by inorganic dissolved solids such as the anions of carbonate, chloride, nitrate, phosphate, and sulfate, and cations such as aluminum, calcium, iron, magnesium, and sodium. Organic substances do not carry electrical current well, and therefore do not significantly affect the conductivity.

The conductivity measurement requires a special meter (salinometer) that applies voltage between two electrodes, 1 cm apart, that are immersed in the solution. The voltage drop, or resistance, is measured in ohms, and the reciprocal of this number (1/ohm) is the conductivity, measured in Siemens per centimeter (S/cm), or sometimes called mhos (ohm spelled backward, as conductivity is the reverse of resistance). Ranges normally found in fresh water are very small, so milliSeimens (mS) or microSiemens (µS) are used. Distilled water has a conductivity of 0.5 µS/cm. Since the ions that produce electrical conductivity are part of the TDS in a solution, the conductivity can be used to calculate the TDS value.

In freshwater without the addition of salt, calcium carbonate ($CaCO_3$) is the greatest contributing mineral to conductivity. Multiply the conductivity reading in µS/cm by 0.4 to get an approximate value of calcium carbonate in mg/L. In typical freshwater conditions, with hardness of 40-250 mg/L $CaCO_3$, the actual conductivity will be 100-600 µS/cm. With the addition of salt, the sodium chloride (NaCl) becomes significantly more important than calcium carbonate in the conductivity measurement. In this case, multiply the conductivity reading by 0.5 to get the approximate mg/L of sodium chloride. With a normal level of added salt in a koi pond from 0.1% to 0.3% (1000-3000 PPM or mg/L), the actual conductivity would be 2000-5800 µS/cm.

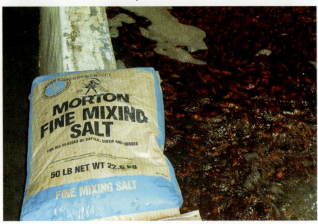

Measuring Pond Volume with Salt

One pound of salt in twelve gallons of water equals 1% salinity. Adding 1 pound of salt per 100 gallons of water raises the salinity 0.12% (1# / 100 Gal = 454g / 378.5 L = 454g / 378,500g = 0.001199 = 0.12%!). Therefore, 1# / 100 Gal x 12 Gal/# [a conversion factor for 1% Salinity] = 0.12 % Salinity, or # Salt / Gal x 12 = % Salinity. So, using a Salinity Meter we can use the formula:

Salt x 12 / % Salinity = Gallons Water.

For example, if a pond had a reading of 0.02% before adding salt (natural salt content) and it was estimated that the pond might hold 1500 gallons, then adding 15 pounds of salt should raise the salinity to 0.14% (0.02% already in the pond plus the added 0.12%) once the salt was completely dissolved and circulated through the pond. Use the pond filtration turnover rate as a guide to know how long to wait before taking a second reading. If the pond filtration pumps 750 gallons per hour, then wait at least 2 hours so that all of the water will have passed through the filter system (in theory) to be sure the salt is evenly dispersed.

After waiting for the dissolved salt to be completely dispersed in the pond, take a second reading of the salinity. If the pond volume, including the plumbing and filtration was exactly 1500 gallons (the estimated volume) the second reading should be exactly 0.14%. If the reading is higher, the pond volume is smaller than 1500 gallons; and if it is a lower reading, then the pond volume is more than 1500 gallons.

To calculate the exact volume in gallons, find the difference between the first and second Salinity % readings (Second Reading - Initial Reading). This is the percent that the added salt actually raised the Salinity. Now multiply the pounds of added salt by the conversion factor 12, then divide this by the change in the salinity just calculated to get the actual volume in gallons.

Salt x 12 / (R2 - R1)% Salinity = Volume of Water in Gallons

Here are the steps summarized:
(1)   Measure Salinity % before adding salt (R1).
(2)   Add 1 pound of salt for each 100 gallons of ESTIMATED pond volume,
        then take a second reading (R2) after salt is dispersed.
(3)   Subtract Initial Reading from the Second Reading for % Salinity changed.
        If the initial reading is zero (no salt in pond), just use the reading from after
        the salt is added to the pond (R2 - 0 = R2).
(4)   Multiply the pounds of salt added by 12.
(5)   Divide this by the % Salinity changed.
(6)   The final result is the Pond Volume in Gallons.

In the example used above, assume the second salinity reading was 0.18%. So the initial reading was 0.02% (Step 1), and (2) 15# of salt was dispersed in the pond, (3) then the actual change of salinity from adding the salt would be 0.18% - 0.02% = 0.16%. (4) Multiply the 15# of salt added by 12 to get 180. (5) Divide 180 by 0.16 to get the actual pond volume of 1125 gallons. This value includes the water in the plumbing and filtration system as well as what you see in the pond!

The formula can also be used to determine how much salt to add to a pond with a known volume to reach a desired salinity percent. For example, if a 2500 gallon pond was to be raised to 0.3% salinity, multiply 2500 gallons by (0.3 % Salinity / 12) to get 62.5 pounds of salt to be added to the 2500 gallon pond for a final salinity reading of 0.30%.

Salt = (Desired % Salinity / 12) x Gallons Water

Hydrogen Sulfide

Under anaerobic conditions, heterotrophic bacteria in pond sediments reduce sulfates in decaying organic matter to produce hydrogen sulfide gas, which is very soluble in water. Hydrogen sulfide is toxic to aerobic organisms because it inactivates the enzyme cytochrome oxidase. Un-ionized hydrogen sulfide (H_2S) is extremely toxic to fish, even at concentrations as low as 0.002 mg/L, and any detectable level should be prevented.

$$CaSO_4 + CH_4 = CaCO_3 + H_2S + H_2O$$

Hydrogen sulfide produces the black ooze in the pond gravel, the soil of potted water plants, and bog areas. It has a foul rotten-egg odor and is toxic to humans as well as to the fish. At high levels, hydrogen sulfide quickly deadens the sense of smell and lethal levels may still exist but go unnoticed. This has caused death in persons exposed to H_2S gas. When strong rotten-egg odors appear while working in the pond, take frequent breaks to areas away from the smell to be sure to not become overwhelmed.

Like ammonia, hydrogen sulfide is toxic to fish in its un-ionized state. Its ionized form is non-toxic. The water temperature and pH levels will control how much will be ionized. Low pH and low temperatures increase the un-ionized state. High pH or high temperatures increase the ionized state. However, due to the extreme toxicity of H_2S to fish, even at higher pH or temperatures, the small percentage of un-ionized H_2S present may still cause fish deaths!

$$H_2S \text{ (toxic)} = HS^- + H^+ \text{ (ionized, nontoxic)}$$

As available hydrogen ions (H^+) increase in acid water (low pH) the above equation shifts from the right to the left, increasing the un-ionized, highly toxic hydrogen sulfide (H_2S) in the pond water.

Do frequent water changes when H_2S is detected, and stir the gravel beds frequently to prevent anaerobic production of H_2S gas. Make sure the filtration has proper water flow and aeration to prevent anaerobic bacterial activity in organic material trapped in the filter. Potassium permanganate added to the pond at 2-6 mg/L removes hydrogen sulfide and reverses its toxicity to fish.

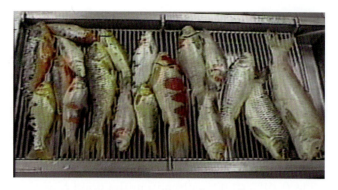

Loss of the inhabitants of a koi pond after hydrogen sulfide was released in cleaning a stagnant filter bed! Rapid fish loss is usually due to water quality problems, not infection.

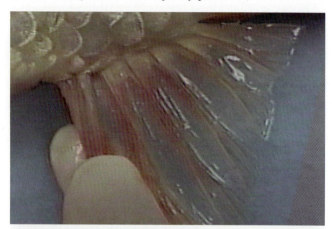

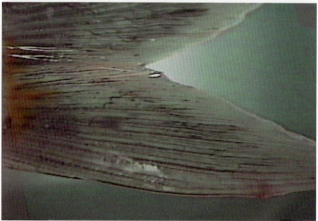

Anal fin and caudal fin blood vessel congestion of a koi exposed to hydrogen sulfide in the pond water.

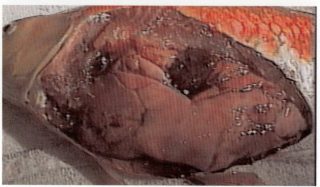

Severe congestion and hemorrhaging in the abdominal organs of a koi exposed to hydrogen sulfide in the pond water.

Biochemical Oxygen Demand (BOD)

This is the amount of dissolved oxygen necessary for the oxidative decomposition of organic material in water by heterotrophic microorganisms. It is measured as the change in oxygen content (in mg/L) of a sealed sample of water incubated in the dark at 68°F / 20°C for 5 days. The greater the difference between the beginning and end oxygen levels (high BOD) the more organic material is in the water. High organic loads can cause rapid depletion of dissolved oxygen from pond water. Frequent pond cleaning to remove dead leaves and other organic material, and periodic partial water changes will lower the BOD.

Total Dissolved Solids (TDS)

This is the dissolved mineral content of the water. It is determined from the total residue remaining after evaporation of a water sample that was previously filtered to remove suspended particles. The residue is weighed and then the TDS is calculated as residue weight divided by water sample volume, and expressed in milligrams per liter (mg/L). Average TDS in natural rivers is about 120 mg/L, but can be considerably higher in ponds. In freshwater ponds the TDS is mostly calcium carbonate, magnesium carbonate, sodium chloride, and sulfates. High TDS will increase the hardness, alkalinity, and conductivity of the water. The US Environmental Protection Agency (EPA) warns that if the TDS exceeds 500 mg/L in drinking water, then this is an indicator of potential concerns.

Total Particulate Matter (TPM)

This is the dry weight of the suspended particles filtered out of a water sample. The water sample is poured through fine filter paper and it is allowed to air dry. Then the original weight of the filter paper is subtracted from the final weight. The difference is the weight of the particulate matter that was suspended in the water sample. This weight in milligrams is divided by the original water sample volume in liters to produce the TPM expressed in milligrams per liter (mg/L). The particulate matter consists of suspended debris, fish wastes, algae, small aquatic organisms, and dust. High particulate matter levels will make the water turbid (cloudy), and can irritate the gills, causing gill epithelial hypertrophy and hyperplasia.

Redox Potential

The "redox" potential is the oxidation and reduction potential (also called ORP) of chemicals in the water. Oxidation originally meant the chemical process of the addition of oxygen (O_2) to a molecule, but now includes any chemical reaction where an electron is lost. The molecule that loses one or more electrons is "oxidized" and is the "reducing agent" for the electron recipient, which is "reduced."

Reduction was originally the removal of hydrogen (H^+) from a molecule, but now is any chemical reaction where an electron is gained (increase in negative charge). The molecule that gains the electron is "reduced" and is the "oxidizing agent" toward the electron donor, which is "oxidized."

In any reaction in which one molecule is oxidized, another must be reduced. Therefore it is always an "oxidation-reduction" reaction. The proportion of oxidized to reduced substances in a solution is called the "redox potential." It is measured with a hydrogen electrode (E_h) as a voltage difference. The redox potential of oxygenated water at pH 7.0 is approximately 0.3 volts (or 300 mV). Normal values for the redox potential (ORP) in a koi pond are 250-400 mV.

Because oxidation-reduction chemical processes provide energy for nonphotosynthetic (heterotrophic) organisms, the redox potential is a guide to available energy production in the water, and hence microbial activity. When it is too low, 3% hydrogen peroxide can be added to the water at 1ml/gallon of water to increase the redox potential, by increasing the oxygen level in the water. Low doses of potassium permanganate may also be added (0.25-0.5 PPM) to oxidize the water and raise the ORP. Low ORP levels result from high organic loads in the pond, algae accumulation, overfeeding, overcrowding, poor filtration and aeration, low oxygen concentration, and from the addition of chemicals to the pond that remove oxygen (e.g., formalin).

The ORP level is increased by the addition of hydrogen peroxide, potassium permanganate, and by the use of ozone, and activated carbon, which removes dissolved organic compounds from the water that lower the ORP. ORP levels above 475 mV for more than a few hours are harmful to the koi and to the nitrifying bacteria in the biological filter, and the ORP value should never be above 550 mV. High ORP levels will irritate or burn the fish's gills, resulting in hyperplasia, necrosis and possibly death.

Water Test Kits

There are many different types of water test kits available (American Marine; Aquarium Pharmaceuticals; Aquarium Systems; Aquatic Eco-systems; Environmental Test Systems; Gilford Instrument Labs; Hach Company; Hagen Corporation; Hanna Instruments; Kordon; La Motte Chemicals; Milwaukee Instruments; and Orion Research are some of the test kit manufacturers and distributors). Check with local petshops and pond supply stores, or search the Internet to find test kit suppliers.

The simplest tests are small plastic strips with chemical pads attached that are dipped into the pond water. The pads change colors which, when compared to a color chart, indicates the level of that substance in the pond. Dry tablet tests are also available where a small tablet is dissolved into a test tube containing the pond water sample. Its color is then compared to a chart to determine the results. Some test kits have solutions that are mixed with the pond water to produce the color reactions. More expensive test kits use a spectrophotometer to electronically compare colors and give more accurate results.

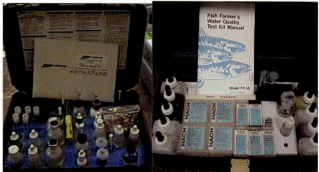

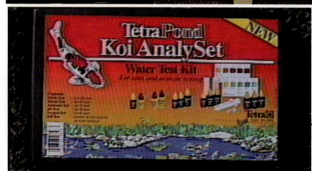

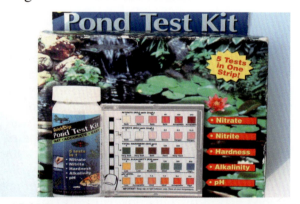

ABOVE: Pond test strips that are dipped into the pond water and measure nitrite, nitrate, hardness, alkalinity, pH.
BELOW: Tests using tablets mixed with pond water.

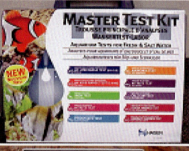

A variety of water test kits from (above) LaMott, Hach, Tetra, (right) Hagen, (left) Jungle and Aquarium Pharmaceuticals.

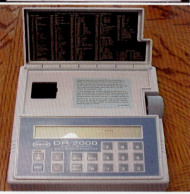

A Hach Spectrophotometer for digitally measuring the results from water tests for greater accuracy.

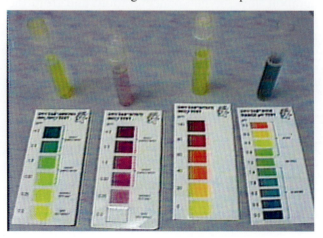

The accuracy of any test kit depends on the quality of chemical components, and the careful following of the test directions. Test reagents must be stored properly, avoiding moisture and temperature extremes. Check for expiration dates on the test reagents to be sure that they are still fresh for the most accurate results. If the manufacturer has not dated the packaging, write the date of purchase on it and replace liquid reagents in 1 year and dry reagents in 2 years. Use a logbook to keep track of the water tests. The following form can be used as a guide for designing your own record.

KOI POND EXAMINATION AND WATER QUALITY ANALYSIS

Dr. Nicholas Saint-Erne

Date: _____

Location: _____

Pond Size: _____

Filtration System: _____

Fish Examination: _____

_____

_____

Water Examination: _____

_____

_____

Water Quality Test Results:	Optimum Range:
Temperature -	65-77°F / 18-25°C
Oxygen Content -	8-12 mg/L
pH -	7.0-8.0 [stable]
Alkalinity -	100-250 mg/L
Hardness -	100-250 mg/L
Ammonia -	0-0.01 mg/L (un-ionized)
Nitrite -	0-0.01 mg/L
Nitrate -	0-20 mg/L
Chlorine -	0 mg/L
ORP -	250-400 mV
Other -	

Recommendations: _____

Treatments: _____

Recheck Date: _____

REFERENCES:

Blasiola, George C. 1984. *Protecting Aquarium Fish and Pond Fish from the Danger of Chloramines,* Metropolitan Water District, Los Angeles, CA.

Boyd, Claude E. 1979. *Water Quality in Warm Water Fish Ponds,* Auburn University, Auburn, AL.

Boyd, Claude E. 1990. *Water Quality in Ponds for Aquaculture,* Auburn University, Auburn, AL.

Cole, Gerard A. 1979. *Textbook of Limnology,* 2nd ed., C.V. Mosby, St. Louis, MO.

Ghadially, Feroze N. 1969. *Advanced Aquarist Guide,* The Pet Library, Harrison, NJ.

Gratzek, John B. (editor). 1992. *Aquariology: Fish Diseases and Water Chemistry,* Tetra Press, Morris Plains, NJ.

Hach. 1997. *Water Analysis Handbook,* 3rd ed., Hach, Loveland, CO.

Hovanec, Timothy A. 1999. "*Nitrospira – not Nitrobacter*" in Aquarium Fish Magazine, vol. 11, no. 4, Fancy Publications, Mission Viejo, CA.

Lagler, Karl F. 1956. *Freshwater Fishery Biology,* 2nd ed., Wm. C. Brown, Dubuque, IA.

Parker, Rick. 1995. *Aquaculture Science,* Delmar Publishers, Albany, NY.

Roberts, Ronald J. 1989. *Fish Pathology,* 2nd ed., Bailliere Tindall, London.

Ruttner, Franz. 1974. *Fundamentals of Limnology,* 3rd ed., University of Toronto Press, Toronto, Canada.

Stoskopf, Michael K. 1993. *Fish Medicine,* W.B. Saunders, Philadelphia.

Warren, Charles E. 1971. *Biology and Water Pollution Control,* W.B. Saunders, Philadelphia.

Wedemeyer, Gary A., Fred P. Meyer, and Lynwood Smith. 1976. *Diseases of Fishes, Book 5: Environmental Stress and Fish Diseases,* T.F.H. Publications, Neptune, NJ.

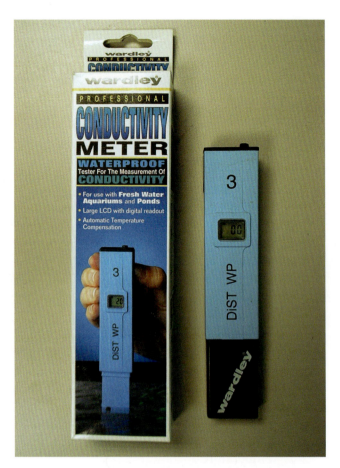

Digital electronic conductivity meter is useful for measuring dissolved minerals in a koi pond.

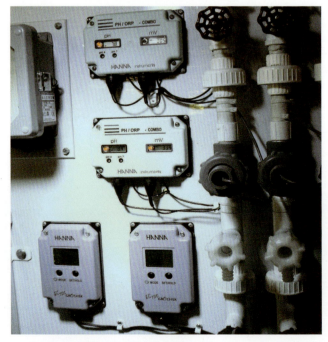

Conductivity, pH, ORP, and temperature probes and meters connected to the filtration system to monitor water parameters in a high quality residential koi pond.

FILTRATION SYSTEMS

Filtration of the pond is what separates an artificial containment of water from a natural environment. With filtration, the artificial pond will be cleaner, the water clearer, and will support a greater density of fish. Without filtration, a pond that doesn't have the natural inflow and outflow of a fresh water source, along with the associated plants, microflora and fauna, and aquatic animals, may stagnate and become a cesspool.

The size of the filter unit should be as large as is practical. It could be summed up as "the bigger the better!" Some pond owners have filtration systems that are as large as, or even larger than, the size of the koi pond. Most filters are small plastic boxes or bins that are connected to the pond by a series of pipes, and water is circulated through them by water pumps. The water passes through various filter media such as foam, gravel, lava rock, plastic beads or rings, and filter brushes. Jacuzzi or swimming pool pressurized sand filters are used as well. For small ponds, submerged box filters, similar to aquarium box filters, can be used, but are much less efficient and require more frequent cleaning than do external filters.

The flow rate of water through the filters should be such that the total volume of pond water passes through the filter every hour. Therefore, a 1000-gallon pond would need a water pump for the filter that pumps 1000 gallons per hour. In highly stocked koi ponds, a greater volume would be even more beneficial; and in low-density ponds, a lower flow rate would suffice. The pipes used in the filter system should be the same diameter as the pump outflow port, or even slightly bigger. Much larger diameter pipes will cause low water pressure in the pipes, resulting in settlement of debris within the pipes. Smaller pipes will cause increased pressure, possibly damaging the pump, or causing gas supersaturation, leading to "gas bubble" disease in the fish. Keep bends in the pipes and total pipe length to a minimum to reduce resistance. Avoid 90 degrees elbows or bends in the pipes to reduce pressure loss.

The water intake for the filters should be near the bottom of the pond for removing debris when the water is warm. In cold weather, the water should be removed near the surface to prevent stirring the denser water at the bottom of the pond, which keeps the bottom water from freezing.

Mechanical Filtration

This is the process of removing suspended solids, detritus, and debris (TPM) from the pond water. Water is pumped from the pond into filter chambers, where it moves by pump pressure or gravity through the filter media and drains back into the pond. The filter media is usually sand, gravel, nylon brushes, foam, or fiber matting. The solid debris is trapped in the filter media, which needs to be cleaned frequently to prevent obstruction of the water flow.

Mechanical filtration clears or "polishes" the water, but does not remove dissolved wastes or toxic chemicals. Water should pass through the mechanical filter before the other filter units to reduce sediment build-up in those filter chambers. Mechanical filters that are separate from the biological filtration units are often called "prefilters."

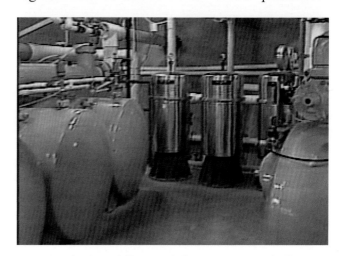

Pressurized sand filters and diatomaceous earth filters (silver canisters in the center) remove solid debris from the pond by mechanical filtration. The diatomaceous earth will filter particles larger than 1 micron in size, so water must pass through it after being filtered by the sand filter to prevent rapid clogging.

Chemical Filtration

This is a process where chemical reactions are used to remove dissolved substances such as ammonia, chlorine, soluble heavy metals, dissolved organic carbon compounds, and other chemicals. The filter medium is placed into a separate chamber of the filter, or placed into a removable mesh bag. Periodically it must be replaced with fresh medium.

One commonly used filter medium is granular activated carbon. It is produced by heating carbonaceous material to 1112°F / 600°C in the absence of air, a process that removes hydrocarbons, then reheating it to 1652°F / 900°C in the presence of an oxidizing gas, which produces the porous internal structures. This allows it to adsorb chemicals such as chlorine, copper, and other heavy metals into microscopic pores on its surface. Eventually all of the pores will be filled and the activated carbon will need to be replaced. Activated carbon will also remove most medications when the pond is treated, so remember to remove it from the filter before treating for diseases. It can be used to safely and quickly remove excess medication when the pond is accidentally overdosed. Activated carbon does not remove ammonia, nitrite, or nitrate from the water.

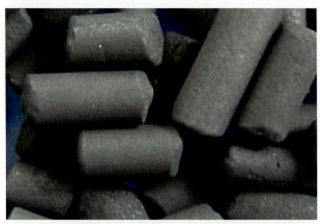

Close-up of activated carbon granules.

Zeolite (clinoptilolite, an alumino-silicate clay) can be used to remove ammonia from pond water by ion exchange. This occurs by the zeolite releasing sodium chloride (NaCl) into the water and absorbing ammonia. Periodically the zeolite must be "recharged" by removing it from the pond and placing it in a plastic container of 3.5% salt water (3 pounds salt per 10 gallons of water). After 24 hours, rinse the zeolite in fresh water and return it to the filter. There it will gradually release the sodium chloride again in exchange for any ammonia. One precaution – if using salt to treat for fish disease, remove the zeolite from the filter first. Otherwise, as the salt concentration in the pond increases, the zeolite will recharge itself, releasing ammonia back into the pond water in exchange for the added sodium chloride.

In locales that have very soft, acid water, using calcium carbonate (crushed oyster shells or limestone) or dolomite [calcium magnesium carbonate, $CaMg(CO_3)_2$] in the filter will increase the hardness and buffering capacity of the pond water. In locales with very hard water, the use of ion exchange resins may be necessary to lower the hardness of the water before adding it into the pond. These units exchange the sodium cation from salt (NaCl) added to the unit for the calcium and magnesium cations in the hard water, producing a softer water.

Biological Filtration

This is the most important filtration process for living organisms. There should be a mechanical filter prior to the biological filter to remove debris that may otherwise clog or impede the water flow through the biofilter. The biofilter requires living aerobic chemolithoautotrophic bacteria to function, so if the water flow is greatly diminished or stopped, even for a few hours, the oxygen levels to the bacteria will be reduced and they will die. This will prevent the nitrification of the toxic ammonia waste in the pond. It may take days or weeks to replace the live nitrifying bacteria and return the biofilter to normal function.

When setting up a new biofilter, it is relatively sterile, without any nitrifying bacteria (*Nitrosomonas, Nitrosococcus, Nitrosospira, Nitrobacter, Nitrospira* and other species). With pond water circulating through the filter, gradually the nitrifying bacteria will grow on the filter media, producing biological filtration. This process can take several weeks to develop at an adequate level to convert all the toxic ammonia

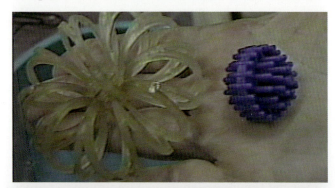

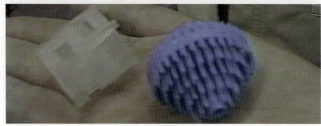

Examples of some of the plastic media with large surface areas for biological colonization that are used in biological filtration systems.

and nitrite into nitrate. In the meantime, toxic conditions can occur in the pond affecting the fish. This is called the "new tank syndrome" in aquaria or "new pond syndrome" in koi ponds. Adding nitrifying bacteria to the biofilter can reduce this stage of inadequate biological filtration.

One way of doing this is to add some filter media (gravel, plastic beads, filter foam) from an established running biofilter. This provides large quantities of live nitrifying bacteria immediately. They will continue to grow and rapidly colonize the new filter media. There is a slight risk in doing this of spreading disease organisms from the old pond into the new filter, however. When changing the biofilter media, do not remove all of the old material at the same time, but leave some to help seed the new material.

Another way of seeding the new biofilter is to add a commercially prepared bacterial supplement. These have bacterial spores or live bacteria in a suspension that become active when added to water in the pond filter. Some of these products work better than others, and all have a limited shelf life before they lose their efficacy. Be sure to buy fresh products that have been stored properly for best results.

The optimum water temperature for biological filtration is 75-95°F / 24-35°C. The rate of nitrification by bacteria decreases as the water temperature drops, and is minimal below 50°F / 10°C. Nitrification occurs most rapidly at pH levels of 8.0–8.5, moderately at 7-8, poorly below 7.0 (ammonia is mostly ammonium at this point) and ceases at pH below 5.0 or above 9.0. Maximum saturation levels of dissolved oxygen are required for most efficient nitrification by aerobic bacteria. Placing airstones connected to aquarium air pumps into the biofilter will ensure adequate oxygen levels. Exposing wet media to air also helps.

An ideal biofilter setup would have shut-off valves on the pipes to the biofilter with a separate air or water pump in the biofilter. This way the biofilter could be bypassed when medicating the koi pond, but it would still be oxygenated to keep the bacteria alive. The main pump would continue moving water through the mechanical filter (bypass the chemical filter as well when medicating) and back to the pond through a waterfall or fountain to aerate the water.

Fluidized Bed Filters

These filters are both biological and mechanical filters in a single unit. They have 0.125" (3.175 mm) diameter polyethylene beads that are "fluidized" in the filter by the flow of water and air bubbles, suspending them within the filter chamber. Each cubic foot of beads has approximately 400-500 square feet of surface area. The beads trap debris acting as a mechanical filter, and nitrifying bacteria colonize the bead surfaces providing biological filtration.

Because of the constant motion of the fluidized beads, no channeling or dead spaces occur, and biological filtration is increased. This results in highly efficient filtration. Regular backflushing (temporary reversal of the flow of water through the filter to flush out waste) of the filter keeps the detritus from accumulating in the beads. Since the plastic beads are not tightly packed, as is the sand in standard sand filters, the bead filters are easier to clean when backflushing, and use less water in the process.

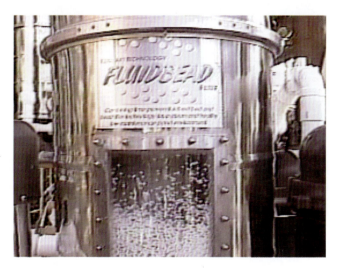

ABOVE: A window into this fluidized bed filter shows the suspended polyethylene beads.
BELOW: Fluidized bed filters come in a variety of sizes and manufacturers for all sizes of koi ponds.

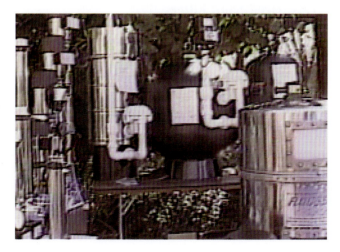

Wet/Dry (Trickle) Filtration

This section of a filtration system increases the air-water interface for improving biological filtration. Air has 21% (210,000 mg/L or PPM) oxygen, while pond water usually has 6-12 mg/L or PPM (0.0006-0.0012%) oxygen, therefore air contains 17,500-35,000 times more oxygen than does the average pond water. By trickling or spraying water onto a biofilter media that is not under the water, but exposed to the high oxygen levels in the air, yet keeping the nitrifying bacteria wet, the bacteria have more accessible oxygen than if they were submerged in the water. This optimizes the aerobic breakdown of ammonia and nitrite wastes in the pond water.

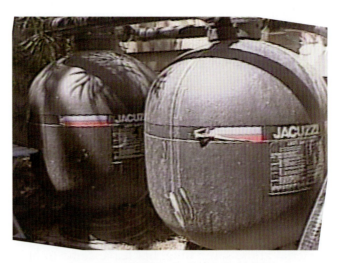
Jacuzzi sand filters used on a koi pond.

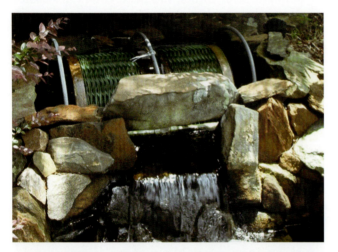
This type of wet/dry biological filter has a spinning drum covered with folded media that rotates in the water. Bacteria colonize the media, and remain wet by the flowing water, which rotates the wet media into the air to expose it to oxygen, increasing the bacteria's biological filtration capacity.

Pressurized Sand Filters

These are the Jacuzzi or swimming pool filters that are often used in koi ponds. They are large, oval fiberglass containers filled with 3-5 mm diameter sand particles. Water is pumped through them under pressure and is filtered mechanically. If the pressure gauge reading increases, then it is time to backflush the unit to remove accumulated waste trapped in the sand. The disadvantage of this system is that it clogs rapidly so it requires frequent checks on the pressure gauge and backflushing. They do keep the water very clear if working properly. Some biological filtration activity also can occur in sand filters, if the water flow is high enough to provide adequate oxygen. Dangerous hydrogen sulfide gas can be produced in dirty sand filters that have reduced flow and inadequate oxygen levels.

Settling Tank

This filtration unit allows sediment and heavy debris to settle out of the water before it flows into the mechanical filter. The water enters from the top, goes under a baffle to reduce turbulence, and overflows into the next filter unit. This leaves behind the heavy particulate matter that settles to the bottom where it can be periodically removed through a bottom drain. The settling tank or chamber must be large enough to slow down the water flow sufficiently to allow the suspended particles to settle out.

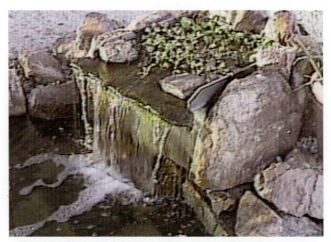
Plants at the top of the waterfall act as a filter by trapping particulate debris and removing nitrates from the water.

Plant Filters and Bogs

This is a separate pond or container that the filtered water flows through before returning to the koi pond. It is filled with aquatic plants like watercress, water hyacinth, water lettuce, or emerging plants like water irises, cattails, and rushes. These plants will remove nitrates, the end result of bacterial biological filtration, from the water. Some phosphates may also be removed. Settling of suspended particles into the soil of the bog filter will also help remove particulate debris from the pond water.

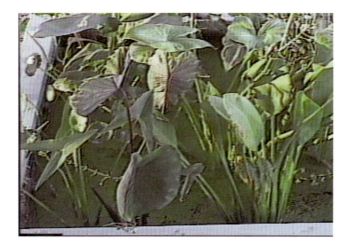

Water flowing through basin of plants to remove nitrates.

Barley Straw Filter

An organic means of unicellular algae control using barley straw has been used in koi ponds. The barley straw is placed into a mesh sack and immersed in the pond in an area where it gets exposure to sunlight and oxygenated water flow (near the filter return outlet or waterfall). As the barley straw aerobically decomposes, after about 6-8 weeks, it produces chemicals (its lignins oxidize into homic acids) that inhibit the growth of planktonic algae. In heavy algae situations, use 1 pound of barley straw for each 100 square feet (50 g per square meter) of pond surface area. One pound of barley straw is sufficient for approximately 1500-20,000 gallons of koi pond water, depending on amount of algae present. Check the barley straw monthly to ensure that it is not becoming anaerobic (smelly). Replace it with fresh barley straw if it is and increase water circulation around it. Otherwise replace it every 6-12 months.

Ultraviolet Sterilizers

An ultraviolet (UV) sterilizer uses a fluorescent low-pressure mercury vapor bulb that produces electromagnetic radiation in the far UV wavelengths of 185-300 nanometers (nm), most often 253.7 nm. This is shorter than visible light wavelengths, which range from violet at 400 nm to red at 700 nm, and infrared light at 800 nm. This bulb is placed into a quartz sleeve that is attached to the water pipes of the filtration system. Water flows outside the sleeve past the UV bulb and any algae, fungi, viruses, bacteria, or protozoa exposed to the UV rays will be killed by irradiation of the microorganism's DNA or RNA. This is helpful in controlling algal blooms and in treating the free-swimming stages of parasites like *Ichthyophthirius*. The quartz sleeve must be kept clean of debris and the bulb needs to be replaced after 12-14 months of continuous operation. After this period of time, the amount of UV light produced will be ineffective, even though the lamp appears to still be working.

The UV dosage is measured in microwatt seconds per square centimeter of surface area ($\mu Ws/cm^2$). The effective dose of UV light varies depending on the organisms. The effective range against bacteria is 2000-22,000 $\mu Ws/cm^2$, yeasts 6000-17,000 $\mu Ws/cm^2$, mold spores 5000-330,000 $\mu Ws/cm^2$, viruses 6000-8000 $\mu Ws/cm^2$, protozoa 22,000-360,000 $\mu Ws/cm^2$, and algae 35,000-40,000 $\mu Ws/cm^2$. The actual dosage level produced by the UV sterilizer is dependent on the power of the UV bulb and the water flow rate. If the water flow rate past the UV bulb is too rapid, the UV sterilizer will be less effective. It is better to use a UV sterilizer rated for a pond larger than for which it is being used, rather than one for a smaller sized pond.

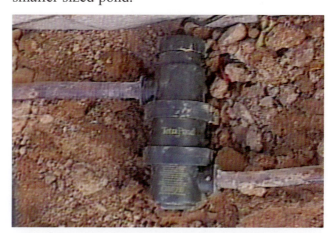

UV Sterilizers come in a variety of sizes and wattages for all sizes of koi ponds.

The optimum operating temperature for the UV lamp is 104°F / 40°C. Direct contact with cooler water will lower the lamp's efficiency. The quartz sleeve insulates the lamp from the water to allow it to operate at a higher temperature, but still allows the UV rays to penetrate through it into the water. Glass blocks penetration of UV rays.

The UV sterilizer should be placed at the end of the filtration circuit so the water passing through it is relatively free of suspended particles that would block the UV rays. The UV sterilizer should be temporarily turned off when adding medications to the pond to avoid loss of the medication's efficacy. It may not be necessary to run the UV sterilizer continuously, but only when disease conditions or algal blooms occur. However, frequent on-off cycles of the UV lamp will shorten its useful life in comparison to continuous operation.

Ozone

The unstable triatomic oxygen molecule ozone (O_3) is a potent oxidizing agent. It is used to prevent diseases by destroying viruses, bacteria, and protozoa, and to improve water quality by oxidizing many organic compounds. An electric ozonator is necessary to produce ozone from air or oxygen. The ozone is added to the water after it has passed through the biological and other filters. It is important that all the ozone dissipates from the filtered water before it returns to the pond to prevent oxidation burns on the gills and skin of the fish. Activated carbon can be used to remove residual ozone from the water. Passing the water through an ultraviolet filter will also break down the ozone. In pure water at 68°F / 20°C, the half-life of ozone is 165 minutes. Ozone is dissociated (broken down) faster in hard water or basic pH water than in soft or acidic water. It also dissociates faster at higher temperatures and in water with high organic loads or inorganic ions.

Ozone is typically used in water at a concentration of 0.01-0.3 mg/L for a short period of up to 2 minutes. It has a distinct odor that can be smelled at concentrations above 0.02 mg/L. At high doses it can be toxic if inhaled, with coughing the first sign to appear. When using an ozone generator, make sure it is in a well-ventilated area or outside. A considerable amount of heat is also produced by the ozonator. Ozone can be used effectively in protein skimmer units, in place of air or oxygen.

Protein Skimmers

Protein foam fractionation is a process where air, pure oxygen (O_2), or ozone (O_3) is injected into a vertical column of water, producing

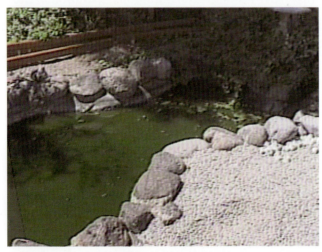

Green water in a koi pond not only makes it hard to see and enjoy the fish, but can be dangerous due to oxygen depletion at night and on cloudy days from respiration by algae, and the possibility of supersaturation of the water on very hot and sunny days from abundant photosynthesis.

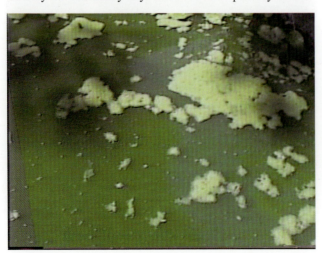

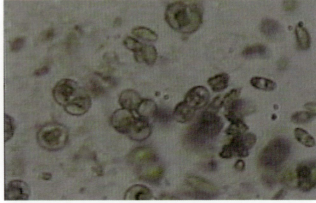

Microscopic, single-cell algae responsible for green water. This is killed by ultraviolet radiation in the UV sterilizer.

foam made of proteinaceous compounds dissolved in the water adsorbing onto tiny bubbles. The foam rises up the vertical tube and is collected in a dry chamber above the water line, which is periodically emptied and cleaned. The treated water is returned from a spout near the top of the vertical tube to the pond. A strong flow of extremely fine bubbles is necessary to efficiently extract dissolved proteins from the water.

The use of foam fractionation removes the dissolved organic carbon (DOC) compounds from the water, which reduces toxic compounds, detritus, and yellow discoloration of the water.

In-Pond Filters

These are the least efficient of the filters, but in small ponds with only a few fish they may be adequate. Basically they consist of a submersible pump which draws water through filter media and pumps it out a fountainhead or to a waterfall. This adds oxygen to the pond by circulating the water. The filter media may be as simple as an attached foam rubber pad, which serves as both mechanical and biological filter, or it may be contained in a plastic box filled with lava rock, plastic balls, or fiber pads. These units must be frequently lifted out of the pond and be rinsed off or otherwise cleaned to keep them working properly. They do work well for hospital tanks or ponds, and for breeding ponds, when only a small amount of fish waste is expected. Frequent partial water changes also help in maintaining these types of ponds.

Channeling

Channeling occurs when the water follows a single path of least resistance around the filter media, or through a small number of channels in media such as pea gravel. This significantly reduces the effectiveness of the filters. In filter media where channeling has occurred, the material that is bypassed may become anaerobic from lack of oxygenated water flow. Hydrogen sulfide production can occur in these areas. Regular back-flushing, cleaning detritus from the filter media, and stirring the sand or gravel to reduce channeling is recommended.

Aeration

Aeration is the movement of water in the pond to provide oxygen absorption and waste gas release through turbulence at the air-water interface. Water that does not flow or move has reduced capacity for exchanging gases, and will often become stagnant and oxygen-depleted. Aerobic bacteria in the biofilter can significantly reduce oxygen levels in the water passing through the filter, so aeration of the water returning to the pond is essential. Additions of fountains, waterfalls, streams, and venturi jets add more oxygen to the water as it returns from the filter. Aquarium airstones, attached to air pumps or compressors, can be placed in the filter canisters or strategically placed in the pond.

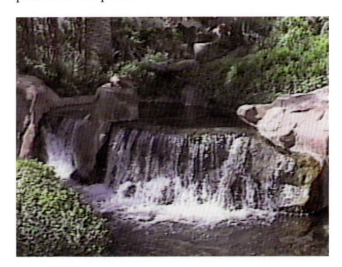

Waterfalls are an excellent source of aeration as well as an aesthetic addition to the koi pond.

Venturi Device

If water flowing through a pipe is passed through a restricted tapered section, a vacuum forms beyond the restricted section. An air inlet pipe attached just beyond the restriction will suck in air and mix it with the flowing water, thus increasing the dissolved oxygen content. The amount of air entering the venturi can be adjusted by a valve on the air inlet pipe. This is commonly used to increase the oxygen in water returning to the pond from the filter system.

Care must be taken to be sure that the air isn't forced through the water under too much pressure in order to prevent supersaturation of the gases into the water.

Surface Skimmer

A skimmer is a prefiltration device where water is taken from the pond surface through the skimmer inlet and passes through a strainer before being pumped into the main filter. This allows floating debris such as leaves to be trapped in a strainer basket or net and be removed from the pond without having the large debris pass into the main filter. The strainer needs to be manually cleaned out frequently.

REFERENCES:

Fruland, R. M. 1977. *Ultraviolet Sterilization and the Serious Aquarist,* Hawaiian Marine Imports, Houston, TX.

Fujita, Grant. 1989. *Koi,* 2nd ed., AKCA, Midway City, CA.

Neaves, Chris. 1994. *Use and Abuse of High Rate Sand Filters on Koi Ponds,* South Africa.

Pool, David. 1993. *Hobbyist Guide to Successful Pond Keeping,* Tetra Press, Blacksburg, VA.

Siegel, Arthur D. 1974. *Ultraviolet Purification of Aquarium Water,* Gull Manufacturing, Cheshire, CT.

Spotte, Stephen. 1970. *Fish and Invertebrate Culture,* Wiley-Interscience, New York.

Spotte, Stephen. 1979. *Seawater Aquariums – the Captive Environment,* Wiley-Interscience, New York.

Summerfelt, Steven T. and John N. Hochheimer. 1997. "Review of Ozone Processes and Applications as an Oxidizing Agent in Aquaculture" in *The Progressive Fish-Culturist,* 59:94-105, The American Fisheries Society, Bethesda, MD.

Tamadachi, Michugo. 1994. *The Cult of the Koi,* 2nd ed., T.F.H. Publications, Neptune, NJ.

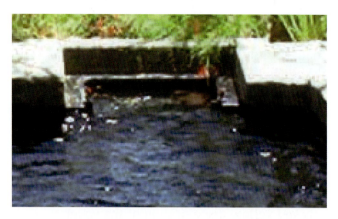

The open top design of this surface skimmer makes it easy to monitor and clean. The water from the surface of the pond overflows into the strainer basket. Leaves and other floating debris are collected in the strainer, and the water goes on through to the filtration system.

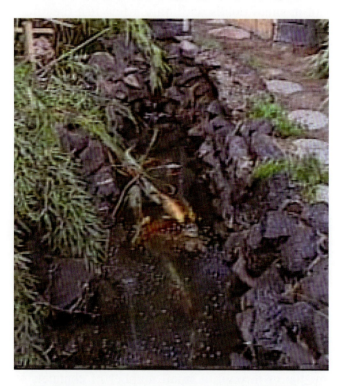

Bubbles, rising from airstones on the bottom of the pond that are attached to an air pump, circulate the water to prevent "dead zones" of poor water circulation in this narrow strip of water that runs along a walkway. Without this extra aeration, this arm off the main pond would be stagnant and have a low dissolved oxygen concentration.

SEASONAL VARIATIONS OF THE KOI POND

Variations in temperature throughout the year will alter a fish's activities and metabolic rate. The immune system becomes less effective at lower water temperatures, and stressful conditions can lead to an increase in diseases. Prevention of stress by proper pond care during each season will help reduce the incidence of disease.

SPRING

In springtime, water temperatures will begin to rise, but will fluctuate between colder and warmer days, sometimes with wide extremes between daytime and nighttime temperatures. Water quality can change rapidly during this time, as bacterial and algal activity increases. This is the time to clean and backflush the pond filter to make sure it is functioning optimally. Make sure the water is being adequately oxygenated as the fish and nitrifying bacteria will utilize more oxygen as the water warms, and warm water holds less dissolved oxygen.

Bacterial decomposition of organic debris (fallen leaves, dead algae, uneaten food) will reduce oxygen and increase ammonia concentrations in the water. Test the water frequently and change 20% of the water if ammonia or nitrite levels are elevated. Remove the debris from the pond as soon as possible (after the ice melts if the pond freezes over). Check aquatic plants, and prune, thin, or repot them as needed.

As the water warms, the nitrifying bacteria in the biological filter will increasingly convert ammonia to nitrite and then nitrate. Below 40°F / 4.4°C there is no nitrifying bacterial activity. At 64°F / 18°C there is about 50% activity of nitrifying bacteria, with rates of nitrification increasing until reaching peak rates above 77°F / 25°C. With greater sunshine in the spring, and higher nitrate levels, algal blooms occur turning the pond green. Again, water changes should be used to reduce the nitrate and algae levels, but the condition often corrects itself when complex plants (water lilies, irises, and parrot's feather) start growing actively and compete for the nitrate.

Gradually the koi will come out of their winter dormant state and become active when the water temperature reaches about 40-45°F / 4.4-7.2°C. They will start feeding at about 45-50°F / 7.2-10°C. Do not overfeed at this point! Uneaten food will increase the ammonia levels in the water, as will the increase in fish waste (urine, feces). Feed the koi in the mornings when the water temperature will be warm during the day, so the food will be properly digested. Do not feed them in the late afternoon or night yet. Fish eating in cold water may be unable to completely digest the food due to decreased digestive enzyme activity at low temperature. Bacterial decay of the ingested food can occur within the digestive tract causing gas formation and bloating.

Pathogenic bacteria also become more active as water warms, and since many fish are weakened during the winter, we see many cases of bacterial diseases in springtime. *Aeromonas salmonicida* infections commonly occur causing red sores on fins and sides, ultimately growing into large ulcers. *Aeromonas* bacteria are inactive below 39°F / 4°C, but increase activity up to water temperatures of 68°F / 20°C. This is why it so frequently occurs in the spring, when fish are weak from winter dormancy and the water temperature is at the optimal level for the bacteria. Feeding antibiotic-medicated food at this time is one way of reducing this disease. A prophylactic treatment of formalin/malachite green solution may also be indicated if the fish have a history of parasitic diseases. Check the salt content of the water and add salt as necessary to maintain the salinity at 0.1-0.3%.

An alternative to letting the fish undergo the spring temperature fluctuation stress is to use a pond heater to raise the water temperature during this time period. The fish can be allowed to go dormant for the winter, but when the water temperature increases in the spring to above 39°F / 4°C, turn on the water heater to raise the temperature above 60°F / 15.5°C. The water temperature should be raised slowly, no more than 2°F / 1°C per day. This will shorten the 4-12 weeks that the fish would naturally be at the stressful temperatures to only 10 days, lessening the risk of bacterial infections. At this temperature, the fish will also be eating, so antibiotic medicated food could be used.

SUMMER

Rising water temperatures (above 63°F / 17°C) will stimulate the koi to spawn in late spring and early summer. Make sure that any fish injured during spawning are treated to prevent secondary bacterial or fungal infections. The spawning mats or plants covered with eggs should be removed to a rearing pond or aquarium if the fry are to be raised. Otherwise, leaving the eggs in the pond will provide food for the adult koi, but if plant growth is heavy, a few fry may survive to add new life to the pond.

The optimum temperature range for koi growth is 66-77°F / 19-25°C. During this time, feed high-energy foods (35-47% protein, 10% fat) for maximum growth. Feed as much food as the koi will eat in a 5-minute period, 2-4 times daily. Overfeeding will pollute the water by increasing ammonia and reducing oxygen. This is even more serious in warmer water, so test the water frequently.

As water evaporates from the pond in the summer, the dissolved minerals (calcium and magnesium carbonates) will remain behind. These minerals form the white chalky residue along the margin of the pond. Over time, they can build up to high levels causing the water to become very hard, resulting in an increase in the pH of the water. Any ammonia in water with a basic pH (greater than 7.0) becomes more toxic to fish. Consequently, it is important to not just replace water as it evaporates from the pond, but to drain out some of the high-mineral–high-pH water and replace it with fresh water. Always use a water dechlorinator when adding city water to the pond. Chlorine in the water will irritate the fish's gills and can lead to respiratory distress, secondary gill infections, or even death.

If summertime temperatures are extreme (water temperature above 86°F / 30°C) the pond may need to be partially shaded. Warmer water not only holds less oxygen, but also increases parasite reproduction that adds to the fish's stress. Treat with appropriate medications if the fish are seen scraping their sides on rocks (flashing), have increased mucus on their skin, or are breathing rapidly at the water surface (due to low dissolved oxygen and gill irritation from parasites). Be aware that many medications may also lower the oxygen level in the water.

Oxygen levels are lowest in the morning, as aquatic plants will use oxygen for respiration at night. During the day they use carbon dioxide (CO_2) for photosynthesis and give off oxygen (O_2), but this process is reversed in the absence of sunlight. Be sure filters, waterfalls, and fountains remain on at night to oxygenate the water, even if no one is there to see them. High levels of carbon dioxide in the water from plant respiration may lower the pH of the water. Adequate water agitation will also cause dissolved CO_2 to dissipate.

AUTUMN

In the fall, prune dead aquatic vegetation, remove fallen tree leaves, and clean out organic debris from pond and filters. Check the koi to make sure all are well fed and healthy. Any thin, injured, or sick fish should be isolated and treated before they become dormant in winter. Treat the pond for parasites if any are still present after the summer treatment. A 2-week course of 0.3% salt is a good preventive treatment against protozoal parasites. Formalin/malachite green solution can also be used in the fall every 2-3 days for a 3-dose preventive treatment. When water temperature drops to 59°F / 15°C decrease the quantity of food, as the fish will become less active. Perform water tests regularly along with partial water changes.

WINTER

Koi should not be fed when water temperatures drop and remain below 45-50°F / 7.2-10°C. Once the temperature is below 40-45°F / 4.4-7.2°C the fish will become dormant. The pond water should be at least 2 ½ feet and preferably 3 or more feet deep. At this depth, the water will remain 39°F / 4°C even if frozen solid at the surface.

Mild surface water agitation will keep the pond from freezing over completely. Solid ice covering the pond can cause damage to the sides of the pond and will trap toxic gasses underneath it. Holes can be drilled in the ice or melted through it, but the ice should never be smashed as this will disturb the fish's slumber, increasing the metabolic demands. Stock tank heaters, floating pond deicers, or similar safe water heaters can be used in locales with extreme winters to keep an area of the pond surface from completely freezing over.

The filtration system should be adjusted so that it does not disturb the water at the bottom of the pond, only the surface water. If the denser water (39°F / 4°C) that settles on the bottom is mixed with the colder water at the surface (32°F / 0°C) it will all chill and can cause the fish to freeze. Cold water holds more oxygen than warm water, so waterfalls and fountains are not necessary for oxygenation during the winter months if the fish are not overcrowded. In ponds heavily planted with submerged aquatic plants, these plants will consume oxygen by respiration if thick ice or snow-covered ice prevents photosynthesis. The resulting low oxygen can cause fish deaths known as "winterkill" to fish farmers. In these cases oxygenation is necessary to avoid hypoxia.

An alternative to winter dormancy for the koi pond is heating the water to keep the koi active all winter. Using a pond heater to keep the water temperature above 60°F / 15.5°C will keep the koi active and eating, preventing winter stress and allowing them to continue to grow through the winter. Temperatures much cooler than this will not increase their metabolic rate adequately. The bacteria in the biofilter must also be at this temperature to process nitrogenous wastes. Some pathogens will still be active at this temperature, so the fish need to be monitored closely and the pond treated as necessary. Covering the pond with a greenhouse type enclosure for the winter months will also prevent heat loss and will keep the gas or electric bill from the pond heater lower.

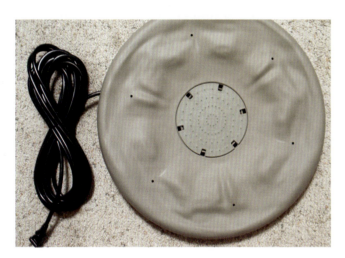

A floating pond deicer will keep an area of the pond surface from freezing over in the winter, but does not heat the pond water.

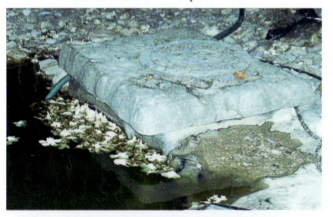

Leaves falling into the pond in autumn, or flowers in the spring, can collect at the surface skimmer or in other filtration areas and cause reduced water flow through the pond's filter, affecting biological filtration.

REFERENCES:

Axelrod, Herbert R., Eugene Balon, Richard C. Hoffman, Shmuel Rothbard, and Giora W. Wohlfarth. 1996. *The Completely Illustrated Guide to Koi for Your Pond,* T.F.H. Publications, Neptune, NJ.

Chien, Luther C. 1999. "Overcoming *Aeromonas* Alley – The Koi Keeper's Nightmare" in *Koi USA*, vol. 23, no. 4, AKCA, Midway City, CA.

McDowall, Anne. 1989. *The Tetra Encyclopedia of Koi*, Tetra Press, Morris Plains, NJ

Nash, Helen. 1994. *The Pond Doctor,* Sterling Publishing, New York.

Saint-Erne, Nicholas. 1994. *Diseases of Koi,* Koi Rx, Las Vegas, NV.

Waddington, Peter. 1995. *Koi Kichi,* Infiltration, Golborne, Warrington, Cheshire, UK.

TRAUMATIC INJURIES AND TOXICITY

TRAUMATIC INJURIES

Electrical Shock

This can occur due to lightning strikes or faulty electrical equipment. Signs include sudden death, paralysis, erratic swimming, and curved spines. Use only products approved for ponds and for outdoor use around the pond. Electrical items should be listed with the Underwriters Laboratory (have a UL tag on them). All outdoor electrical outlets should have safety measures such as circuit breakers and ground fault circuit interrupter (GFCI) outlets. These will disconnect power to any pumps or electrical appliances that may become flooded or short circuit. Use a professional electrician for installing electrical wiring to the pond.

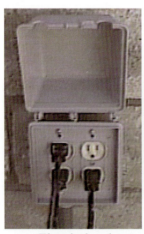
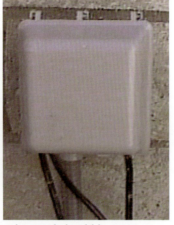

Electrical outlets around a pond should be on a GFCI and be protected from pond water and rain.

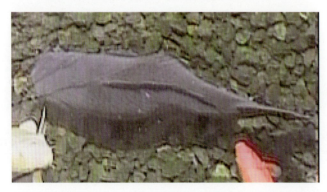

Electrical shock is one of the causes of spinal deformities in koi, the sharp muscle contraction injures the vertebrae.

Jumping out of the Pond

New koi sometimes will jump out of the pond while exploring their new environment. During heavy rainstorms, the pond level may rise allowing fish to jump out of the pond. Prevent this by lowering the water level prior to rainstorms. While spawning, koi may become so vigorous that they make their way up the side of the pond and out onto the ground. Anytime a koi leaves the water for dry land it is an emergency! If the fish is still flopping, use a net, wet towel, or even wet hands to scoop it up and place it back into the pond. If it swims away normally, chances are good that it will be fine. If it is lethargic, swims irregularly, or is not respiring, it may need artificial respiration and observation in a hospital tank. If it is not moving when found, and even appears slightly dry on the skin, do not give up hope yet. Lift the opercula (gill covers) and see if the gills are still moist and pink. If they are, there may still be a chance even if the fish is not moving. Placing it in water (preferably a hospital tank) and giving artificial respiration has revived many fish that seemed dead.

To provide artificial respiration, use the net or your hands to gently move the fish forward through the water. If possible insert the thumb into the bottom of the gill slit to open the operculum, and the tip of the forefinger into the corner of the mouth to open it. Then water will flow through the mouth and across the gills. Periodically stop moving the fish to see if it shows any gill, mouth, or fin movement on its own. If there is no movement after the tissue has had time to rehydrate, then the fish is most likely deceased. Fish that do resuscitate should be treated for topical skin wounds if present, and salt should be added to the pond water to 0.3% to reduce osmotic stress.

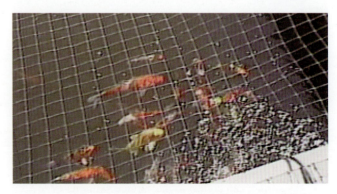

A removable screen over the pond will keep the fish in.

Overfeeding

In addition to making the koi fat, overfeeding can also cause hepatic lipidosis (fat infiltration of the liver) and water pollution (ammonia build-up). The best prevention is to feed a good quality, fresh koi food three or four times a day for young koi, and one to two times daily for mature koi. Give only as much food as they will consume within 5 minutes.

Vacation time is notorious for overfeeding problems. Well-meaning fish-sitters often grossly overfeed their wards and the owner returns to dead or dying fish and toxic water conditions. The best prevention of this is to prepare in advance each meal in a sealed container such as a zip-lock bag. Label each container with feeding time and date and any specific instructions. Give the fish slightly less per meal than would normally be given just to be on the safe side. Leave an emergency telephone number with the fish-sitter where the owner or the veterinarian can be reached, or the number of a local koi club member or koi dealer who can be consulted if a problem occurs.

Overstocking

Large numbers of koi swimming together make a dazzling collage of colors that is hard to resist, but the pond volume and filtration system must be adequate to handle the stocking density of fish. If the fish are overcrowded, oxygen content may be depleted and ammonia toxicity can occur. Overstocked ponds will be more easily devastated by contagious diseases, poor water quality, or problems such as pump or filter failures. Also, a pond that may contain a stable population of young koi may gradually become overstocked as the koi grow larger. Then, the pond's filtration capacity is finally overwhelmed and catastrophe occurs suddenly in a pond that appeared to be stable previously.

Predators

Dogs, cats, raccoons, herons, and neighboring children can all take their tolls on the koi pond population. Fencing around the pond may be necessary to keep out dogs and children, and netting over the pond is required to deter raccoons, cats, and herons. Deep ponds with straight sides make it harder for predators to reach koi than it is with shallow sloping-sided ponds. Various bird-scaring devices are available such as air cannons, metallic ribbons, noisemakers, fake owls, and big predator-eye balls. Another useful device is a motion-activated water sprayer that attaches to the garden hose. When an intruder gets near the pond in the motion-detection zone the sprayer is activated and sprays a fan of water to scare off the predator.

Baby koi can be preyed upon by larger koi, frogs, water turtles, aquatic snakes, birds, and aquatic insects. Keep them in netted fry-rearing ponds for protection until they are large enough to safely go out in the main pond with the bigger fish.

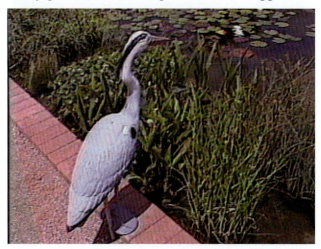

ABOVE: Heron statues are often used to deter real herons from feeding on koi as herons are territorial and will avoid other herons.

BELOW: Water turtles such as red-eared sliders can make interesting additions to koi ponds if the koi are large and the turtles kept well fed with prepared diets. They can be predators to small fish, or turtles like snapping and soft-shelled turtles can be a danger if they take up residence in a koi pond.

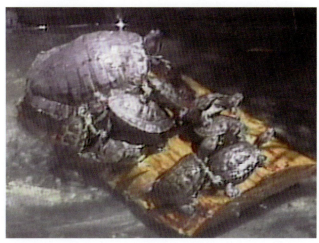

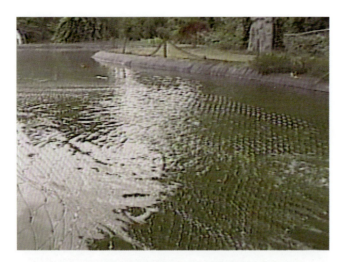

This entire pond is covered with netting to protect the fish from predators. A shade cloth could also be draped across a pond to provide shade in a situation where the fish were getting sunburned, or the water was overheating.

Sunburn

Koi in shallow water (less than 2 feet deep) that is in direct sunlight for extended periods of time each day (no shade) may suffer from sunburn. The lesions appear as hyperemia (redness) of the skin, usually the white parts, and blistering along the margins of the scales on the back. Severe cases may result in ulceration of the skin.

Treatment is to increase the depth of the water if possible, and to provide shade over the pond. Temporarily using large pieces of styrofoam or other floating objects in the pond will provide immediate sources of shade. Floating plants such as water lilies will also provide some shade for the fish. Antibiotic or antifungal treatments may be needed if secondary infection of the skin occurs.

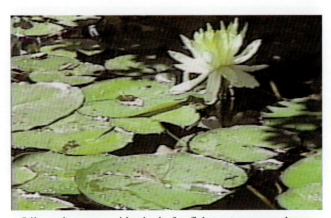

Lily pads can provide shade for fish to prevent sunburn.

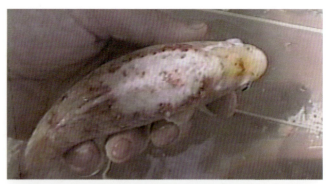

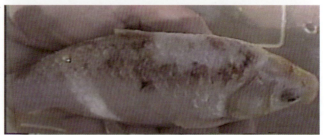

A light colored koi in a shallow pond in July with severe sunburn of the dorsum. The center of the lesion has sloughed its epidermis and scales, the edges are erythematous.

Supersaturation

"Gas bubble disease" occurs when water is supersaturated with dissolved gases. Water pumped from a deep well may have a high level of dissolved carbon dioxide or nitrogen. If not aerated or agitated when added to the pond to release the pressurized gas, the fish will absorb the supersaturated gas from the water and get gas emboli in their gills and blood vessels. This can cause the eyes to bulge out (exophthalmos) or bubbles to appear in the vessels of the fins.

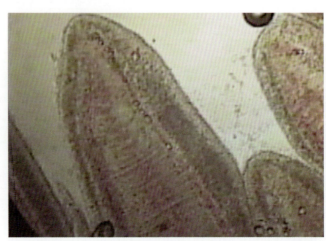

Gas bubbles visible within the gill lamellae on a gill biopsy of a koi with gas bubble disease from supersaturation.

Running a garden hose submerged in the pond, which prevents gases from being released into the atmosphere, may also cause this problem. Faulty water pumps can pressurize gas in the water and lead to gas emboli formation. Water agitation such as a waterfall will help to release dissolved gases and prevent supersaturation.

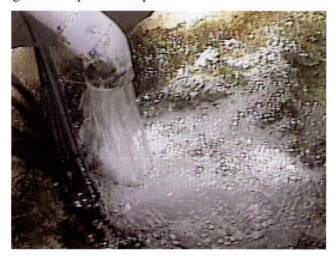

Water pumped into a very shallow pond under high pressure on a hot day caused the water to accumulate excess dissolved gases and resulted in supersaturation of the water and the koi developed gas emboli.

Occasionally supersaturation can be a result of excess unicellular algae in the pond water. In direct sunlight the algae produce an abundance of dissolved oxygen, increasing the partial pressure of the gas in the water, and therefore in the fish's blood. When the sunlight decreases, so does the algae's oxygen production, lowering the partial pressure of the gas in the pond water. Young koi especially have trouble equalizing the gas pressure in their blood, and the "bends" or trapped gas bubbles can occur in their bloodstream. Strong water agitation and shading the pond will prevent supersaturation from algae photosynthesis.

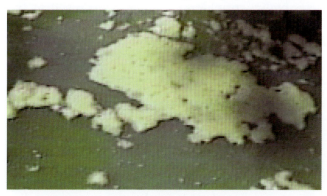

Froth on the surface of the pond from oxygen production by the green algae in the pond.

Temperature Shock

When koi are transferred from water at one temperature to water that is significantly higher or lower in temperature, it can cause thermal shock. The best way to avoid this is to place the koi into polyethylene bags containing their original water and float these in the new pond until the water temperatures are equal. Then remove the fish from the bags and place them into the new pond. It is best not to dump the old water from the bags into the pond. Temperatures can also fluctuate widely while koi are being transported, so the bags containing the fish should be placed in sturdy cardboard or styrofoam boxes, or in ice chests to insulate them from temperature changes.

TOXICITY

When constructing a pond, be sure to use appropriate and safe materials. Swimming pool liners may be coated with algacides. Roofing rubber liners may also be coated with chemicals. Be sure to use only liners that are labeled as safe for fish. The best liners currently are made from ethylene-propylene-diene-monomer (EPDM) rubber. These will usually last 20 years or more.

Concrete ponds must be coated with a nontoxic sealing agent to prevent the gradual leaching of toxic lime into the water. After the concrete has hardened, scrub and rinse it several times, fill it with water and let it sit for a few days, drain, rinse again, and let air-dry. Then apply a nontoxic pond sealant to the concrete surface. Refill the pond after the sealant is completely dry.

Garden fertilizers, weedkillers, and insecticides are toxic if sprayed where they can land on the water or run into the pond when it rains or when the lawn is watered. Use caution when working in a garden near the pond, especially on windy days. Be sure neighbors aren't spraying in a manner that could blow toxins into your pond.

Oils, gasoline, and antifreeze can poison ponds near areas where automobiles are parked. The carbon monoxide exhaust is also toxic if sucked into air pumps and then released into the pond aerators. Constructing ponds away from garages or driveways will avoid these hazards.

Wood preservatives used for outdoor decking can be toxic, and chemically treated lumber should not be used around the pond. Rainwater running off the wood and into the pond can leach out the chemicals and poison the fish. Creosote used as preservative on telephone poles and railroad ties is very toxic, so these types of wood should not be used around ponds. Consult an experienced lumber dealer about suitability of available wood when doing construction around ponds.

Heavy metals (e.g., aluminum, copper, iron, lead, and zinc) can be dissolved in water supplies and cause toxicity to the fish. A low pH increases the solubility of metal ions in the water, increasing toxicity. Hard water helps reduce the toxic effects by causing the metal to precipitate out of solution. Copper containers or pipes, and galvanized tubs should not be used for fish ponds as copper and zinc metal poisonings may occur. Do not use wire mesh screens in the ponds or filters because of possible metal poisoning. Use plastic mesh screen if needed for the pond.

Many submersible water pumps used in filters have oil within their housings. Sometimes cracks in the housing, or leaks around gaskets will allow oil to leak into the pond. It will form an oil film on the water surface. Immediately turn off and remove the faulty pump. Let the water surface calm and then suck out the oil slick with a waterproof shop vacuum. If that is not available, a clean plastic bucket can be pushed into the water so that the surface water overflows into it, skimming the oil into the bucket. Dump the bucket before it is full and repeat until the oil slick has been removed. Where feasible, without risk to the environment, the pond can be overfilled so that the surface water with the oil slick overflows out of the pond. Paper towels can be used to wipe off the pond edge and plants. After extracting the oil, do a 50% water change in the pond, adding dechlorinator to the new water. Replace the pump immediately to provide oxygen to the fish and to maintain biological filtration.

Using inappropriate materials as filter media is an often overlooked cause of poisonings. Fiber mats used in air filters or evaporative coolers can have antifungal agents added to them, so they should not be used as filter materials for the pond.

Ammonia toxicity is discussed at length in the water quality section, but one interesting form of ammonia toxicity deserves mention here. When a new fish is purchased and sent home in a plastic bag with oxygen and a little bit of water, and the fish is in the bag for a considerable period of time, ammonia will accumulate in that water. The pH of the water often lowers because of the fish's respiration producing dissolved carbon dioxide. This lower pH keeps the ammonia from being as toxic because it is ionized to a large extent to the ammonium ion. Do not open the bag until ready to remove the fish because, if it is opened and the carbon dioxide is released, the pH will increase making the ammonia more toxic.

When the koi finally reaches its new pond, the bag is floated in the pond to equalize the water temperatures before the fish is released. Many people recommend adding pond water to the bag with the fish before releasing the fish into the pond. This can be very dangerous for the fish! The pond water will likely raise the pH of the water in the bag, converting the ammonium ion back to toxic ammonia! If the fish is left in the bag now, it may be exposed to high levels of toxic unionized ammonia.

The best technique is to float the sealed bag (in the shade or covered with a cloth) for about 15 minutes to equalize temperatures, and then open the bag and lift or net the koi out of the bag and release it into the pond (or preferably quarantine unit). Do not dump the water from the bag into the pond. Ideally, the water temperature change should be less than 5°F / 3°C and the pH difference should be less than a 0.5 change in pH units. The most important factor, though, is to get the koi out of the transport water containing a high ammonia level as soon as possible.

Overdosage of fish medications such as trichlorfon, formalin, potassium permanganate, and copper sulfate can be highly toxic to fish. Trichlorfon or other organophosphate chemicals can cause seizures, muscle spasms, and even spinal injury when overdosed. Atropine sulfate injections will counteract the toxicity if given soon after the overdosage occurs. Be sure to always follow label directions carefully, measure the medication accurately, AND KNOW HOW MANY GALLONS OF WATER THE POND REALLY HOLDS! Don't guess – it may cost the lives of the fish! Use a flowmeter on the garden hose when initially filling the pond, or use the domestic water meter, making sure all other water uses (sinks, toilets, baths, sprinklers) are not being used at the same time. Write down the exact gallon volume for future reference. When estimating gallons in a filled pond, make accurate measurements of the pond dimensions and water depths. Draw the pond to scale with the dimensions indicated. Then use a calculator to make an accurate calculation of the total volume of water in the pond. The water volume contained in the filter and connecting pipes must also be considered if the filtration system will be used during treatments.

Feeding moldy fish foods containing mycotoxins produced by the fungus *Aspergillus flavus* can cause neoplastic changes. The neoplasia consists of an invasive malignant trabecular hepatocarcinoma. The mycotoxin also induces hepatic necrosis, branchial edema, and generalized hemorrhages. Death occurs from liver failure and hemorrhaging. Diagnosis can be made by examining the food and by microscopic examination of the histopathological changes in the liver cells. Always keep foods cool and dry in airtight containers, and don't use old, rancid, or moldy fish food.

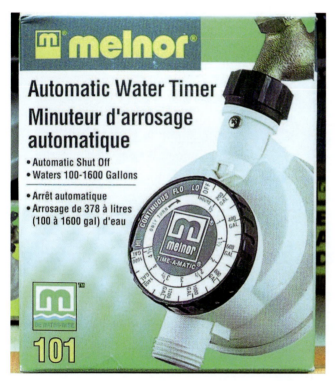

An inexpensive automatic water timer from a hardware store can be used to measure water as it is added to the pond to determine pond volume. Set the volume of water to add to the pond in increments, recording the amount of each increment added. Adjust to smaller increments as the pond gets closer to being filled. Be sure to keep track of all the incremental additions, and then the sum of all these is the total amount of water added to the pond. Keep this information stored in a safe place for future reference when calculating medication dosages.

Always use a dechlorinator when adding tap water to a koi pond to prevent toxicity!

REFERENCES:

Francis-Floyd, Ruth. 1998. *Fish*, in *The Merck Veterinary Manual*, 8th ed., Merck, Whitehouse Station, NJ.

Fujita, Grant. 1989. *Koi,* 2nd ed., AKCA, Midway City, CA.

Meyer, Stephen A. 1999. "Oil Slick" in *Aquarium Fish Magazine,* vol. 11, no. 1, Fancy Publications, Mission Viejo, CA.

Penzes, Bethen and Istvan Tolg. 1983. *Goldfish and Ornamental Carp*, Barron's Educational Series, Woodbury, NY.

Roberts, Ronald J. 1989. *Fish Pathology,* 2nd ed., Balliere Tindall, London.

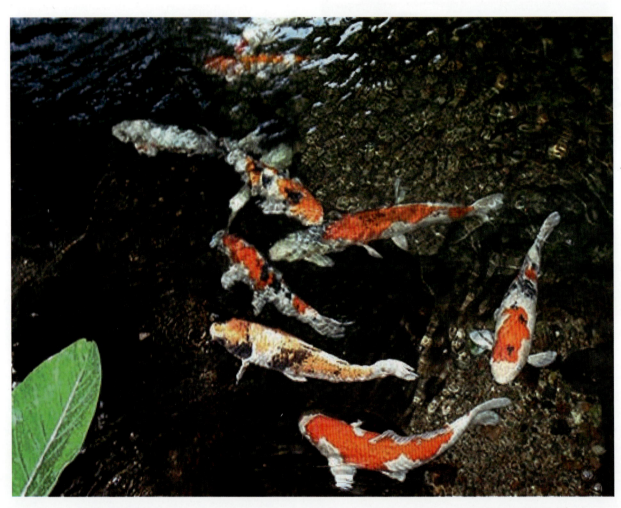
Good water quality is essential for disease prevention, and healthy koi are a joy to behold.

CHAPTER 6:
DISEASE PREVENTION

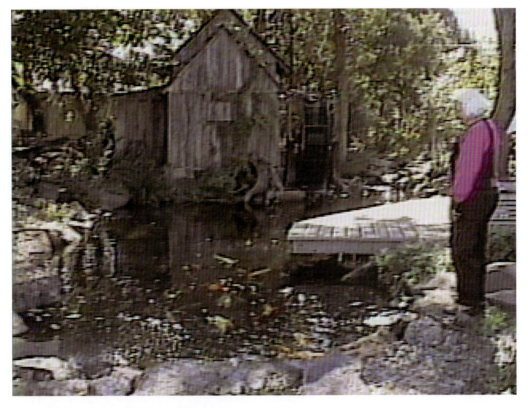

Adequate pond size, reasonable stocking densities, and proper filtration and aeration
(note the water wheel in the background) as in this beautiful koi pond in Wichita, Kansas
will go a long way in reducing disease situations.

STRESS AND DISEASE IN KOI

Stress is the term used to describe the sum of the physiological changes an organism incurs in response to adverse external influences. Those external influences are called stressors and include such things as injury, illness, environmental contamination, fear, medications, nutritional deficiency, overcrowding, parasitism, predation, reproduction, temperature extremes, transportation, or other similar factors. In many instances, more than one stressor is present at the same time.

The stress response in most vertebrate animals is to increase the release of endogenous catecholamines (epinephrine, or adrenaline) and cortisol from the adrenal glands, or in fish, interrenal tissue. This in turn stimulates a release of glucose (gluconeogenesis) by the liver. The blood glucose level elevates, providing more energy for a flight response or immune system response. The blood also shows neutrophilia (increased neutrophils) and lymphopenia (decreased lymphocytes). While causing an initial increase in protection, long-term effects of stress are a decrease in immune response (decreased antibody production and reduced phagocytosis ability) and therefore a decreased resistance to disease.

In order to prevent diseases in koi, you must provide a stress-free environment (as much as possible) by ensuring proper water quality and feeding a nutritious diet. Regular partial water changes will keep wastes from accumulating in the pond. Frequent water testing is vital in monitoring the status of the pond water. The actual frequency will vary depending on the age of the pond, how well established and regulated it is, the type of filtration provided, and the number of fish in the pond.

Nutritional deficiencies, especially of amino acids, fatty acids, and vitamins C, A, and E, have been shown to reduce the amount of globulin and antibody an animal can produce in response to an infection. This would reduce the animal's resistance to the disease. In a malnourished state, the effect of multiple stressors would further exacerbate the disease. Proper nutrition, with adequate vitamin, mineral, and fatty acid supplementation, is essential in maintaining optimum koi health.

Koi for sale at an auction are often displayed in plastic tanks, then once sold are individually bagged in plastic bags filled with oxygen and labeled with the lucky purchaser's name, and floated in the water until taken home.

DISEASE PREVENTION

By using routine preventive measures, many of the previously mentioned disease conditions can be avoided. Begin with healthy koi, protect them from stress and exposure to diseases, test them for parasites and pathogens, and treat them periodically with preventive medications.

Koi Acquisition

First of all, obtain koi from only reputable sources. Check to see that the fish is free of injury or signs of disease before bringing it home. Also check the other fish in the pond or aquarium. Some may be showing signs of disease before they all do. Is the water clear and clean? Are any medications being added to the water? What kind of filtration system is being used? Where were the fish originally bred, and how long have they been at the current facility?

Look for good body conformation, clear eyes, perfect fin condition. The fish should be alert, active, and swim smoothly, and eat readily when fed. Avoid fish with damaged skin or scales, excess mucus on the body, ragged fins, sunken muscles on the back, or bloated abdomen. If it sits on the bottom, or swims only when prodded, it may be weak or diseased. Healthy koi are precise and graceful swimmers.

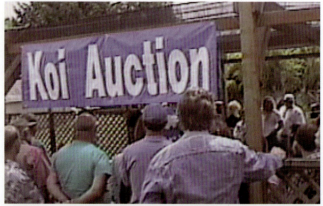

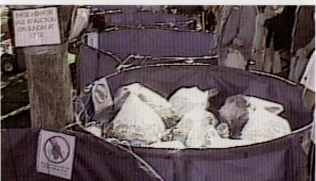

Transportation

Always handle and transport the fish safely. Be sure it is netted carefully, using a koi net of appropriate size and mesh or a one-way koi sock. Do not frantically chase it with the net; use two nets if possible, one to guide the fish into the other. Once netted, a good practice is to place the fish into a plastic koi bowl without lifting it out of the water. Place the bowl in the water under the net, and release the koi into it. Use this to carry the koi, rather than the net. Place the net over the bowl to keep the koi from jumping out.

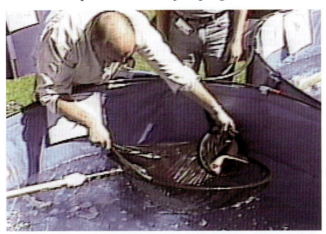

After the koi is caught with the large koi net, it is scooped out of the net with the koi sock, a fine mesh net that won't injure the koi's skin, scales, or fins. The sock net is twisted at each end (below) to keep the koi securely inside. Then the koi is lifted out of the water and transferred to another container, where it is released from the opening at the bottom end of the net, head first, so it isn't injured.

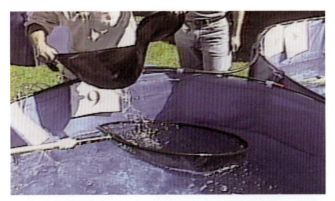

The koi should be placed individually into doubled plastic bags with just enough water to comfortably cover it. The remainder of the bag is filled with air or preferably pure oxygen. Noniodized salt can be added to the transport water at one teaspoonful per gallon. One aspirin tablet (325 mg) per gallon of water can also be added to reduce transportation shock. If the trip is extensive or more than one fish is placed in a bag, adding an ammonia detoxifier such as AmQuel (sodium hydroxymethanesulfonate, $HOCH_2SO_3^- Na^+$) will help to reduce ammonia toxicity by binding ammonia as nontoxic aminomethanesulfonate.

$$NH_3 + HOCH_2SO_3^- + Na^+ \Rightarrow$$
$$H_2NCH_2SO_3^- + Na^+ + H_2O$$

The plastic bags of fish should then be placed on their sides in a cardboard box and insulated or packed with newspapers to maintain constant temperature and prevent the bags from rolling around in the box. In hot weather, frozen gel-packs or frozen plastic bottles of water can be placed outside of the bag in the boxes to keep the koi cool. For long trips, they should be packed into styrofoam boxes or ice chests to maintain the constant temperature for a longer period. Handle these boxes carefully to avoid dropping them or jarring unnecessarily.

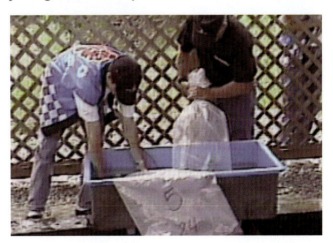

Koi are placed into strong plastic bags with just enough water to cover them completely. The bags are filled with pure oxygen and sealed. Using cardboard boxes (below) insulated with styrofoam will ensure the water temperature remains constant during transportation.

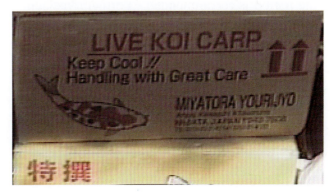

Quarantine

Once the fish arrive safely at home, they should not be placed into the pond! This is a common mistake made by most koi keepers. Instead they need to go into a previously prepared quarantine pond or tank. This environment must be large enough to adequately hold the new fish. It should have an established filtration system separate from that of the main pond. It should be deep enough or covered to prevent the new fish from jumping out. A large aquarium, a plastic water tank, or similar container may suffice for the quarantine facility. It should be of a known water volume for accurate medication dosing. Canister or box filters of appropriate sizes can be used for filtration and oxygenation. Plan on performing frequent, even daily, water changes on the quarantine facility.

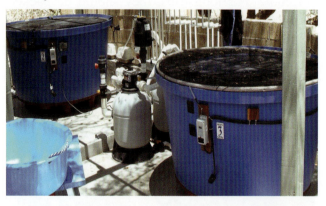

Covered 300-gallon quarantine tanks that each have their own filter, heater, and airstones for aeration.

Newly acquired fish are often stressed from transportation. Adding salt to the quarantine pond will reduce the osmoregulatory effort needed by these fish. Use 2-3 pounds of salt per 100 gallons of water to produce 0.2-0.3% salinity. Maintain this level during the quarantine period, adding the appropriate amount of salt to the new water when doing the partial water changes. The use of preventive medications during the quarantine period is recommended. Formalin/malachite green solution can be used every other day for 3-5 doses to reduce fungus and protozoa. Trichlorfon can be used once weekly against anchor worms, fish lice, and susceptible flukes. A good regimen is to use it once weekly for 4 weeks, and use formalin/malachite green on weeks 1 and 3, treating every other day during those weeks. Perform frequent water changes, measuring ammonia, nitrite, nitrate, and pH to determine how often. Remember to use a dechlorinator when adding new water to the quarantine facility. Always keep the salt concentration up to the 0.2-0.3% level. The quarantine period should run a minimum of 2 weeks, ideally 4 or more. The word "quarantine" originally meant 40 days isolation.

Other treatments during quarantine can include feeding medicated fish foods or adding antibiotics to the water. Injections of antibiotics can be given to fish with skin lesions. This is also a good time for vaccinations such as Furogen to protect against *Aeromonas salmonicida* infections. Skin, fin, and gill biopsies can be examined to check for parasites. Once the fish are eating well and acting normally, with no obvious lesions or parasites, then they can be introduced into their permanent home. Compare water quality, pH, and temperature between the two ponds when transferring them. Disinfect the nets and other quarantine facility equipment with diluted chlorhexidine solution after use.

Koi Shows

One final precautionary note about problems associated with koi shows needs to be addressed. In the Japanese-style koi show, all fish of the same size (Bu) and color variety are mixed together in one plastic show pond. The judges can then look at all of the fish being judged in that class in a single location. This makes it easier for the judges in comparing the merits of each fish. It also makes it easy to spread diseases from one fish to another. One may bring home more than just a ribbon – possibly diseases!

In the English-style show, each koi owner is assigned one or more show ponds in which only their own fish are placed, never exposing them to other people's koi. The judges then have to look

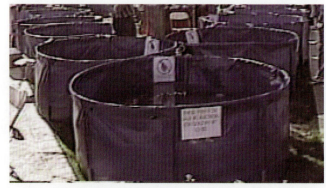

The safest style of koi show is the English-style where each koi owner has their fish isolated in individual show tanks, and use their own nets and show bowls, to avoid the possible spread of infectious diseases.

at koi of each category spread out in many different show ponds, making their job much more arduous, but reducing the health risk to the koi. While this is the preferred method for the safety of the koi, it is not always possible. With either style of koi show, the wise koi owner will still quarantine their koi upon returning home, as well as any newly purchased koi, before placing them into the main koi pond. Always bring your own net, koi bowl, water test kit, and other needed equipment to the koi show for use with only your own fish!

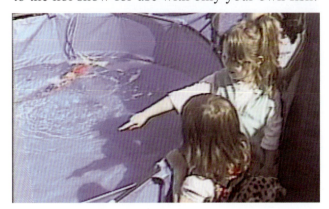

Everyone loves the beautiful koi at a koi show!

REFERENCES:

Anderson, Douglas P. 1974. *Immunology,* T.F.H. Publications, Neptune, NJ.

Dixon, Beverly A. 1990. "Stress and Fish Disease" in *Aquarium Fish Magazine,* vol. 2, no. 4, Fancy Publications, Irvine, CA.

Stoskopf, Michael K. (editor). 1988. "Tropical Fish Medicine" in *The Veterinary Clinics of North America – Small Animal Practice,* vol. 18, no. 2, W.B. Saunders, Philadelphia.

Wedemeyer, Gary A., Fred P. Meyer, and Lynwood Smith. 1976. *Diseases of Fishes,* Book 5*: Environmental Stress and Fish Diseases,* T.F.H. Publications, Neptune, NJ.

Disease Prevention Summary:

Quarantine new fish for 14-28 days. The longer the better, to assure no disease enters into an established pond.
Whenever koi are kept in a small container for examination, treatments, or temporary holding, always provide adequate aeration to prevent hypoxia and fish losses.
Monitor water quality frequently. Poor water quality makes fish more susceptible to diseases.
Do partial water changes regularly. This prevents nitrate and mineral buildup in the water.
Keep filters clean and functioning properly. This provides high levels of oxygen in the pond and eliminates wastes.
Feed a nutritionally balanced diet. Store food in airtight containers away from heat and light.
Antibiotics or other medications can be added to the food.
Remove detritus from pond.
High organic load increases growth of pathogens and reduces medication effectiveness.
Use proper hygiene (disinfection) on nets and other equipment.
Preferably have a separate set of equipment for the quarantine facility.
Ultraviolet light will kill free-swimming stages of many parasites and microorganisms.
Clean the UV light often to prevent reduction of irradiation capacity.
Activated carbon will adsorb chemicals from the water, so it should be removed when medicating the pond.
Filtration should continue in order to provide oxygenation.
Check the koi regularly for signs of disease.
Annual veterinary fish and pond examinations may diagnose a problem early.
Remember: an ounce of prevention is worth a pound of cure!
Preventive medications against parasites can be added to the pond on a periodic basis.
Join a koi club, subscribe to koi and pond magazines, read koi and pond books!
Knowledge is power, but a little knowledge is a dangerous thing – so learn as much as you can from multiple sources, and share your findings and experiences with others.

APL VETERINARY LABORATORIES

4230 S. BURNHAM AVE., SUITE 250
LAS VEGAS, NEVADA 89119
(702) 733-7866
TOLL FREE (800) 433-2750

JAMES K. KLAASSEN, DVM Ph.D.
DIRECTOR

PATIENT WALLACE, FISH ORANGE	REFERRED BY AD-V 335 ANIMAL MEDICAL HOSPITAL/NV
AGE/SEX 1Y M ACCESSION NO. 01398896	1914 E SAHARA AVE
COLLECTED 03/27/1990 18:00 MED. RECORD NO. 0000264303	LAS VEGAS, NV 89104
RECEIVED 03/27/1990 19:23	

TEST	RESULTS	FLG	REFERENCE RANGE	UNITS	LOW	NORMAL	HIGH
DR SAINT ERNE							

03/27/90 18:00 CULTURE (KIDNEY)

AEROMONAS SPECIES

SENSITIVE : AMIKACIN, CEPHALOTHIN, CHLORAMPHENICOL, GENTAMICIN

INTERMEDIATE : ERYTHROMYCIN

RESISTANT : AMPICILLIN, CARBENICILLIN, CLINDAMYCIN, METHICILLIN, PENICILLIN, TETRACYCLINE, TRIMETHOPRIM/SULFAMETHOXAZOLE

AEROMONAS SPECIES IDENTIFIED AS AEROMONAS SOBRIA.

LIGHT GROWTH AEROMONAS HYDROPHILIA

SENSITIVE : AMIKACIN, CEPHALOTHIN, CHLORAMPHENICOL, GENTAMICIN

INTERMEDIATE : ERYTHROMYCIN

RESISTANT : AMPICILLIN, CARBENICILLIN, CLINDAMYCIN, METHICILLIN, PENICILLIN, TETRACYCLINE, TRIMETHOPRIM/SULFAMETHOXAZOLE

PRINTED DATE/TIME: 04/01/1990 04:06

CHAPTER 7:

CASE STUDIES

```
                        ADVANCED VETERINARY HOSPITAL
------------------------------------------------------------------------
 11/05/98        P a t i e n t   C h e c k - I n   R e p o r t        Page   1
------------------------------------------------------------------------
         Name: FISH                    Ident:          FISH
      Species: FISH               Owned by: Perry & Cyndi
        Breed: KOI FISH                         Ginger Cr
        Color: TANCHO                     Las Vegas NV
     Birthday: 0/00/00
          Sex: F                               89108
  Rabies Tag:                        Tele: (702) 656-
  Ani. Notes:                     Balance:      .00
  C11. Notes: CELL# 682              Curr:      .00      30Day:        .00
  C12. Notes:                       60Day:      .00      90Day:        .00
     Reminder:                     Weights:
------------------------------------------------------------------------
  Date    Invoice    Description                              Code Prov
------------------------------------------------------------------------
 04/27/98 Note==) CALLBACK-) DOING GOOD.                            OF
 04/23/98 0033134 EXOTIC ANIMAL EXAM                        EOV     NS
                  PHONE MESSAGE                             PHO     NS
                  CYTOLOGY- FISH                            NECF    NS
                  ALBON 40% INJECTION                       IM      NS
 04/23/98 Note==) PE:UPPER TAIL ERODED AWAY                         NS
                    ALSO AFFECTING DORSAL FIN                       NS
                    AND CAUDAL PEDINCLE                             NS
                  BIOPSY-)GILL HYPERPLASIA +                        NS
                       MICRO- ABCESSES                             NS
 03/12/97 Note==) SEVERAL FISH HAVE DIED.  TWO GOLDFISH HAVE AREAS OF SCALE  NS
                  LOSS AND REDDENED LESIONS, SUGGESTIVE OF AEROMONAS  NS
                  SALMONICIDA INFECTION.  TX: AMIKACIN INJECTIONS, MEDICATED  NS
                  FISH FOOD.                                        NS
 06/11/96 Note==) CALLBACK - PER OWNER DOING OKAY-GIVING MEDS FINE
 06/08/96 Note==) MISSING SCALES ON (L) SIDE OF BODY. RAISED ORANGE BUMP ON
                  (L) SIDE.
                  MICROSCOPIC EXAM -) BACTERIA ON SKIN SCRAPING, NO PARASITES
                  IN FECES. SEVERE HYPERPLASIA OF GILLS - NO PARASITES SEEN.
                  REC: ANTIBIOTIC FEED.
 06/08/96 0012683 EXOTIC ANIMAL EXAM                        EOV     NS
                  PHONE MESSAGE                             PHO     NS
                  TETRACYCLINE 500mg                        DD      NS
```

Sample medical records (above) and
laboratory test results (left) from koi patients.

134

NEOPLASIA IN KOI

Neoplasia, or cancer, occurs occasionally in koi. Most cases involve skin tumors, fin tumors, and intra-abdominal tumors associated with the gonads. These usually occur as a slow-growing mass that can get quite large. With internal tumors, damage can occur to other organs by constant pressure from the tumor. Surgery is the best treatment for tumors. The removed tissue should be fixed in 10% buffered neutral formalin and submitted for histopathology.

Case 1

History – A large female Ki Utsuri koi was presented to the clinic for having a bloated abdomen for a long period of time. Because of its poor condition, the owner elected euthanasia rather than exploratory surgery. It came from a large (38,000 gallons) pond that contained hundreds of very big koi.

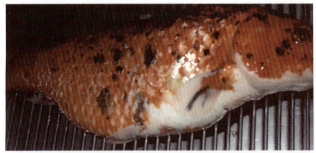

Koi with a severely bloated abdomen.

Examination – Necropsy examination revealed fish lice (*Argulus*) on the skin and gill flukes (*Dactylogyrus*). No protozoa were found on skin scrapings or fin and gill biopsies. The abdominal organs appeared normal except for the neoplastic ovaries. There were no normal ova present. The neoplastic tissue was sectioned and submitted to a veterinary laboratory for histopathology.

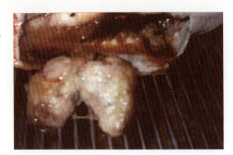

Ovarian tumor found in the abdomen of this koi.

Histopathology – Sections of what appear to be tissue from the reproductive tract are present. Some of the sections are lined by a simple columnar ciliated epithelium and may be sections of the genital pore. Within the lumina of the sections is deeply eosinophilic, homogeneous, and often degenerative material containing basophilic particulate matter that may represent degenerative yolk. In some areas there is an inflammatory process evident within the mucosa and submucosa that is made up of variable numbers of neutrophils with fewer mononuclear cells. Many of the macrophages contain abundant eosinophilic, golden, phagocytosed material. The granulomatous process in the tissue is so severe that identification of it is impossible. No infectious agents are seen with H & E stains, however acid-fast stains to rule out *Mycobacterium* may aid in a definitive etiology.

Diagnosis – Ovarian granuloma of unknown etiology.

Comment – The pond was treated with formalin/malachite green solution every 3 days for 3 treatments, and then trichlorfon once weekly for 4 weeks to control the external parasites.

Case 2

History – Twelve months later, a female Kohaku koi from the same pond was presented with a bloated abdomen. It was euthanized for necropsy.

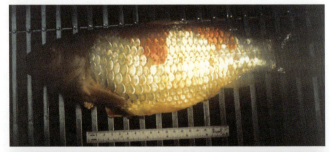

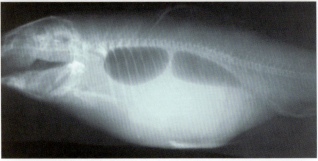

Kohaku koi with abdominal tumor, visible on radiograph.

Examination – Because of its lethargic condition, it had acquired a large number of fish lice (over 100). It also had gill flukes. Necropsy revealed a large abdominal mass, causing pressure necrosis on the adjacent organs. The mass was sectioned for histopathology.

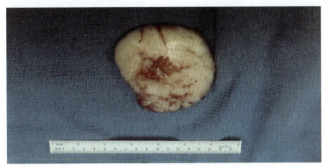

Tumor (9 cm) that was compressing abdominal organs.

Histopathology – Sections of a solidly cellular mass are examined. The mass consists of interlacing streams and sheets of closely packed, mildly to moderately atypical spindloid cells. Nuclei are round to oval and generally vesiculate with a small nucleolus. The cells have eosinophilic fibrillar cytoplasm and occasional mitotic figures are seen. Much of the mass is degenerate and necrotic with areas of hemorrhage and mixed leukocytic infiltrates present throughout. The tumor appears to be of mesenchymal origin. No infectious agents, including myxosporidian protozoa, are identified.

Diagnosis – Abdominal sarcoma of unknown etiology.

Case 3

History – Three years later, a large Orenji koi from the same pond died. It also had a bloated abdomen. Other koi in the pond appeared normal.

Examination – This fish had fish lice on its skin and gill flukes. No other parasites were detected. Necropsy revealed a large (10 x 15 cm) fluid-filled multilobar cyst in the abdomen. Fluid taken from the cyst was clear and had a specific gravity of 1.012, and a total protein content of 0.2 g/dL. All other organs appeared normal, including egg-filled ovaries. There were no signs of septicemia or peritonitis present.

Histopathology – Multiple sections were examined. One consists of recognizable ovarian tissue containing numerous normal developing ova. Adjacent to the ovary is a large, poorly demarcated mass of tissue that is largely necrotic and composed of degenerate cellular aggregates separated by dense streams of fibrocollagenous connective tissue/stroma. The cells are closely packed and round/oval to polygonal-shaped. Leukocytes are present throughout the necrotic areas. There are a few areas where the cells appear somewhat spindloid and/or streaming. In other areas they form solid sheets. No infectious agents are seen. Special stains for *Mycobacterium* are suggested to rule out granulomatous inflammation from this bacterium.

Diagnosis – Malignant periovarian carcinoma

Comment – It may be unusual to have multiple fish from the same pond present with abdominal tumors, however this is a large pond with many mature koi, and the fish's age may be a factor. All of the koi were females, and the mass involved ovarian tissue in at least two of the cases. This may be an age-related ovarian cancer. Another possibility could be Mycobacteria, but none of the koi exhibited any of the common signs of this infection, and there was no generalized peritonitis or granulomatous reaction to any other abdominal organs.

Case 4

History – This male Doitsu koi lived in a beautiful 4000-gallon backyard pond that was heavily planted, and filtered with a pressurized sand filter, an upflow biological filter, and had a large waterfall flowing into a stream area of the pond. All of the fish were active and eating well, and this one had an obvious bulge on one side of the abdomen.

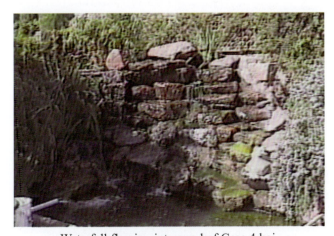

Waterfall flowing into pond of Case 4 koi.

Examination – No parasites were found and the fish appeared healthy except for the abdominal bulge.

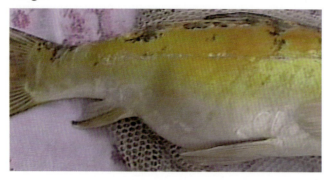

"Choman" belly - hard bulge in abdomen of a koi.

Treatment – The koi was anesthetized in a plastic container of water that had 1 ml/L of isofluorane anesthetic added to it. Once anesthetized, it was placed on its back in rolled wet towels to position it, and anesthetic solution was pumped across its gills. A ventral midline incision was made to expose its abdominal cavity. A large (161 g) abdominal mass associated with the testis was isolated, ligated with hemoclips, and removed. The abdomen was flushed with sterile saline. The other organs appeared normal. The skin was sutured with nonabsorbable nylon suture material. An injection of Baytril antibiotic was given and the fish was placed in fresh water where it recovered from anesthesia normally.

Diagnosis – Undifferentiated gonadal sarcoma

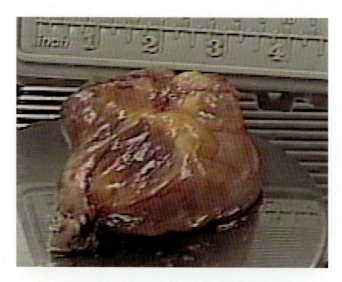

Gonadal sarcoma removed from abdomen of this koi. It was 8 cm in diameter and weighed 161 grams.

Comments – The occurrence of gonadal tumors in koi seems quite high, and they are frequently reported in the literature. Not all abdominal swellings are tumors however. Ascites (dropsy) can cause swollen abdomens, as can granulomas from *Mycobacterium,* and bloated kidneys from *Hoferellus (Mitraspora).* Once I performed surgery expecting to remove an abdominal tumor, and found a grossly enlarged, irregularly shaped, hemorrhaged caudal lobe of the swim bladder. I ligated and excised the caudal lobe, distal to the pneumatic duct, and the koi did fine. It may have been damaged due to a traumatic blow and stretched abnormally, or there could have been an underlying bacterial infection, but the cranial lobe of the swim bladder appeared normal. Radiographs would have helped make a diagnosis prior to surgery.

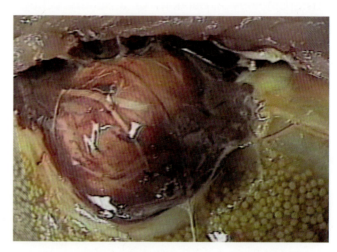

Bloated kidney seen on necropsy from another koi must be differentiated from abdominal tumors. Causes of kidney enlargement may include bacterial infection (*Mycobacterium*) or protozoa (*Mitraspora*).

Case 5

History – A large Shiro Bekko koi had a pink mass on the ventral half of the caudal fin, attached to the distal end of the caudal peduncle and extending bilaterally. It was in a 110,000-gallon pond that was fortunately shallow enough to wade into it to catch the fish. The water quality tests measured temperature at 73°F / 23°C, pH 7.8, total ammonia 0.6 mg/L (at this temperature and pH there would be approximately 2.95% un-ionized ammonia, or 0.0177 mg/L), nitrite 0.09 mg/L, total hardness 393 mg/L as $CaCO_3$, alkalinity 136.8 mg/L, chlorine 0.0 mg/L, and copper 0.04 mg/L. These values are within acceptable limits, although a partial water change would lower the hardness and reduce the ammonia and nitrite levels.

Examination – Other than the obvious mass, there were no abnormalities noted on physical examination or biopsies.

Treatment – The koi was placed in a plastic container of water with 100 mg/L of MS-222 anesthetic. Once anesthetized, the caudal peduncle and fin were cleaned with Betadine solution. A scalpel was used to excise the ventral portion of the caudal fin, extending the incision into the base of the caudal peduncle to remove the total skin mass. The caudal peduncle was cauterized with Kwik Stop styptic powder to control hemorrhaging. The koi was then placed into fresh water where it recovered normally. The bilateral masses were sent to a veterinary laboratory for histopathology.

Histopathology – The two masses were gray to light tan with focally hemorrhagic and necrotic areas. One measured 3.5 x 2.5 x 1 cm, the other 3 x 2 x 1.5 cm. Microscopic examination revealed a fairly well-demarcated, nonencapsulated mass which in one area is actively invading between the scales of the caudal peduncle. The mass extends from recognizable squamous epithelial cells in some areas with anastomosing sheets, streams, and clusters extending deeply into the dermis. The neoplastic cells are moderately pleomorphic and closely packed. They are generally polygonal-shaped with round to oval vesiculate nuclei with a small nucleolus. The cytoplasm is eosinophilic and faintly granular and intracellular bridges are often recognizable. The mitotic rate is less than 1 per every 6 or 7 high-powered fields. Occasional entrapped mucus cells are seen and a moderate number of mixed hemocytes are interspersed. Moderate to large numbers of mixed hemocytes are also present within the opposite epidermis with similar cells extending into the dermis. Neoplastic cells extend to the deep presumptive resection margin.

Diagnosis – Cutaneous squamous cell carcinoma.

Comments – Because the tumor extended to the deep margin of the excision, local occurrence is possible from remaining tumor cells in the caudal peduncle. This type of tumor also has a metastatic potential, possibly spreading to other areas of the body.

Follow-up – The koi was kept in a hospital tank for 6 days, and fed Tetracycline medicated fish food. Then it was returned to the pond. Two months later it was rechecked and found to have the ventral portion of the caudal fin regrowing normally. Examinations at 3 and 6 months post-surgery showed normal regowth of tail fin tissue, but no return of the tumor.

Case 6

History – A koi had a moderately large mass on its right cheek that had slowly grown over several months. It was in a pond with waterfall falling into a stream that then flowed into a round pond of sufficient size. Other koi were not affected.

Examination – In addition to the cheek mass, there was some discoloration of the skin on the left side of the head.

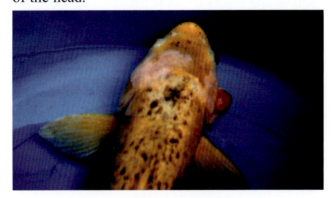

Mass on right cheek prior to surgery.

Treatment – The koi was anesthetized with Isoflourane added to the water, and the mass was debrided and removed as best as possible. Topical antibiotic ointment was applied on the lesion

Diagnosis – Fibrosarcoma

Comments – The tumor gradually regrew at the periphery of the original surgical removal site.

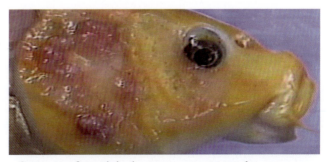

One year after original surgery some tumor has regrown.

BACTERIAL INFECTIONS

Bacterial infections in koi frequently occur secondarily to environmental stress, such as with poor water quality, awakening from winter dormancy, overcrowded conditions, and parasitic infestations. When bacterial infections are diagnosed, prompt treatment is required for both the bacterial infection and the underlying stressors.

Case 7

History – A Ki Bekko koi had erythematous lesions on its sides. It was in a 250-gallon pond. The owner had checked the water and said that it was normal.

Examination – *Argulus* were visible on the skin. Skin scrape revealed motile bacillus bacteria. Gill biopsy revealed *Ichthyobodo* and gill hyperplasia. A culturette swab was taken from the skin wound and submitted for bacterial culture and antibiotic sensitivity (C & S) testing. The wound was then swabbed with diluted Betadine solution. The fish was injected with chloramphenicol antibiotic intraperitoneally (IP). The owner was prescribed a chloramphenicol-medicated fish pellet, formalin/malachite green for the *Ichthyobodo*, and trichlorfon to treat the fish lice.

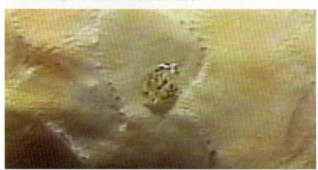

Fish louse (*Argulus*) can cause skin damage that may become secondarily infected by bacteria.

C & S Results – Two species of bacteria were cultured from the skin wound:

Aeromonas sobria – Sensitive: amikacin, amoxicillin/clavulinic acid, cephalothin, chloramphenicol, enrofloxacin, sulfisoxazole, gentamicin, nitrofurantoin, trimethoprim/sulfamethoxazole
Resistant: ampicillin, carbenicillin, tetracycline

Pseudomonas putrefaciens – Sensitive: amikacin, ampicillin, amoxicillin/clavulinic acid, carbenicillin, cephalothin, chloramphenicol, enrofloxacin, sulfisoxazole, gentamicin, nitrofurantoin, trimethoprim/sulfamethoxazole
Resistant: tetracycline

Comment – The culture proved that not all cases of ulcer disease are caused by *Aeromonas salmonicida* or even *Aeromonas hydrophila*. The skin scrape showed motile bacteria, and both of the isolated bacteria are motile, but *A. salmonicida* is not. The sensitivity test showed that chloramphenicol was an effective antibiotic in this case. In addition to the antibiotic, the pond needs to be treated for the fish lice and *Ichthyobodo,* which were the primary stressors that compromised the koi's skin and allowed the bacteria to enter and proliferate. Remember to have the laboratory always incubate fish swab cultures at 68-77°F / 20-25°C.

Case 8

History – A new shipment of koi arrived at a retail pond store with multiple skin lesions.

Examination – Some of the koi were very emaciated, as well as having skin ulcers. Anchor worms (*Lernaea*) were found on a few of the koi. The fish were anesthetized with MS-222 for examination and biopsies. Microscopic examination of biopsy tissues revealed skin flukes (*Gyrodactylus*), and the protozoa *Ichthyobodo* and *Ichthyophthirius*. A culturette swab was taken from a skin lesion and then the lesions were cleaned with diluted Betadine solution. The fish were injected with gentamicin, and the owner was instructed to use formalin/malachite green solution every other day for 3 treatments, followed by weekly doses of trichlorfon.

C & S Results – Two species of bacteria were cultured from the skin lesion:

Pseudomonas putida – Sensitive: amikacin, ampicillin, amoxicillin/clavulinic acid, carbenicillin, chloramphenicol, enrofloxacin, sulfisoxazole, gentamicin, nitrofurantoin, tetracycline, trimethoprim/sulfamethoxazole
Resistant: cephalothin

Enterobacter species - Sensitive: amikacin, amoxicillin/clavulinic acid, carbenicillin, chloramphenicol, enrofloxacin, sulfisoxazole, gentamicin,

nitrofurantoin, tetracycline, trimetho-prim/sulfamethoxazole
Resistant: ampicillin, cephalothin
Comments – Here is a case of skin ulcers with no species of *Aeromonas* present, but numerous primary skin parasites. Both bacteria were sensitive to the gentamicin antibiotic. The abundance of parasites on these fish at the koi dealer underlines the importance of quarantine of all new fish prior to adding them to an existing pond!

Case 9

History – A large dead koi with severe necrotic lesions on its sides was presented for necropsy. It came from a large densely-populated pond. No water was submitted for analysis.

Examination – In addition to the ulcerated lesions, fish lice were found on the skin. No other parasites were seen on biopsy. Necropsy exam showed serosanguinous abdominal fluid and organ adhesions, signs of bacterial septicemia. A culturette of the inside of the kidney was taken and sent to the lab.

C & S Results – Two species of bacteria were cultured from the kidney tissue:

Aeromonas hydrophila - Sensitive: amikacin, amoxicillin/clavulinic acid, carbenicillin, chlor-amphenicol, enrofloxacin, sulfisoxazole, gentam-icin, nitrofurantoin, tetracycline, trimetho-prim/sulfamethoxazole
Resistant: ampicillin, cephalothin

Vibrio fluvialis - Sensitive: amikacin, chloram-phenicol, enrofloxacin, sulfisoxazole, gentamicin, nitrofurantoin, tetracycline, trimetho-prim/sulfamethoxazole
Resistant: ampicillin, amoxicillin/clavulinic acid, carbenicillin, cephalothin

Comment – *Aeromonas hydrophila* is the bacteria most commonly associated with hemorrhagic septicemia as seen in this fish. *Vibrio* species of bacteria are common marine fish pathogens, but are infrequently seen in freshwater fish. The fish lice not only cause primary skin lesions that become bacterially infected, but also spread the bacteria to each fish they parasitize. The remaining fish were treated with koi pellets medicated with tetracycline. The pond was medicated with trichlorfon for the fish lice.

Case 10

History – An orange Doitsu koi that had died the previous night was presented for necropsy.

Examination – This koi had severe erosion of the lips and ulcers on its sides. The gills were pale and mucousy. Skin, fin, and gill biopsies showed motile bacilli bacteria, *Ichthyophthirius, Ichthyobodo*, and *Dactylogyrus*. The abdominal organs appeared normal and a culturette swab was taken from the interior of the kidney tissue.

C & S Results – Two bacteria species were cultured from the kidney tissue, indicating septicemia was present:

Klebsiella pneumoniae – Sensitive: amikacin, ampicillin, carbenicillin, chloramphenicol, enrofloxacin, sulfisoxazole, gentamicin, nitrofu-rantoin, tetracycline, trimetho-prim/sulfamethoxazole
Resistant: amoxicillin/clavulinic acid, cephalexin

Enterobacter species - Sensitive: amikacin, car-benicillin, chloramphenicol, enrofloxacin, sul-fisoxazole, gentamicin, nitrofurantoin, trimetho-prim/sulfamethoxazole
Resistant: amoxicillin/clavulinic acid, ampicillin, cephalexin, tetracycline

Comment – *Klebsiella* and *Enterobacter* are both Gram-negative bacteria and are common pathogens of terrestrial animals, but not of fish. They may indicate poor water conditions existing in the pond, or decreased resistance of the koi due to immunosuppression from the parasites.

Klebsiella occurs naturally in decaying wood, and in the organic debris in the water. They also reduce nitrate back into nitrite and ammonia, so large populations of these bacteria can reverse the effects of the biological filter! Because they have a mucoid capsule around their cell walls, they are resistant to environmental extremes, and produce a creamy or yellowish slimy growth when abundant. Removing decaying organic debris from the pond will reduce the incidence of these bacteria.

The pond was treated with formalin/malachite green solution to eliminate the protozoal parasites. Maintaining a salt concentration of 0.1-0.3 % will also help reduce protozoal parasites. Monogenean trematodes may not respond to these treatments and may require trichlorfon or Dimilin treatments.

140

ENVIRONMENTAL PROBLEMS

Sometimes the fish are healthy and the pond looks good, and everything seems to be going right, but then disaster strikes. In general, when fish gradually appear to become ill and die a few at a time, parasitic or infectious diseases should be suspected. When many fish become ill or die suddenly, a water quality or other environmental concern usually is involved.

Case 11

History – A client had about 80 large koi in a 26,000-gallon pond with two Jacuzzi pressurized sand filters, and a separate upflow lava rock biological filter. Venturi jets were placed on some of the return outlets to the pond for oxygenation. The water was clear and water tests were normal. He had recently purchased an expensive female Kohaku koi for breeding purposes and had it in a separate filtered holding pond for quarantine. It had showed no signs of illness, but he found it dead one morning.

Examination – The fish measured a total length of 15.4 in. / 39 cm. It showed no apparent lesions. No parasites were seen on biopsy. Necropsy showed an icteric (jaundiced) liver, and yellow ascitic fluid in the abdomen. A fluid sample was sent to the lab for analysis.

Fluid Analysis Results – Color: yellowish brown, appearance: turbid, viscosity: watery, protein: 2.0 g/dL, specific gravity: 1.026, WBC: 4200/µL, neutrophils: 90%, lymphocytes: 10%, RBC: 5150/µL.

Cytology – Microscopic examination of the cells in this fluid shows predominantly degenerating cellular debris. Many of them appear to be histiocytes where the nuclei are pyknotic and eccentric. Also seen are small numbers of mononuclear inflammatory cells admixed with neutrophils. Occasional larger, also degenerating cells resembling mesothelium are noted. No pathogens nor malignant cells are seen.

Diagnosis – Inflammatory degeneration of the liver.

Comment – As opposed to an infectious agent, in this case the cause of death was liver failure. Through questioning the owner, it was determined that he had just sprayed an olive tree next to and growing over the quarantine pond with a chemical to keep it from fruiting. This must have fallen into the water and the resulting toxicity caused acute liver degeneration. Be aware of all activities occurring both in and around the pond!

Case 12

History – A 1500-gallon pond containing about 30 koi and goldfish had a UV sterilizer added about a week earlier. It already had a Jacuzzi sand filter plus a separate pump that returned its flow through a 10-foot-tall rock cascade waterfall. The pond was heavily planted with potted water lilies and irises. Other than an abundance of filamentous algae, the owner had not noted any problems. Water test results were within normal limits. The owner had left town for the Labor Day weekend, and when she returned home, she found all her fish were dead.

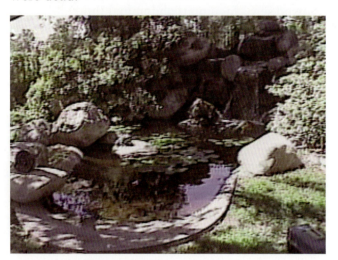
Pond where sudden koi deaths occurred.

Examination – The refrigerated dead fish showed postmortem autolysis, eliminating the ability to get an accurate bacterial culture. No parasites were seen on the tissue samples. There was pale discoloration of the gills.

Diagnosis – Hypoxia.

Comment – The missing information here is what happened while the owner was gone on that hot summer weekend! The lawn caretaker had shut off the waterfall because "no one was there to see it," not realizing that it was essential for aerating the pond. The recent addition of the UV filter indicated that algae had been a concern in this pond.

With an abundance of plants and algae, even without a dense population of fish, there can be a significant oxygen demand for respiration at night, when plants respire using O_2 rather than photosynthesize using CO_2 and sunlight. This is a problem especially at the hottest time of the summer, when elevated water temperatures hold decreasing amounts of oxygen. By dawn, the level of dissolved oxygen can be lethally low. The fish are seen gasping at the surface, and often die with their mouths open. The gills usually are pale-colored from hypoxia. Always ensure adequate aeration to the pond and to the biological filter, which requires oxygen for the bacterial conversion of ammonia to nitrite and then nitrate.

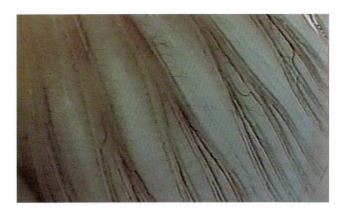

Capillary congestion in anal fin of a koi that died of hydrogen sulfide toxicity.

Case 13

History – This unlucky pond owner noticed a foul odor when cleaning his filter. The next day 6 koi and 3 goldfish were found dead. A water sample tested ammonia: 0, nitrite: 0.1, nitrate: 0, pH: 8.0.

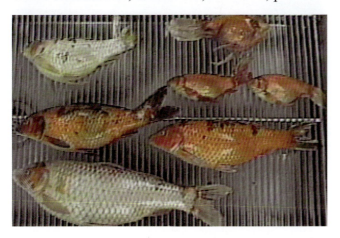

Sudden death of many fish is usually caused by a water quality issue, rather than an infection. These koi and goldfish were exposed to hydrogen sulfide.

Examination – External exam found no skin lesions, but did find redness at the base of the fins, pale gills, and a few gill flukes. Internal exam revealed vasocongestion of the swim bladder and necrosis of the liver and kidneys.

Diagnosis – Hydrogen sulfide toxicity.

Comment – The key here is the odor noticed by the owner when cleaning his filter. Hydrogen sulfide has a rotten-egg smell and is highly toxic to people, as well as other animals. It is a gas that accumulates under anaerobic conditions due to bacterial reduction of organic sulfates. Anywhere that debris accumulates without adequate water flow can be a site of H_2S gas production. Once released from an accumulated pocket, it quickly dissolves in the water. It causes cyanosis, or lack of the ability for blood to carry oxygen. Because of its high toxicity, do a complete water change when its odor is detected in the water. Clean the filter or other source of the gas in an outdoor area, away from the pond if possible. Adding potassium permanganate to the water will oxidize the H_2S, reducing its toxicity. It is also less toxic as temperature and pH increase. Frequent cleaning of filters and debris removal will prevent the development of anaerobic conditions that produce hydrogen sulfide.

PARASITE INFESTATIONS

Parasites are a frequent cause of koi keeping problems. In a natural environment, fish can carry parasites without significant morbidity. When placed in artificial environments, the number of abnormal conditions (diet, water quality, competition, population density, increased exposure to pathogens) reduces their resistance and immunity to diseases. In many cases the same symptoms can be attributed to several different parasites that may require different modes of treatment. Some parasites are rather difficult to completely eradicate and treatments seem only to keep their numbers in check. Anything that can be done to eliminate stress will help increase the fish's own ability to fight disease.

Case 14

History – This client had a 1500-gallon backyard pond with a Jacuzzi sand filter and a waterfall that split into two streams that each ran into his pond. The fish had been dying over the last week, with no visible lesions on them. The water tests revealed temperature: 78°F / 25.6°C, pH: 8.4, total ammonia: 0.5 mg/L (times 12.5% un-ionized ammonia concentration equals 0.0625 mg/L), oxygen: 8 mg/L (at saturation), total hardness: 410 mg/L $CaCO_3$, and no chlorine detected.

Examination – Microscopic examination of skin scrapes revealed *Trichodina* protozoa, and skin flukes (*Gyrodactylus*). Fin biopsies showed *Ichthyophthirius, Ichthyobodo,* and *Trichodina* protozoa, plus skin flukes (*Gyrodactylus*). Gill biopsies showed *Ichthyobodo* and *Trichodina* protozoa, and gill flukes (*Dactylogyrus*).

Diagnosis – Heavy parasite burden and ammonia toxicity resulting in gill hyperplasia and hypoxia.

Comments – This case shows what can happen when standard precautions are not followed. In addition to the high ammonia content, the high pH and hardness can occur by not doing periodic water changes. As water evaporates, it leaves minerals behind. Only replacing lost water will gradually increase the hardness and pH, making any accumulated ammonia more toxic. Removing pond water periodically and then replacing it, using a dechlorinator, will remove ammonia and concentrated minerals. The variety of parasites indicates that fish from many sources were mixed together, each bringing in a parasite, which gladly coexisted on the koi. If each fish had been quarantined and treated before adding it to the pond, it would have reduced the occurrence of this situation. Interestingly, the gill flukes were on the gills and the skin flukes were on the skin, although frequently they are found in either location, but obviously they do have a preference!

Case 15

History – Several light-colored koi were presented for dorsal skin lesions. Other koi in the pond and the goldfish did not have any lesions.

Examination – The lesions were erythematous and the epithelium was sloughing. Algae were growing on the damaged skin. There were no lesions on the sides of the fish. Microscopic examination of a skin scraping revealed large amounts of cellular debris, green algae, nematodes, and nematode ova.

Diagnosis – Opportunistic parasitism of damaged epithelium by algae and normally free-living nematode worms. The cause of the skin lesion was not determined at the clinic, but became obvious when visiting the client's pond: sunburn.

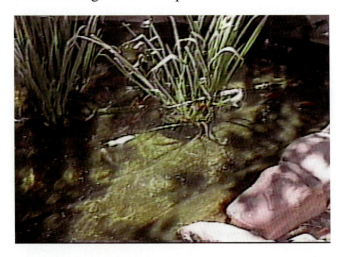

The koi spent much time on a shallow shelf at pond edge.

Comments – Upon examination of this client's cement pond, it was found to be in full sun (in the summer in Las Vegas) and very shallow. A wide shelf around the edges was less than 1 foot deep, yet most of the fish were in this area. The white koi had the dorsal skin lesions, but the pigmented koi and goldfish did not. The lesions were determined to be caused by sunburn, and the algae and worms were taking advantage of the nutritive value of the sloughing skin. So the original diagnosis of parasites was secondary to an environmental problem. Temporary shade was constructed over the pond to protect the fish. Ultimately the pond was deepened as a permanent solution.

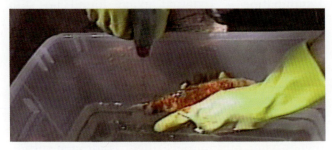

The backs of the sunburned koi were sprayed with Betadine solution to kill superficial microorganisms.

Case 16

History – A client called because numerous fish had died in her 600 gallon pond. She had koi, goldfish, mosquitofish (*Gambusia affinis*), and two western painted turtles in her pond. The turtles had been with the fish in the pond for years and did not bother them. No recent additions or changes had been made. Water tests results were temperature: 62°F / 17°C, pH: 8.2, ammonia: 0 mg/L, nitrite 0 mg/L, nitrate 3 mg/L. The overall condition of the pond looked good, the water was clear and had good aeration with fountains at each end of the small formal pond, and good filtration.

Examination – Necropsy on the dead koi revealed flukes on the gills (*Dactylogyrus*), with gill hyperplasia.

Diagnosis – Heavy parasite burden resulting in gill hyperplasia and hypoxia, with possible secondary bacterial infection causing acute septicemia.

Comments – Since nothing had changed with this pond recently, the parasites had to be with the koi for a long period of time, without causing previous disease conditions. Cooler water in October, when this occurred, may have lowered the fish's immune response, allowing the flukes or bacteria to proliferate.

The pond was treated with Trichlorfon, 0.25 mg/L of pond water, once weekly for 4 weeks. Since the commercial Trichlorfon powder is only 80% active Trichlorfon this needs to be considered in dosing the pond. The dose for this pond would be 0.25 mg Trichlorfon/L x 1 mg Powder/.80 mg Trichlorfon [i.e., 80% active Trichlorfon] = 0.3125 mg commercial powder/L. Convert this to a dose per gallon by multiplying it by 3.8 L/gallon to get 0.3125 mg/L x 3.8 L/gallon = 1.1875 mg/gallon. So a 600 gallon pond would get 600 gal x 1.1875 mg/gallon = 712.5 mg. Always double check calculations and be sure of pond volume accuracy.

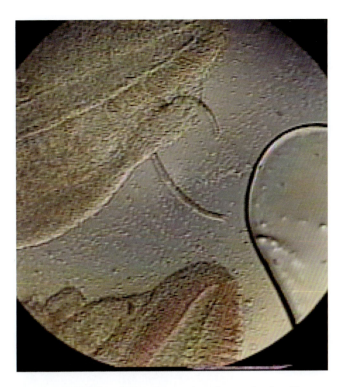

Two gill flukes (*Dactylogyrus*) on hyperplastic gills.

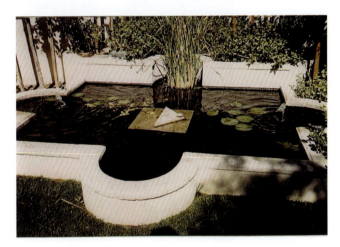

This is the pond that housed the koi and other fish with the two water turtles.

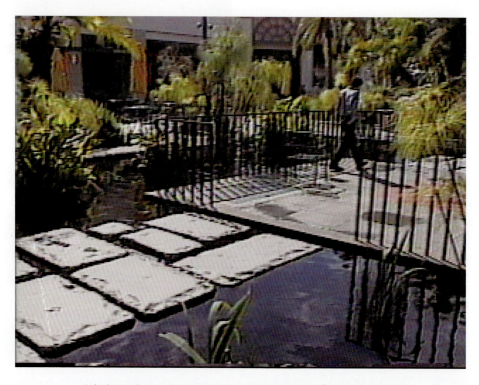

A koi pond at a shopping center in Newport Beach, California.

CHAPTER 8:
FORMULARY

FLUID VOLUME EQUIVALENTS:

milliliter (ml = cc)	liters (L)	teaspoon (tsp)	tablespns (tblsp)	ounces (fl. oz)	cups (C)	pints (pts)	quarts (qts)	gallons (gal)
1	0.001	0.2028	0.0676	0.0338	0.0042	0.00212	0.0011	0.000265
4.93	0.005	**1**	0.333	0.167	0.021	0.0104	0.0052	0.0013
14.787	0.015	3	**1**	0.5	0.0625	0.0312	0.0156	0.0039
29.574	0.03	6	2	**1**	0.125	0.0625	0.0312	0.0078
59.147	0.06	12	4	2	0.25	0.125	0.0625	0.0156
118.295	0.12	24	8	4	0.5	0.25	0.125	0.03125
236.59	0.24	48	16	8	**1**	0.5	0.25	0.0625
473.18	0.48	96	32	16	2	**1**	0.5	0.125
946.36	0.95	192	64	32	4	2	**1**	0.25
1000.0	**1**	203	67.6	33.84	4.23	2.11	1.0567	0.2642
1892.72	1.9	384	128	64	8	4	2	0.5
3785.43	3.79	768	256	128	16	8	4	**1**

1 gallon = 230.9 cubic inches = 0.134 cubic feet = 8.34 pounds
1 cubic foot = 7.48 gallons = 62.4 pounds of water

1 liter = 1000 cubic centimeters (cc) = 0.001 cubic meters
1 cubic meter = 1000 liters = 1000 kilograms of water

APPLICATION OF CHEMICALS TO THE POND

Before applying any chemicals or medications to the pond, be sure an accurate measurement of the water volume has been made. Underdosage of medications will reduce the effectiveness of the treatment and overdosage can cause additional stress to the fish, or even death.

Pond volume can be calculated in a rectangular pond by multiplying the length times the width of the pond, and then multiply by the average water depth. Circular pond volumes are calculated by the pond's surface area (πr^2) times the average depth. That is the radius [1/2 of the diameter] squared ($r^2 =$ radius x radius) times 3.14 (π, or pi) times the average depth. The average depth can be calculated by measuring the depth of the water in the pond at regular intervals throughout the pond's surface area, adding the depth measurements together, and then dividing the sum by the total number of depth readings taken. Irregularly shaped ponds can be measured in small sections at a time and these calculations added together for the total pond volume. The final result will give you the total volume of water in the pond in cubic feet (if measured in feet) or cubic meters (if measured in meters).

After measuring the pond, multiply the volume of water in cubic feet by 7.48 to get the total gallons of water in the pond. Multiply the measured pond volume in cubic meters by 1000 to get total volume in liters. Be sure to add to the volume of pond water the amount of water that is in the filtration system for the total volume of water!

A more accurate way of measuring the volume of water in the pond is to use a flow meter when initially filling it up. One may be obtained from some hardware stores that attaches to the end of the garden hose. If the house has a water meter on the main waterline, its initial reading can be subtracted from the final reading after filling the pond to measure the water volume. Be sure no other water is running in the house while filling the pond. write down the pond volume and save it for future reference.

Another method of determining pond volume makes use of a salinity meter and adding a known volume of salt to the pond. If a reading is taken in the pond before adding salt, and another is taken after adding an accurately measured and dissolved amount of salt, the difference in salinity can be used to determine pond volume. The advantage of this method is that it takes into account the water in the filters and plumbing, which measurements of the pond do not.

One pound of salt in twelve gallons of water equals 1% salinity. Adding 1 pound of salt per 100 gallons of water raises the salinity 0.12% (1 #/100 gal = 454 g/378.5 L = 454 g/378,500 g = 0.001199 = 0.12%!). Therefore, 1 #/100 gal x 12 gal/# [a conversion factor for 1% salinity] = 0.12% salinity, or # salt/gal x 12 = % salinity. So, using the salinity meter we can use the formula: # salt x 12 / % salinity = gallons water.

For example, if a pond had a reading of 0.02% before adding salt (natural salt content) and it was estimated that the pond might hold 1500 gallons, then adding 15 pounds of salt should raise the salinity to 0.14% (0.02% already in the pond plus the added 0.12%) once the salt was completely dissolved and circulated through the pond. Use the pond filtration turnover rate as a guide to know how long to wait before taking a second reading. If the pond filtration pumps 750 gallons per hour, then wait at least 2 hours so that all of the water will have passed through the filter system (in theory) to be sure the salt is evenly dispersed.

After waiting for the dissolved salt to be completely dispersed in the pond, take a second reading of the salinity. If the pond volume, including the plumbing and filtration, was exactly 1500 gallons (the estimated volume) the second reading should be exactly 0.14%. If the reading is higher, the pond volume is smaller than 1500 gallons; and if it is a lower reading, then the pond volume is more than 1500 gallons.

To calculate the exact volume in gallons, find the difference between the first and second salinity % readings (second reading – initial reading = salinity difference). This is the percent that the added salt actually raised the salinity. Now multiply the pounds of added salt by the conversion factor 12, then divide this by the change in the salinity just calculated to get the actual volume in gallons.

 # salt x 12 / (R2%– R1% salinity) = volume of water in gallons

Here are the steps summarized:

Measure salinity % before adding salt.
Add 1 pound of salt for each 100 gallons of ESTIMATED pond volume, then take a second reading after salt is dispersed.
Subtract initial reading from the second reading for % salinity changed. If the initial reading is zero (no salt in pond), just use the reading from after the salt is added to the pond (R2 – 0 = R2).
Multiply the pounds of salt added by 12.
Divide this by the % salinity changed.
The final result is the pond volume in gallons.

Once the total pond volume is known, calculate the appropriate dosage of medication to apply. Double-check calculations carefully. Start with the pond volume, and the recommended dose of the medication, then calculate the quantity of medication that needs to be added to the pond.

For example, assume the pond volume is 2550 gallons (and we know that because a water meter was used when the pond was initially filled with water, and the information was written down and carefully stored for future reference). If we wanted to treat a gill fluke infestation with Chloramine-T (see chart on next page) we would also need to know the water pH and hardness. If the pond had a pH of 7.6 and a hardness of 150 mg/L, then the dose of Chloramine-T most appropriate would be the 18 mg/L. So now we know the pond volume and the recommended dose of the medication. Multiply these together, using conversion factors (see Fluid Volume Equivalents chart) as necessary, to calculate the amount of chemical to add to the pond.

2550 gallons x 18 mg Chloramine-T / L of pond water x 3.79 L / 1 gallon

Pond volume x drug dose x conversion for liters to gallons (1 gallon = 3.79 L, from chart).
Since liters (L) is the denominator (bottom) of the first equation, it is the numerator (top - above or before the slash) on the second equation. This makes the units cancel each other out.

So now we have 2550 x 18 mg Chloramine-T x 3.79.
Gallons and liters have cancelled themselves out, leaving only the units for the drug.
When this is the case, then the formula is correct, as the drug dose is what we are seeking.

Multiply this all out to get: 173,961 mg Chloramine-T, which equals 173.961 grams.
Since 1000 milligrams = 1 gram, or 173,961 mg x 1 gram/1000 mg = 173,961 x 1 gram/1000 (the mg units cancel each other out) = 173.961 grams - rounded off to 174 grams.
Then use a gram scale to measure out the calculated dose to add to the pond.

Dilute mixtures with distilled water or with pond water prior to application and distribute them uniformly throughout the pond to avoid areas of high concentration of medication. Be sure adequate aeration is available, as many treatments will lower the dissolved oxygen level in the water. Remove any activated carbon from the filtration system if it is present. Carbon will adsorb the chemical or medication from the water preventing its effectiveness. Ultraviolet lights should also be turned off temporarily when medications are in the pond. Use proper caution when handling chemicals and wear protective clothing, gloves, and goggles as necessary.

The following instruction sheets may not be used for commercial purposes without written permission from the author.

CHLORAMINE – T

n-Chloro-para-toluene Sulfonamide Sodium Salt

($C_7H_7SO_2N$ NaCl $\langle 3H_2O$)

Usage:
Chloramine-T is used to treat bacterial gill disease and other bacterial infections. It can also be used to control monogenean trematodes (skin and gill flukes).

Dosage:
It is important to know the pH and total hardness of the pond water before treating with chloramine-T. Soft water and low pH increase the toxicity of chloramine-T, and high pH and hardness reduce its effectiveness. Use the following chart to determine appropriate dose:

pH	Soft Water	Hard Water
6.0	2.5 mg/L	7.0 mg/L
6.5	5.0	10
7.0	10	15
7.5	15	18
8.0	20	20

Treatment Procedure:
Dissolve the appropriate amount of chloramine-T in a plastic container of deionized water, making sure it is well mixed. Then disperse it evenly over a large area of the pond surface so that spots of high concentration are avoided. After 4 hours, perform a 25-50% partial water change. Be sure to add dechlorinator to the new water. Repeat treatment every 1-2 days for up to 4 times if needed.

For treatment of an individual koi, remove it from the pond and place it into a large plastic container of pond water. Use an air stone and pump to provide adequate aeration. Add the appropriate amount of chemical to the water and mix thoroughly. After 4 hours, remove the fish and return it to the pond. Repeat every 1-2 days for up to 4 times.

Caution:
For ornamental fish pond use only. Do not apply to ponds containing fish for food use.
Do not use in combination with formalin or benzalkonium chloride.

Safety Data:
Keep out of reach of children!   May be harmful if swallowed. Do not breathe dust.
Wear protective gloves and clothing when handling chemicals. Use a mask for dust.
Wash thoroughly after handling or in case of skin contact. Flush eyes with water for 15 minutes in case of eye contact. If swallowed get medical aid immediately.

COPPER SULFATE
($CuSO_4$, Anhydrous)

Usage:
Copper sulfate is used to treat certain bacterial (*Flexibacter columnaris*) and protozoal (*Oodinium, Ichthyobodo, Ichthyophthirius, Chilodonella, Epistylus*) diseases. It can also be used to control algae growth.

Dosage:
It is important to know the total alkalinity of the pond before treating with copper sulfate. Low alkalinity water increases the toxicity of copper sulfate and high alkalinity reduces its effectiveness. A safe level to use can be determined by dividing the total alkalinity in mg/L (= parts per million, PPM) by 100. This gives the PPM of $CuSO_4$ that can be safely used.

$$\text{Total alkalinity (PPM)}/100 = CuSO_4 \text{ dose (PPM)}$$

If the total alkalinity is less than 50 PPM, copper sulfate treatments are not recommended because of the higher risk of fish losses. Greater than 250 PPM alkalinity causes copper to form an insoluble salt and precipitate out of solution.

After calculating the safe dose of copper sulfate in PPM, multiply that by 14.9 milligrams $CuSO_4$ per gallon of water [a conversion factor for 1 PPM of copper sulfate]. For example, a safe dose of 2.0 PPM (from a water with alkalinity of 200 PPM/100) times 14.9 mg/gal equals 29.8 mg $CuSO_4$ per gallon water.

Treatment Procedure:
Dissolve the appropriate amount of copper sulfate in deionized water, making sure it is well mixed. Then disperse it evenly over a large area of the pond surface so that spots of high concentration are avoided. Maintain desired copper level in the water for 2 weeks. Use a copper test kit daily to determine the current copper level and add an additional 149 mg $CuSO_4$ per 100 gallons of water for each 0.10 PPM copper needed to maintain the desired concentration.

Caution:
For ornamental fish pond use only. Do not apply to ponds containing fish for food use.
In ponds with algae, copper treatments can cause oxygen concentrations to drop. Be sure adequate water aeration is available, especially in warm weather.

Effectiveness of copper sulfate is reduced with increased pH, alkalinity, hardness, salinity and with dissolved or suspended organic matter in the water. Potassium increases the toxicity of copper sulfate. Copper is toxic to invertebrates in the pond.

Safety Data:
Keep out of reach of children! Poison! May be fatal if swallowed.
Wash thoroughly after handling or in case of skin contact. Flush eyes with water for 15 minutes in case of eye contact. If swallowed get medical aid immediately.

FORMALIN SOLUTION

Ingredients: Formaldehyde (HCHO) 37%
                     Water (H$_2$O) 51%
                     Methanol (HCOOH) 12%, to inhibit paraformaldehyde formation

Usage:

Formalin can be used in ornamental fish ponds for the treatment of external protozoal parasites (*Chilodonella, Trichodina, Trichophyra, Ichthyobodo, Ambiphyra,* and *Ichthyophthirius*) and monogenean trematodes. Do not confuse this 37% solution with the 10% buffered neutral formalin used for tissue preservation.

Dosage:

Use one milliliter (1 ml) formalin per 10 gallons of pond water (see chart) to achieve a dosage of 25 PPM (mg/L) formalin.

Application	Pond Water
1 ml (20 drops)	10 gallons
10 ml (2 teaspoons)	100 gallons
30 ml (1 ounce)	300 gallons
100 ml (3.3 ounces)	1000 gallons
120 ml (4 ounces)	1200 gallons

Treatment Procedures:

Pour appropriate amount of solution into pond near a water inlet so that it quickly disperses in pond. Continue to vigorously circulate the water in the pond to prevent oxygen level decrease, as 25 mg/L of formalin may lower the dissolved oxygen in the water by as much as 5 mg/L. Repeat treatment every 2-3 days for a total of 3 applications.

Caution:

For ornamental fish pond use only. Do not apply to ponds containing fish for food use. If fish become stressed during treatment, make a partial or complete water change. Decrease dose by half in water above 80°F / 27°C. Do not use in water less than 40°F / 5°C. Always store solution at temperatures above 40°F / 5°C to prevent the formation of toxic paraformaldehyde, which appears as a white precipitate in formalin solutions.

Safety Data:

Keep out of reach of children!
Avoid eye or skin contact. Avoid inhaling vapor. Harmful if inhaled or absorbed through skin. Wash thoroughly with soap and water after handling.

First Aid:

In case of contact, immediately flush eyes or skin with plenty of water. If inhaled, move to fresh air. If swallowed, give water then induce vomiting immediately and get prompt medical aid.

FORMALIN/MALACHITE GREEN SOLUTION

Ingredients: Formaldehyde (HCHO) 36.87%
Malachite Green   0.36% (14 grams / gallon formalin)
Water 50.77%
Methanol 12%

Usage:
Formalin/malachite green solution can be used in ornamental fish ponds for the treatment of external protozoal parasites (*Chilodonella, Trichodina, Trichophyra, Ichthyobodo, Ambiphyra,* and *Ichthyophthirius*) and monogenean trematodes.

Dosage:
Use one milliliter (1 ml) formalin/malachite green solution per 10 gallons of pond water (see chart) to achieve a dosage of 25 PPM formalin and 0.10 PPM malachite green.

Application	Pond Water
1 ml (20 drops)	10 gallons
10 ml (2 teaspoons)	100 gallons
30 ml (1 ounce)	300 gallons
100 ml (3.3 ounces)	1000 gallons
120 ml (4 ounces)	1200 gallons

Treatment Procedures:
Pour appropriate amount of solution into pond near a water inlet so that it quickly disperses in pond. Continue to vigorously circulate the water in the pond to prevent oxygen level decrease. Repeat treatment every other day for a total of three applications.

Caution:
For ornamental fish pond use only. Do not apply to ponds containing fish for food use. If fish become stressed during treatment, make a partial or complete water change. Do not use galvanized containers as zinc increases the toxicity of malachite green and its solutions. Decrease dose by half in water above 80°F / 27°C. Do not use in water less than 40°F / 5°C. Always store solution at temperatures above 40°F / 5°C to prevent toxic paraformaldehyde formation.

Safety Data:
Keep out of reach of children!
Avoid eye or skin contact. Avoid inhaling vapor. Harmful if inhaled or absorbed through skin. Wash thoroughly with soap and water after handling. Malachite green may be carcinogenic at high doses.

First Aid:
In case of contact, immediately flush eyes or skin with plenty of water. If inhaled, move to fresh air. If swallowed, give water then induce vomiting immediately and get prompt medical aid.

HYDROGEN PEROXIDE
(H_2O_2)

Usage:
Hydrogen peroxide is active against a wide variety of organisms – bacteria, fungi, viruses, protozoa, and monogenean trematodes. It is also used to prevent fungal growth on fish eggs. Hydrogen peroxide is environmentally safe because its decomposition products are oxygen and water ($2H_2O_2$ $2H_2O + O_2$). It is also used to temporarily increase oxygen levels in the pond due to hypoxia from overcrowding, filter malfunction, and formalin or potassium permanganate treatments.

Dosage:
Pond Treatment –
For adding directly to the pond, the dosage of 3% hydrogen peroxide is 1 ml/gallon of pond water, or 1 cup/240 gal (or 0.26 ml/L = 7.9 mg/L). Mix in the water and circulate thoroughly.

Bath Treatment –
For a short-term bath or dip, the dosage is 0.50 ml H_2O_2 (100% active)/liter water (= 500 mg/L). This equals 1.9 ml 100% H_2O_2/gallon water.
Divide the dose of hydrogen peroxide by the percent dilution being used.

For example: If using a 3% peroxide solution,
1.9 ml (100%)/(3%) = 63.3 ml.
Then use 63.3 ml of the 3% solution per gallon water.

If using 35% commercial grade hydrogen peroxide,
1.9 ml (100%)/(35%) = 5.4 ml.
Then use 5.4 ml of the 35% solution per gallon water.

Treatment Procedure:
Calculate the appropriate amount of hydrogen peroxide to use. If treating fish in short-term bath, place the fish in a plastic container with the diluted hydrogen peroxide solution for 15 minutes. Treat every other day until the condition heals.

If treating fish eggs, dip the eggs or spawning mat containing the eggs in the diluted hydrogen peroxide solution for 15-60 minutes.

Safety Data:
Keep out of reach of children!
Wear rubber gloves and eye protection when handling hydrogen peroxide at concentrations higher than 3%. Wash hands after handling hydrogen peroxide. If it gets in the eye, flush with plenty of water. Ingestion of hydrogen peroxide may produce gastrointestinal irritation and vomiting.

IODINE SOLUTION

(Iodine 0.1%)

Ingredients: 1% iodine in poloxamer complex   10%
0.9% sodium chloride in water   90%
Total diluted iodine solution (1:9) 100%

Usage:

Iodine antiseptic solutions have a wide spectrum of microbial activity. Apply to skin lesions to prevent bacterial and fungal infections. Use on skin ulcers caused by *Aeromonas* infections ("hole in side disease"). Commercial polyvinyl pyrilidone iodine solutions (Betadine) can be diluted with 0.9% saline solution to reduce risk of irritation to fish.

Dosage:

Use a cotton swab to apply a small amount of iodine solution topically on skin and fin wounds. Treat daily until wounds heal.

Treatment Procedures:

Carefully net fish and bring to surface of water. Squirt iodine solution onto cotton swab and apply gently to skin lesions. Replace fish into water after application.

Caution:

For ornamental fish pond use only. Do not use on fish intended for human consumption.
Do not apply to gills or allow to run onto gills.

Safety Data:

Keep out of reach of children!
Wash thoroughly with soap and water after handling.
Avoid contact with eyes.

First Aid:

In case of eye contact, flush immediately with plenty of clean water. Get medical attention if irritation occurs. If swallowed, give water then induce vomiting and get prompt medical aid.

METRONIDAZOLE

1-(2-hydroxyethyl)-
2-methyl-5-nitroimidazole

Usage:
Metronidazole may be used as a protozoacide, and is especially effective against intestinal protozoa (*Hexamita, Spironucleus*).

Dosage:
Use one tablet (250 milligrams) per 10 gallons of water in an isolation aquarium; or add one tablet per ounce of fish food (250 mg/28 g food). Treat daily for 5 days.

Treatment Procedures:
Bath Treatment - Crush and dissolve appropriate number of tablets in a small quantity of water. Then add to quarantine aquarium. Change 10-25% of the water each day before adding more medication.

Food Treatment - Place fish food pellets in a plastic bowl. Use slightly less food than would normally be fed to ensure that all medicated food will be eaten quickly. Mix in the white of an egg until the food is lightly moistened. Crush the appropriate amount of metronidazole tablets and add to food, mixing thoroughly. Then briefly heat the mixture in a microwave just long enough so that it is dry. Keep medicated food covered in refrigerator until used.

Caution:
For ornamental fish pond use only. Do not apply to ponds containing fish for food use.

Safety Data:
Keep out of reach of children!
Avoid eye or skin contact.
Wash thoroughly with soap and water after handling.
If swallowed, get medical aid as necessary.

POTASSIUM PERMANGANATE
($KMnO_4$)

Usage:
Potassium permanganate is used to treat ectoparasites (protozoa, flukes, and fish lice) and bacterial infections in freshwater fish. It also aids in algae control and pond water clarification. It acts as an oxidizing agent in the oxidation of organic and inorganic matter in the pond, and will oxidize toxic hydrogen sulfide (H_2S) to make it nontoxic.

$$4KMnO_4 + 3H_2S \circledR 2K_2SO_4 + S + 3MnO + MnO_2 + 3H_2O$$

Dosage:
Use at an initial concentration of 2 mg/liter (2 PPM) of pond water. This will color the water purple if it is low in organic matter, or pinkish if the organic load is high. As the permanganate ion (MnO_4^-) is reduced to nontoxic manganese dioxide (MnO_2) the color will fade. Repeat the 2 mg/L dose the next day if the color fades lighter than pink. If the color stays darker than pink, no more potassium permanganate is added. Treat daily for up to 4 days. Apply chemical in the morning so the fish can be monitored throughout the day. Overdose results in burns on the skin and gills of the fish, and can be fatal. Do a partial water change to dilute the potassium permanganate if the fish show signs of toxicity. Toxicity increases in colder water, hard water, or high pH water.

One level teaspoonful contains about 6 grams of potassium permanganate powder. At a dose of 2 mg/L (7.6 mg per gallon) this would be one level teaspoonful for each 3000 liters (789.5 gallons) of pond water, or 1¼ teaspoons per 1000 gallons.

Treatment Procedure:
It is best to use finely powdered $KMnO_4$ rather than crystals. In either case, dissolve the required amount in a plastic container of water first, then add this solution to the pond. Disperse uniformly throughout the pond, and maintain adequate water circulation to oxygenate the water. Decaying algae and other organic matter will lower the dissolved oxygen in the water. In water with low organic content, the concentration of potassium permanganate can remain high enough to kill the beneficial bacteria in the filter system. It may help to shut the biofilter off for a few hours immediately after treatment. Do not shut off biofilters for more than 6 hours or the nitrifying bacteria will die from anoxia. Maintain water circulation and aeration in the pond even though the biofilter is temporarily bypassed.

Caution:
For ornamental fish pond use only. Do not apply to ponds containing fish for food use.

Safety Data:
Keep out of reach of children!
Wear gloves, safety goggles, and dust mask when applying this product to the pond.
Avoid eye or skin contact. Wash thoroughly with soap and water after handling.
If swallowed, get medical aid as necessary.

SIMAZINE, 0.60% SOLUTION

2-Chloro-4,6 bis (ethylamino)-s-triazine

Usage:
Simazine solution is used to control algae growth in fish ponds and aquariums. It is safe for use with most aquatic plants, however some water plants (water hyacinth, water fern) may begin to turn brown and die with continued use of product.

Dosage:
Use 0.65 milliliters (ml) simazine solution per 1 gallon of pond water (see chart) for a final dilution of 1 mg/L (PPM). Double this dose for heavily affected ponds.

Application	Pond Water
0.65 ml	1 gallon
5 ml (1 teaspoon)	7 gallons
15 ml (1 tblspoon)	20 gallons
30 ml (1 ounce)	40 gallons
120 ml (4 ounces)	160 gallons
473 ml (1 pint)	640 gallons
946 ml (1 quart)	1280 gallons
3785 ml (1 gallon)	5120 gallons

Treatment Procedure:
Pour appropriate amount of solution into pond whenever algae begin to grow. Circulate the water in the pond to mix. Algae should start to disappear within a week. If no improvement is seen after a week, repeat application. Retreat when algae begin to reappear. For best results, remove as much excessive algae growth as possible before treating. This will reduce the amount of organic matter left to decay in the pond, which could increase the ammonia, nitrite, and nitrate levels, and reduce the oxygen content in the water. It is best to treat before the pond water reaches 75°F / 24°C.

Caution:
For ornamental fish pond use only. Do not apply to ponds containing fish for food use.

Safety Data:
Keep out of reach of children!
Avoid eye or skin contact. In case of eye contact, flush for 15 minutes with plenty of water and get medical attention. For skin contact, wash with soap and water. If swallowed, give water then induce vomiting immediately and get prompt medical aid.

Do Not Use Treated Water For Irrigation Purposes.

SIMAZINE GRANULES, 90%

2-Chloro-4,6 bis (ethylamino)-*s*-triazine

Usage:

Simazine is used to control algae growth in fish ponds and aquariums. It is safe for use with most aquatic plants, however some water plants (water hyacinth, water fern) may begin to turn brown and die with continued use of product.

Dosage:

The concentration of simazine in the pond water should be 1-2 mg/L (PPM). The following table provides levels of 1 mg/L. Double the dose in heavily affected ponds to produce a level of 2 mg/L.

Application	Pond Water
5 cc (1 level teaspoon) = 3grams	800 gallons
15 cc (1 level tablespoon)	2400 gallons
30 cc (1 ounce) = 18 grams	4800 gallons
120 cc (4 ounces)	19,200 gallons
240 cc (1 cup) = 150 grams	38,400 gallons

Treatment Procedure:

Pour appropriate amount of granules into pond whenever algae begin to grow. Circulate the water in the pond to mix. Algae should start to disappear within a week. If no improvement is seen after a week, repeat application. Retreat when algae begin to reappear. For best results, remove as much excessive algae growth as possible before treating. This will reduce the amount of organic matter left to decay in the pond, which could increase the ammonia, nitrite, and nitrate levels, and reduce the oxygen content in the water. It is best to treat before the pond water reaches 75° F / 24° C.

Caution:

For ornamental fish pond use only. Do not apply to ponds containing fish for food use.

Safety Data:

Keep out of reach of children!
Avoid eye or skin contact. In case of eye contact, flush for 15 minutes with plenty of water and get medical attention. For skin contact, wash with soap and water. If swallowed, give water then induce vomiting immediately and get prompt medical aid.

Do Not Use Treated Water For Irrigation Purposes.

SODIUM CHLORIDE

(NaCl)

Usage:
Sodium chloride, or salt, is used to treat some bacterial and parasitic diseases of fish. It also minimizes osmoregulatory stress in fish, prevents nitrite toxicity (methemoglobinemia), and stimulates mucus production to protect the skin.

Dosage:
Use noniodized, food-grade salt for medicating fish. Artificial marine aquarium salt mixes can be used, which provide other important minerals as well. If using water softener salt, make sure that it does not contain anticaking or rust-inhibiting agents (such as yellow prussic acid) which could be harmful to fish. Do not confuse potassium chloride (KCl) water softening salt for sodium chloride, as it is toxic at doses used for salt in koi ponds.

For continuous treatment, add 1 gram salt per liter of pond water (1 g/L = 1 PPT = 0.12% = 3.8 g/gallon = 1 level teaspoonful per gallon = 1 pound/100 gallons). One cup of packed granular salt weighs about 252 grams, or 0.56 pounds. Therefore, 1 pound of granular salt would fill 1.8 measuring cups, or 14.3 ounces.

Repeat dose in 1-2 days, bringing total salt concentration to 0.2%. If fish are not showing signs of stress, a third dose may be added in another 1-2 days bringing the total salt concentration to 0.3%. For short duration pond treatments (24 hours) the salt content in the koi pond can be raised to as high as 0.5%. After 24 hours at this dose, add fresh water to dilute the salt to the normal 0.3% or less.

For short-term bath treatment in a hospital tank or plastic container, use a 3% salt solution (30 g/L = 30 PPT = 3.8 ounces/gallon = 1 cup salt/2.5 gallons) for 5-10 minutes. If the fish loses its equilibrium and rolls over, remove it from the salt solution and place it in fresh water immediately.

For young fish or ones that appear sick, use a 1-2% solution (10-20 g/L, 1.3-2.6 ounces/gallon) for 10-20 minutes, or less if fish show signs of stress.

Treatment Procedure:
Dissolve required amount of salt in a plastic container of warm water, then evenly disperse solution throughout the pond.

Caution:
High salt concentrations may occur from water evaporating from the pond, as salt does not evaporate. Add water as necessary to prevent concentration of the salt. Dilute salt solutions in the pond by removing some pond water and replacing it with fresh water.
Salt solutions may be toxic to aquatic plants at concentrations above 0.3%.

Safety Data:
Keep out of reach of children!
In case of eye contact, flush with plenty of fresh water.

SODIUM THIOSULFATE, 20%

($Na_2S_2O_3 + 5H_2O$)

Usage:

Sodium thiosulfate solution is used to remove chlorine from water that is added to the fish pond or aquarium. Most municipal waters contain from 0.5 up to 1.5 mg/L (PPM) of added chlorine. Much of this is lost by the time the water reaches the faucet, but even doses as low as 0.02 mg/L can be toxic. Untreated chlorinated water can cause gill and skin irritation in fish, and even death.

Dosage:

To completely dechlorinate water, it is necessary to use 7.4 mg of sodium thiosulfate for each 1 mg of chlorine. The following chart doses a 20% sodium thiosulfate solution (760 grams sodium thiosulfate / gallon distilled water) at 1.0 mg/L (sufficient for residual chlorine concentrations up to 0.15 mg/L).

Application	Pond Water
1 drop	2 gallons
1 ml (20 drops)	50 gallons
5 ml (1 teaspoon)	250 gallons
30 ml (1 ounce)	1500 gallons
120 ml (4 ounces)	6000 gallons

*** *Sodium thiosulfate will remove the chlorine from water containing chloramine, but does not remove the ammonia.* ***

Treatment Procedure:

Pour appropriate amount of solution into pond whenever adding new water to the pond. Circulate the water in the pond to mix, and the sodium thiosulfate will reduce the chlorine (Cl_2 or HOCl) in the water to nontoxic chloride (Cl^-) as sodium chloride (NaCl).

$$Cl_2 + 2(Na_2S_2O_3 \cdot 5H_2O) = Na_2S_4O_6 + 2NaCl + 10H_2O$$

Caution:

For ornamental fish pond use only. Do not apply to ponds containing fish for food use.

Safety Data:

Keep out of reach of children!

Avoid eye or skin contact. In case of eye contact, flush for 15 minutes with plenty of water and get medical attention. For skin contact, wash with soap and water. If swallowed, give water then induce vomiting immediately and get prompt medical aid.

TETRACYCLINE HYDROCHLORIDE, USP

($C_{22}H_{24}N_2O_8$,HCl)

Usage:
Tetracycline HCl is used to treat coccidia and bacterial infections in fish. It acts as a bacteriostatic antibiotic by inhibiting protein synthesis in susceptible organisms. Bacterial culture and sensitivity testing is recommended to ascertain that any bacteria present are susceptibleto tetracycline antibiotic.

Dosage:
Bath Treatment - Use one capsule (500 mg) per 10 gallons of water. Treat daily for 7-10 days.

Food Treatment - Use one capsule (500 mg) in 200 g (7 ounces) of fish food. Feed fish the medicated food for 7-10 days.

Treatment Procedure:
Bath Treatment - Dissolve appropriate number of capsules in a small quantity of warm water and add to pond or quarantine aquarium. Change 10-25% of the water each day before adding more medication.

Food Treatment - Place fish food in a plastic bowl. Use slightly less food than would normally be fed to insure that all medicated food will be eaten quickly. Then mix in the white of an egg, enough to lightly moisten the food. Add the appropriate amount of antibiotic (see dosage above) to the food by opening the capsules and mixing thoroughly with food. Then briefly heat the mixture in a microwave just long enough so that it is dry. Keep medicated food covered in refrigerator until used.

Caution:
For ornamental fish pond use only. Do not apply to ponds containing fish for food use.

Safety Data:
Keep out of reach of children!
Avoid eye or skin contact. In case of eye contact, flush for 15 minutes with plenty of water. For skin contact, wash with soap and water. If swallowed, get medical aid as necessary.

TRICHLORFON, 80% Active

(2,2,2- Trichloro-1-hydroxy ethyl)-
Phosphonic acid dimethyl ester

($C_4 H_8 Cl_3 O_4 P$)

Usage:
Trichlorfon may be used to control gill flukes (*Cleidodiscus, Dactylogyrus, Gyrodactylus*), anchor worms (*Lernaea*), and fish lice (*Argulus*) in ornamental fish ponds. It can be toxic to invertebrates such as snails, clams, and aquatic insects.

Dosage:
Since the commercial Trichlorfon powder is only 80% active ingredients, this must be taken into account when calculating the amount to use. The dose of the active ingredient is 0.25 mg/L. For the commercial powder, it is 0.25 mg Trichlorfon/L x 1 mg powder/0.80 mg Trichlorfon (because it is only 80% active) = 0.3125 mg commercial powder/L (this gives 0.25 PPM active Trichlorfon). Then, 0.3125 mg/L x 3.8 L/gallon = 1.19 mg/gallon or 1 mg/0.84 gallons. Convert from mg to grams (multiply the numerator and denominator both by 1000), and it becomes 1 gram / 840 gallons. There is approximately 3.58 grams of commercial Trichlorfon powder in one level measuring teaspoonful. So, 3.58 grams/ 1 teaspoonful x 840 gallons/1 gram = 3007 gallons/teaspoonful of commercial Trichlorfon powder. In other words, use 1 level teaspoonful of Trichlorfon powder for every 3000 gallons of pond water. Hard water may require double or even triple the dose. Treat once weekly for 4 weeks.

Treatment Procedures:
Dissolve required amount of powder in a cup of deionized water before using for best results. Then distribute evenly over pond surface. For small ponds, dissolve one-quarter teaspoonful in 1 cup (8 ounces.) of deionized water, and then use 1 ounce of solution per 93 gallons of pond water. Treatment of ponds should be completed before the water temperature reaches 80°F / 26.6° C. It is best to treat the ponds in the mornings when the pH and temperature are lower.

Caution:
For ornamental fish pond use only. Do not apply to ponds containing fish for food use. Do not apply to ponds used as a source of drinking water for animals.

Safety Data:
Keep out of reach of children!
Avoid eye or skin contact. Do not inhale powder. Harmful if inhaled or absorbed through skin. Wash thoroughly with soap and water after handling. Wash contaminated clothing with soap and hot water before reusing. Wear gloves when handling powder.

May be fatal if swallowed. Do not contaminate food; do not use utensils for food purposes after contact with this medication.

If poisoning occurs, get prompt medical aid.
Prolonged exposure will result in cholinesterase depression.

To Physician - Atropine sulfate and/or 2-PAM are antidotes.

Discard remaining mixed solution carefully as it is toxic to humans, pets, and wildlife.
Do not store solution for further use as product degrades rapidly when mixed in solution.
Keep trichlorfon powder dry during storage – humidity decreases its effectiveness.

QUICK REFERENCE GUIDE TO CHEMOTHERAPEUTICS FOR KOI

ANESTHETICS – See topic under CLINICAL PROCEDURES, page 50.
Amikacin – 5 mg/kg IM, IP every 72 hours (q72h)
Atropine – 0.1 mg/kg IM, IP for treatment of organophosphate toxicity
Aztreonam (Azactam) – 100 mg/kg IM, IP every 2-5 days
Butorphanol – 0.1 mg/kg IM for pain control postsurgically
Ceftazidime (Fortaz) – 20 mg/kg IM q72h
Chloramine-T – 5-20 mg/L for a 4-h bath, repeat in 1-2 days
Chloramphenicol – 25-50 mg/kg IM, IP q3-7d
Dexamethasone – 1-2 mg/kg IM, IP q12h
Dipterex – 0.25 mg/L (1 ml/ 400 gallons pond water) every 4 days for 4 doses
Difluorobenzuron (Dimilin) – 0.06 mg/L once weekly for 3 doses
Enrofloxacin (Baytril) – 10-14 mg/kg IM, IP q48h, or PO q24h
Epinephrine (1:1000) – 0.2-0.5 ml IM, IP, IC
Fenbendazole (Panacur) – 50 mg/kg orally for 2 days, repeat in 2 weeks; 2 mg/L water q7d x 3 doses
Formalin (37% formaldehyde) – 25 mg/L (1 ml/10 gal) in pond every other day
Florfenicol (NuFlor) – 30-50 mg/kg IM, IP, PO q24-72h
Fumagillin (Fumidil B) – 1 g/kgof food (0.1%) fed daily for 3-8 weeks
Furosemide – 2-3 mg/kg IM, IP q12-72h
Gentamicin – 3 mg/kg IM once only due to kidney toxicity
Hydrogen peroxide – 250-500 mg/L dip to prevent fungal growth on eggs
Itraconazole – 1-5 mg/kg q24h in food for 7 days
Levamisole – 10 mg/L for 12-24h bath; 50 mg/L for a 2h bath
Lufenuron (Program) – 0.13 mg/L in pond as needed to control crustacean parasites
Malachite green – 0.1 mg/L in pond every 3 days for 3 doses
Mercurichrome – swab onto skin lesions
Methylene blue – 1-3 mg/L bath q24-48h
Metronidazole – 50 mg/L bath, daily for 3-10 days, 10 mg/g of food daily for 5 days
Minocycline – 2 mg/kg orally
Nitrofurpirinol (Furanace) – 0.25 mg/L in pond, 1-4 mg/L bath for 60 min
Oxolinic acid – 1 mg/L bath for 24 h
Oxytetracycline (Terramycin) – 50-75 mg/kg BW, added to food daily for 10 days
Potassium permanganate – 2-5 mg/L bath
Povidone-iodine – 0.1% solution topically, 100 mg/L for 10-min dip to disinfect eggs
Praziquantel (Droncit) – 5-25 mg/kg IM, IP, PO, 10 mg/L for 6-24h bath
Prednisolone – 1 mg/kg IM, IP
Rifampin – 6 mg/100 g of food
Sodium chloride (salt) – 20-30 g/L for short-duration bath, 1-3 g/L in pond
Sulfadimethoxine-ormetoprim (Romet, Primor) – 50 mg/kg IM or added to food
Tetracycline – 250 mg/100 g of food
Trichlorfon (Masoten, Dylox) – 0.25-0.5 mg/L in pond, every 5-7 days
Trimethoprim sulfa – 30 mg/kg IM, IP, PO q24-48h
Vitamin C – 3-5 mg/kg IM, PO q24h

IC = intracardial,
IM = intramuscular,
IP = intraperitoneal (actually intracoelomic in fish)
PO = per os (by mouth),
BW = body weight of fish
q = each
h = hour

REFERENCES:

Fowler, Murray E. and R. Eric Miller (editors). 1999. *Zoo & Wild Animal Medicine* 4, W. B. Saunders, Philadelphia.

Francis-Floyd, Ruth. 1992. *Use of Formalin to Control Fish Parasites,* Cooperative Extension Service, University of Florida, Gainesville, FL.

Francis-Floyd, Ruth. 1993. *The Use of Salt in Aquaculture,* Cooperative Extension Service, University of Florida, Gainesville, FL.

Francis-Floyd, Ruth. 1998. *"Fish"* in *The Merck Veterinary Manual,* 8th ed., Merck, Whitehouse Station, NJ.

Herwig, Nelson. 1979. *Handbook of Drugs and Chemicals Used in the Treatment of Fish Diseases,* Charles C. Thomas, Springfield, IL.

Lazur, Andrew. 1992. *The Use of Potassium Permanganate in Fish Ponds,* Cooperative Extension Service, University of Florida, Gainesville, FL.

Lewbart, Gregory A. 1999. "Pet Fish Formulary" in *Veterinary Syllabus,* Wild West Veterinary Conference, Reno, NV.

Mashima, Ted Y. and Gregory A. Lewbart. 2000. "Pet Fish Formulary" in *The Veterinary Clinics of North America – Exotic Animal Practice,* 3:1, W.B. Saunders, Philadelphia.

Noga, Edward J. 1996. *Fish Disease: Diagnosis and Treatment,* Mosby, St. Louis, MO.

Stoskopf, Michael K. 1993. *Fish Medicine,* W.B. Saunders, Philadelphia.

Stoskopf, Michael K. 1999. "Fish Pharmacotherapeutics" in *Zoo and Wild Animal Medicine* 4, W.B. Saunders, Philadelphia.

Watson, Craig. 1994. *Use of Copper in Aquaculture and Farm Ponds,* Cooperative Extension Service, University of Florida, Gainesville, FL.

Whitaker, Brent. 1999. "Preventive Medicine Programs for Fish" in *Zoo and Wild Animal Medicine* 4, W.B. Saunders, Philadelphia.

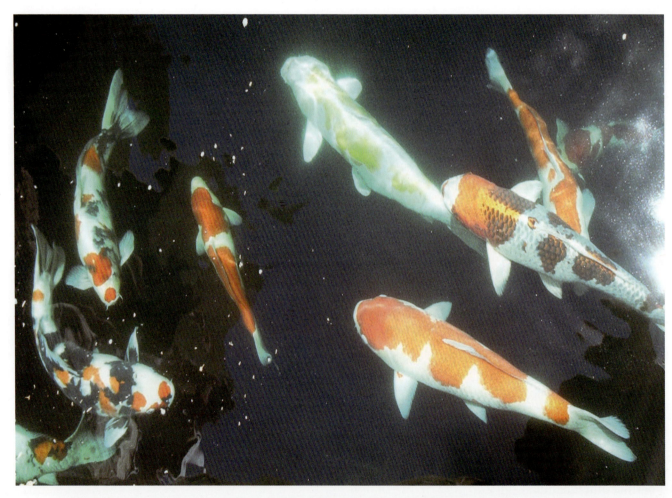

Use the Japanese Terminology Glossary and the information in the Koi Varieties section to identify which of these koi is the Hariwake, Showa Sanshoku, Inazuma Kohaku, Taisho Sanke, Nidan Kohaku, and Kujaku.

GLOSSARY

MEDICAL TERMINOLOGY

Acute - recent occurrence of clinical signs of a disease

Aerobic - requires the presence of oxygen

Anaerobic - occurs in the absence of oxygen

Anoxia - total lack of oxygen

Antibody - a specific serum protein (immunoglobulin) that is produced by an organism's immune system in response to the presence of an antigen

Antigen - a foreign substance that evokes a specific immune response in an animal

Autotrophic - organisms that obtain energy from solar radiation (photosynthetic) or from inorganic substances (chemosynthetic)

Chronic - persistent state of disease

Clinical sign - observable evidence of a disease state

Communicable - capable of being transmitted from one organism to another (contagious)

Congestion - abnormal accumulation of blood within an organ or peripheral blood vessel

Cuticle (or Glycocalyx) - the mucus or slime (mucopolysaccharides and glycoproteins) on the fish's skin, which is secreted by epithelial cells and goblet cells in the epidermis covering the scales

Debride - to clean a wound of all foreign material and injured or infected tissue

Definitive host - the host that harbors the adult stage of a parasite

Denitrification - the process where a nitrogen-based compound is broken down into its basic elements

Detritus - decomposing organic material in an ecosystem

Disease - any deviation from the normal structure or function of any part of the body

Environment - all of the conditions, circumstances, and influences surrounding and affecting the development of an organism

Epithelium - the surface layer of cells covering cutaneous, mucous and serous surfaces

Erythema - reddening of the skin

Etiology - the specific cause of a disease

Euthanasia - causing a painless death

Fishes - the plural of "fish" when referring to more than one species of fish

Genotype - the inheritable genetic code of an organism

Hematocrit - also called packed cell volume (PCV), is the proportion of blood volume that is occupied by red blood cells, expressed as a percent

Hemorrhage - the abnormal loss of blood from a blood vessel

Heterotrophic - organisms that obtain energy from preformed organic compounds

Host - a plant or animal that harbors or nourishes another organism

Hyperemia - excess blood in an organ or tissue

Hyperplasia - an abnormal increase in the normal number of cells of an organ or tissue

Hypertrophy - an abnormal enlargement of the individual cells of an organ or tissue

Hypoxia - a deficiency of oxygen below physiologically required levels

Infection - invasion and multiplication of pathogenic microorganisms in body tissues

Infestation - invasion of the body tissues by parasites (protozoa, helminths, arthropods)

Inflammation - a response to tissue injury to effect removal of the cause

Intermediate host - a necessary host that harbors a larval stage of a parasite

Lethargic - deficient in alertness or activity

Milt - a white solution that contains the spermatozoa of male fish (semen)

Moribund - dying from a disease

Necropsy - the examination of a dead body

Neoplasm - abnormal growth of new tissue

Neotenic - an organism that never develops into the adult stage of the life cycle, but is capable of reproduction in its larval form

Ovum - plural ova; the egg produced by the female, prior to fertilization

Operculum - plural is opercula; the bony plate covering the gills

Parasite - a plant or animal that lives upon or within another living organism at whose expense it obtains some advantage

Paratenic host - an intermediate host in a parasite's life cycle in which the parasite lives without undergoing further development, and is not a necessary host in the parasite's life cycle

Pathogen - any disease-producing microorganism (viruses, bacteria, fungi)

Percent (%) - parts per hundred

Phenotype - the physical characteristics of an organsm

Physoclistous - swimbladders lacking a connection to the pharynx

Physostomous - having a pneumatic duct between the swimbladder and the pharynx

PPM - parts per million, or 1 milligram per liter (mg/L)

PPT - parts per thousand, or 1 gram per liter (g/L), or 1 milliliter per liter (ml/L)

Quarantine - from the Latin word "quarant" meaning forty, the period of days that one was originally isolated to prevent the spread of bubonic plague; this is the isolation of new or sick fish in a separate pond or aquarium until such a time as they are free from contagious diseases

Respiration - oxygen uptake for use in cellular activities

Roe - the eggs (ova) in the abdominal cavity of a female fish

Selective breeding - a breeding program where the breeder choses which fish to breed on the basis of some predetermined criteria

Septicemia - the presence of living and reproducing bacteria in the blood stream

Stress - the sum of all biological phenomena elicited in an organism by adverse external influences

Symbiosis - the relationship between two species of organisms living intimately together that each obtain some benefit from the other

Telangiectasis - dilatation of the capillaries in the gill lamellae with pooling (microthrombi) of the red blood cells

Total Length - the measured length of a fish from the tip of its snout to the end margin of the tail fin held in a natural position

Toxin - a chemical produced by an organism that causes disease or death when introduced into the body tissues

Vector - a temporary host that is responsible for transmitting a parasite between primary hosts

Virulence - the disease producing power of a microorganism

Viscera - the internal organs

Zoonosis - any animal disease that can be transmitted to humans

Zygote - the fertilized ovum

JAPANESE TERMINOLOGY USED WITH KOI

Japanese Vowel Pronunciations: **a** - short a as in saw; **e** - short e as in vet; **i** - long e as in see; **o** - long o as in toe; **u** - long u as in Sue; **ai** - long i as in pie; **ei** - long a as in say.

Most Japanese words are accented on the first syllable when pronounced.

Ai – (pronounced as eye) indigo blue color

Aigoromo – a variety of koi that has indigo blue edging on the red scales

Ago Sumi – black mark on the gill plate

Aka – red color

Aka Muji – solid red koi with no pattern and normal scales (also called Higoi)

Asagi – light blue

Bekko – tortoise shell

Beni – deep red color

Benigoi – truly solid-red colored koi

Boke Sumi – blurred or faded black markings

Bozu – no red on the head of a Kohaku (an undesirable trait)

Bu – size division used in koi shows

Budo – grape

Cha – tea, or tea brown-colored

Chagoi – a brown koi with normal scale pattern

Dan – a step, used in counting the major spot patterns on koi. "San Dan" means three steps, or three major spots on the dorsum

Doh – the main body or trunk of a koi

Doitsu – the Japanese word for "Deutsche" which means German, and refers to carp introduced from Germany that have fewer than normal scales

Fukurin – (pronounced who'-ku-reen) area of skin around a scale in mature koi

Gin – (pronounced with a hard g, as in gun, and rhymes with keen) silver metallic

Go – five

Gosai – five years old

Goi – the Chinese word for carp, carried over to Japan along with the fish

Goromo – robed

Gosanke – the "Big Three Families" of koi varieties: Kohaku, Taisho Sanke, and Showa Sanshoku

Hada – skin

Hana – flowery

Hara – abdomen (belly)

Hariwake – white metallic body with gold patterns

Hi – (pronounced with a long e, as in he) red

Higoi – an early 1800s red color mutation of the wild carp

Hikari – metallic luster

Hoo Aka – red marking on the gill plate of a Kohaku

Ichi – one

Ichimatsu – checkerboard pattern

Ike – pond

Inazuma – lightning, referring to a long zigzag red color pattern on the dorsum of a Kohaku

Iroage – the practice of feeding koi special foods to enhance color development

Ji – skin

Jihada – texture of the skin

Jyami – small undesirable Sumi dots on Sankes or Showas that detract from the main Sumi markings

Kabuto – a helmet, used for markings on the head

Kagamigoi – the mirror carp, a German-scaled (Doitsu) koi with a row of scales only on either side of the dorsal fin and larger than normal scales along the lateral line

Kage – shadow

Kanoko – the Hi appears on individual scales, producing a dappled effect

Karasu – (Japanese for crow) an all-black koi

Kasane Sumi – a black Sumi mark on the red Hi marking of a Sanke

Kawagoi – the leather carp, a German-scaled (Doitsu) koi with no scales, or only a few scales along the dorsal fin

Kawari – different, changing

Ki – (pronounced as key) yellow

Kin – gold metallic

Kiwa – sharpness of the edge of a red or black color pattern

Kohaku – red and white color pattern

Koi – a colored variety of domesticated common carp (*Cyprinus carpio*)

Koishi – Nishikigoi breeders

Kokesuki – an orange area in the Hi color pattern due to an injury or scale damage

Koromo – robed (goromo when preceded by a color: aigoromo = blue-robed)

Kuchi – mouth

Kuchibeni – lipstick (red mouth), a koi with red lips

Kujaku – peacock

Kumonryu – nine-crested dragon, a name given to Doitsu black koi with white head and fins

Magoi – wild common carp

Maki – wrapped, referring to a color pattern that wraps down the side of a koi to the belly

Maru – round

Maruten – a round patch of color on the head

Matsuba – pinecone pattern

Menkaburi – red mask, too much red on the face of a Kohaku

Menware – head region divided in color; black dividing the red pattern on a Showa

Mesu – female

Midori – green

Mizu – water

Motoaka – Hi spot at the base of the pectoral fins

Motogoro – Sumi spot at the base of the pectoral fins

Moyo – pattern

Mudagoke – wasted scales, used for extra scales on Doitsugoi that detract from the pattern

Muji – literally "no pattern," meaning solid color, or one color

Nezu – gray

Ni – two

Nidan – two steps

Nisai – two years old

Nippon (or Nihon) – the native word for Japan

Nishiki – a colorful brocaded silk cloth

Nishikigoi – literally "brocaded carp," the Japanese name for colored carp, or koi

O – tail

Obire – caudal fin

Odome – the white area after the last red patch and before the caudal fin on a Kohaku

Ogon – metallic gold

Orenji – orange

Osu – male

Otsutsu – tail tube; the caudal peduncle, or narrow tail section of the body, between the dorsal and caudal fins

Purachina – the whitest color of the platinum Ogons

Rin – scales

Sakura – cherry blossom

San – three

Sandan – three steps

Sanke – three families, used for the three colors red, white, and black

Sansai – three years old

Sanshoku – three colors (used as Showa Sanshoku, rarely as Taisho Sanshoku)

Sarasa – white body with alternating red and white on back

Sashi – the leading edge of a black or red color pattern against the white shiroji

Sebire – dorsal fin

Sekoke – a nutritional disease caused by oxidized (rancid) fat in the diet that results in an α-tocopherol deficiency, causing muscular dystrophy and a wasting away of body muscles

Shimi – undesirable black spots on a koi with no other black markings

Shiro – white

Shiro Muji – a white koi with no pattern

Shiroji – the white background color of the skin

Shitsu – quality of color

Shusui – autumn water

Sora – sky

Soragoi – blue-gray koi

Sumi – black (from the name for black ink)

Taikei – body conformation

Tancho – a koi whose only Hi is a mark on the top of the head, from the Tancho crane or Manchurian crane (*Grus japonensis*), which has a red circle on top of its head

Tategoi – a koi with perceived potential to improve its color pattern with age

Tebire – pectoral fin

Tejima – black stripes that may appear on the pectoral fins of a Sanke

Tobi – the stronger, faster-growing individuals in a batch of koi fry

Tobihi – an undesirable red spot or scale

Toh – head

Toh Hi – red on the head

Tosai – one year old

Ushirogiwa – the back edge of a color pattern

Utsuri – reflection

Wagoi – normally scaled koi (not Doitsu-scaled)

Yamabuki – a metallic yellow Ogon koi named after a bright yellow flower

Yogyoen – a koi farm

Yon – four

Yondan – four steps

Yonsai – four years old

Yoroigoi – armored koi, a Doitsu scale pattern with large scales irregularly scattered around the body like a coat of mail armor

Zukinkaburi – literally "weaving a scarf," meaning a red pattern on the forehead

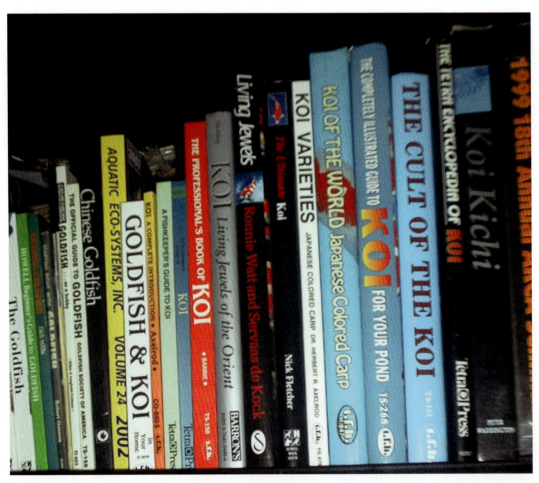
One can never have too many koi books.

BIBLIOGRAPHY

KOI BOOKS AND MAGAZINES

As the primary purpose in writing this book is to provide current information on disease prevention and treatment of koi fish, there is a great amount of material that is not included in this work. Topics such as pond design and construction, aquatic plants, judging koi shows, pond fish other than koi, and aquatic wildlife are not covered in this book. See the following books and magazines for more information on these and other topics. Also, the Associated Koi Clubs of America (AKCA) maintains an excellent Internet website '**koiusa.com**' that contains much valuable information, and has links to several hundred other koi-related websites.

Koi Books:

Amano, M. 1968. *Live Jewels*, Kajima Shoten Publishing, Tokyo, Japan.

Amano, M. 1971. *Fancy Carp, the Beauty of Japan*, Kajima Shoten Publishing, Tokyo, Japan.

Andrews, Christopher and Angela Riley. 1986. *Koi and Fancy Goldfish,* ADI 43, Tetra Press, Morris Plains, NJ.

Axelrod, Herbert R. 1973. *Koi of the World – Japanese Colored Carp,* T.F.H. Publications, Neptune, NJ.

Axelrod, Herbert R. 1983. *Koi and Garden Ponds,* T.F.H. Publications, Neptune, NJ.

Axelrod, Herbert R. and William Vorderwinkler. 1984. *Goldfish and Koi in Your Home,* T.F.H. Publications, Neptune, NJ.

Axelrod, Herbert R. 1987. *A Complete Introduction to Koi and Garden Pools,* T.F.H. Publications, Neptune, NJ.

Axelrod, Herbert R. 1988. *Koi Varieties: Japanese Colored Carp - Nishikigoi,* T.F.H. Publications, Neptune, NJ.

Axelrod, Herbert R., Eugene Balon, Richard C. Hoffman, Shmuel Rothbard, and Giora W. Wohlfarth. 1996. *The Completely Illustrated Guide to Koi for Your Pond,* T.F.H. Publications, Neptune, NJ.

Axelrod, Herbert R. 1997. *Healthy Pond Fish,* T.F.H. Publications, Neptune, NJ.

Ballou, Burt (editor). 1996, 2000. *AKCA Guide to Koi Health,* Associated Koi Clubs of America, Midway City, CA.

Ballou, Burt (editor). 1997. *AKCA Guide to Koi Nutrition,* AKCA, Midway City, CA.

Ballou, Burt (editor). 1998. *AKCA Guide to Pond Construction,* AKCA, Midway City, CA.

Ballou, Burt (editor). 1999, 2000. *AKCA Guide to Filters and Pre-Filters,* AKCA, Midway City, CA.

Barrie, Anmarie. 1992. *The Professional's Book of Koi,* T.F.H. Publications, Neptune, NJ.

Blasiola, George C. 1995. *Koi,* Barron's Educational Series, Hauppauge, NY.

Brewster, B., et al. 1989. *The Interpet Encyclopedia of Koi,* Salamander Books, London.

Caddock, Nigel. 1997. *Nishikigoi – Still Waters*, Nishikigoi International, Warrington, Cheshire, UK.

Chang Chien-Te. 1596. *The Book of the Cinnabar Fish,* China.

Cole, Peter. 1997. *The Art of Koi Keeping,* The Blandford Press,

Copperfield, Alison. 1994. *Keeping Koi in Australia,* Koi Society of Australia, Fairfield West, Australia.

Fan Li. 475 BC. *Fish Breeding*, China.

Fletcher, Nick. 1999. *The Ultimate Koi,* Howell Book House, New York.

Fujita, Grant. 198-. *Textbook of Nishikigoi,* AKCA, Midway City, CA.

Fujita, Grant. 1989. *Koi,* 2nd ed., AKCA, Midway City, CA.

Hickling, Steve. 2002. *Koi - Living Jewels of the Orient,* Barron's, Hauppauge, NY.

Hirooka, Hyohei. 1964. *The Care and Training of Koi,* Hawaii.

Horvath, L., G. Tamas, and C. Seagrave. 1992. *Carp and Pondfish Culture,* Fishing News Books, Oxford, UK.

James, Barry. 1985. *A Fishkeeper's Guide to Koi,* Tetra Press, Morris Plains, NJ.

James, Barry. 1986. *An Interpet Guide to Koi,* Salamander Books, London.

Johnson, Erik L. 1997. *Koi Health and Disease,* Johnson Veterinary Services, Marietta, GA.

Kataoka, M. 1989. *Nishikigoi Dangi,* Takayoshi Kataoka, Kumagayashi, Japan.

Kelsey-Wood, Dennis. 1997. *Koi as a New Pet*, T.F.H. Publications, Neptune, NJ.

Kelsey-Wood, Dennis. 1997. *Koi as a Hobby*, T.F.H. Publications, Neptune, NJ.

Kelsey-Wood, Dennis. 1997. *Proper Care of Koi*, T.F.H. Publications, Neptune, NJ.

Kodama, Mamoru. 2002. *Kokugyo,* Shin Nippon Kyoiku Tosho, Shimonoseki, Japan.

Kuroki, Takeo. 1966. *Koi,* Japan.

Kuroki, Takeo and Tokumitu Iwago. 1970. *The Japanese Colored Carp: Nishiki- Goi,* Kodansha LTD, Tokyo, Japan.

Kuroki, Takeo and Tokumitu Iwago. 1971. *Encyclopedia of Nishiki-Goi,* Kodansha LTD, Tokyo, Japan.

Kuroki, Takeo. 1980. *Nishikigoi and Ponds,* Zen Nippon Airinkai, Oita, Japan.

Kuroki, Takeo. 1981. *Manual to Nishikigoi,* Shin Nippon Kyoiku Tosho, Shiminoseki City, Japan.

Kuroki, Takeo. 1987. *Modern Nishikigoi*, Shin Nippon Kyoiku Tosho, Shiminoseki City, Japan.

Ladiges, W. 19—. *Coldwater Fish in the Home and Garden,* Tetra Press, Morris Plains, NJ.

Mills, Dick. 19—. *Coldwater Fishes,* Salamander Fishkeepers Guides, Tetra Press, Morris Plains, NJ.

Miya, Sadaichiro. 1967. *The 100 Best Nishikigoi,* Miyakoya, Ojiya City, Niigata, Japan.

McDowall, Anne (editor). 1989. *The Interpet Encyclopedia of Koi*, Salamander Books, London.

McDowall, Anne (editor). 1989. *The Tetra Encyclopedia of Koi*, Tetra Press, Morris Plains, NJ.

Penzes, Bethen and Istvan Tolg. 1983. *Goldfish and Ornamental Carp*, Barron's Educational Series, Woodbury, NY.

Pool, David. 1991. *Hobbyist Guide to Successful Koi Keeping*, Tetra Press, Morris Plains, NJ.

Randolph, E. 1990. *Coldwater Fish in the Home and Garden,* Tetra Press, Morris Plains, NJ.

Ranson, Stan (editor). 1987. *Practical Koi Keeping*, vol. 1, Koi USA, Midway City, CA.

Ranson, Stan (editor). 1995. *Practical Koi Keeping*, vol. 2, Koi USA, Midway City, CA.

Ranson, Stan (editor). 1997. *Practical Koi Keeping*, vol. 3, Koi USA, Midway City, CA.

Roe, Colin and Anthony Evans. 1967. *Koi, Keeping the Fancy Pond Carp of Japan,* Petfish Publications, London. [First English book about Koi].

Rothbard, Schmuel. 1997. *Koi Breeding,* T.F.H. Publications, Neptune, NJ.

Saint-Erne, Nicholas. 1994. *Diseases of Koi,* Koi Rx, Las Vegas, NV.

Saint-Erne, Nicholas. 2002. *Advanced Koi Care*, Erne Enterprises, Glendale, AZ.

Sakai, Hiroji. 2001. *Homeland of Nishikigoi,* Sakai Fish Farm, Hiroshima, Japan.

Skomal, Gregory. 1999. *Koi: An Owner's Guide to a Happy Healthy Fish,* Howell Book House, New York.

Takeshita, Glenn Y., 1969. *Koi for Home and Garden,* T.F.H. Publications, Neptune, NJ.

Tamadachi, Michugo. 1994. *The Cult of the Koi,* 2nd ed., T.F.H. Publications, Neptune, NJ.

Tamaki, Takehiko. 1977. *Nishikigoi Fancy Koi*, Tamaki Yogyoen, Hiroshima, Japan.

Valley of the Sun Koi Club. 1984. *Koi Pond Construction Ideas and Suggestions,* VSKC, Phoenix, AZ.

Vrbova, Zuza. 1990. *Junior Pet Care – Koi for Ponds,* T.F.H. Publications, Neptune, NJ.

Waddington, Peter. 1995. *Koi Kichi,* Infiltration, Golborne, Warrington, Cheshire, UK.

Watt, Ronnie and Servaas de Kock. 1996. *Living Jewels – Koi Keeping in South Africa*, Delta Books, Jeppestown, South Africa.

Wisner, Nancy Cooper and Frederick Albert Simon. 1996. *Keeping Koi,* Sterling Publishing, New York.

Pond and Water Garden Books:

Allison, James. 1991. *Water in the Garden,* Tetra Press, Morris Plains, NJ.

Archer-Wills, Anthony. 1993. *The Water Gardener,*

Archer-Wills, Anthony and Helen Woodhall. 1999. *Designing Water Gardens*, Conran Octopus, London.

Archibald, David. 1990. *Water Gardens,* Harrowsmith,

Arnoux, Jean-Claude. 1997. *The Ultimate Water Garden Book,* Taunton Press, Newtown, CT.

Atkinson, Scott. 1965 (revised 1997). *Garden Pools, Fountains and Waterfalls*, Sunset Publishing Corp., Menlo Park, CA.

Axelrod, Herbert R., Albert Spalding Benoist, and Dennis Kelsey-Wood. 1992. *The Atlas of Garden Ponds,* T.F.H. Publications, Neptune, NJ.

Axelrod, Herbert R. 1997. *Designing Your Garden Pond,* T.F.H. Publications, Neptune, NJ.

Axelrod, Herbert R. 1997. *Stocking Your Garden Pond,* T.F.H. Publications, Neptune, NJ.

Barrett, Jim. 1999. *Quick Guide: Ponds & Fountains*, Creative Homeowners, Upper Saddle River, NJ.

Barrie, Anmarie. 1997. *Your New Garden Pond,* T.F.H. Publications, Neptune, NJ.

Bauer, O.N., et al. 1969. *Diseases of Pond Fishes,* National Science Foundation, Washington, DC.

Beaulieu, Ed and Dave Kelly. 2002. *Pond Builder's Bible*, Aquascapes Designs, Batavia, IL.

Beedell, Suzanne. *Water in the Garden,*

Binsacca, Rich. 2001. *Garden Pools, Fountains and Watercourses,* Black & Decker

Bird, Richard and Lucy Huntington. 2001. *Water Gardens: Everything You Need to Create a Garden,* Cassell Academic,

Beneke, Jeff. 2001. *Sunset Garden Pools, Fountains & Waterfalls,* Sunset Books, Menlo Park, CA.

Bird, Richard and Lucy Huntington. 2002. *Water Gardens: Instant Reference to More Than 250 Plants,* Cassell Academic,

Booth-Moores, Andrew. 1992. *Garden Pools: Waterfalls & Fountains*, Practical Gardening,

Boyd, Claude E., et al. 1997. *Dynamics of Pond Aquaculture,* Lewis Publishers,

Bridgewater, Alan and Gill Bridgewater. 2001. *Outdoor Water Features,*

Brown, Ron. *Rock and Water Gardens,*

Buczacki, Stefan T. 2000. *Best Water Gardens*, Hamlyn, UK.

Calkins, Carroll. 1984. *Gardening with Water, Plantings and Stone,*

Case, David. 1994. *Water Garden Plants – the Complete Guide,* The Crowood Press, UK.

Claflin, Edward. 1988. *Garden Pools and Fountains*,

Clarke, Ethne. 2002. *Water Features for Small Gardens*, Cassell Academic

Clevely, A. *The Water Garden: Month by Month*,

Coborn, John. 1997. *Garden Ponds as a Hobby*, T.F.H. Publications, Neptune, NJ.

Conrad, Roseanne D. 1998. *An Owner's Guide to the Garden Pond*, Howell Book House, New York.

Cooper, Guy. 1987. *English Water Gardens*,

David, Al. 1987. *Garden Ponds: A Complete Introduction*, T.F.H. Publications, Neptune, NJ.

Dawes, John. 1989. *John Dawes's Book of Water Gardens*, T.F.H. Publications, Neptune, NJ.

Dawes, John. 1998. *The Pond Owner's Handbook*, Ward Lock, London.

Dawes, John. 1998. *The Pond Owner's Problem Solver*, Tetra Press, Blacksburg, VA.

Dimmock, Charlie. 2001. *Water Garden Workbook*,

Druse, Ken. 1993. *Water Gardening*, Burpee

Dunn, Teri. 2002. *Water Gardens: A Guide to Creating, Caring For, and Enjoying Aquatic Landscapes*, Metro Books,

Dutta, Reginald. 1977. *Water Gardening Indoors and Out*,

Ellis, Barbara. 1997. *Water Gardens: How to Plan and Plant a Backyard Pond*, Taylor,

Fell, Derek. 2001. *Water Gardening for Beginners*,

Fisher, Kathleen. 2000. *Complete Guide to Water Gardens*, Creative Homeowners, Upper Saddle River, NJ.

Francis, Allison. *Easy Water Gardens*, Time-Life,

Fowler, Veronica Lorson and Jamie Beyer. 1999. *Ortho's All About Garden Pools & Fountains*, Meredith Books, Des Moines, IA.

Gilmer, Maureen. 2002. *Water Works: Creating a Splash in the Garden*,

Glattstein, Judy. 1994. *Waterscaping*, Storey Communications, Pownal, VT.

Greenoak, Francesca. 1996. *Water Features for Small Gardens*, Sterling Publishing, New York.

Grinstain, Dawn. 1992. *Pools, Ponds, and Waterways for Your Garden*,

Hale, Gill. 1999. *The Feng Shui Garden*, Storey Communications, Pownal, VT.

Halls, Steve. 2000. *Your Healthy Garden Pond*,

Heriteau, Jacqueline and Charles Thomas. 1996. *Water Gardens*, Houghton Mifflin, New York.

Herritage, Bill. 1986. *Pools & Water Gardens,* 2nd ed., Sterling Publishing, New York.

Herritage, Bill. 19—. *The Lotus Book of Water Gardening,* Lotus

Hervey, George. *The Book of the Garden Pond,*

Hessayon, D.G. 1993. *The Rock & Water Garden Expert*, Expert Books, London.

Jantra, Helmut. 1995. *Garden Pool Design,* T.F.H. Publications, Neptune, NJ.

Jekyll, Gertrude. 1983. *Wall and Water Gardens,*

Kramer, Jack. 1971. *Water Gardening: Pools, Fountains, and Plants,*

Kelsey-Wood, Dennis. 1998. *Landscaping Your Garden Pond,* T.F.H. Publications,   Neptune, NJ.

Ladiges, W. 1983. *Coldwater Fish in the Home and Garden,* Tetra Press, Morris Plains, NJ.

Lambert, Derek. 1999. *English Garden Ponds,* T.F.H. Publications, Neptune, NJ.

Lambert, Derek. 1999. *Gardener's Guide to Water Gardens,* T.F.H. Publications, Neptune, NJ.

Lambert, Derek. 1999. *Fishkeeper's Guide to Water Gardening,* T.F.H. Publications, Neptune, NJ.

Ledbetter, Gordon. 1982. *The Better Water Gardens Book of Patio Ponds,* Alphabet and Image, Ltd., Sherbourne, UK.

Leverett, Brian. 1991. *Water Gardens: Step by Step to Success,* Crowood, UK.

Lewis, Eleanore (editor). 2001. *Water Gardens*, Better Homes and Gardens,

Love, Gilly. 2001. *Water in the Garden: Inspiring Ideas and Designs for Beautiful Water Features,*

Lovgren, Gosta H. 2000. *The Ponder's Bible,* Carolelle Publishing, Lavallette, NJ.

Matson, Tim. 1997. *Earth Ponds Sourcebook*, Countryman Press, Woodstock, VT.

May, Peter J. 1997. *The Perfect Pond Recipe Book,* T.F.H. Publications, Neptune, NJ.

May, Peter J. 1999. *The Perfect Pond Detective* Book 1*: The Biological Balance,* T.F.H. Publications, Neptune, NJ.

May, Peter J. 1999. *The Perfect Pond Detective* Book 2*: Physical and Mechanical Problems,* T.F.H. Publications, Neptune, NJ.

McHoy, Peter. 1986. *Water Gardening,* Blandford,

McRae, Jim, et al. 1998. *Water Gardens,* Sunset Publishing Corp., Menlo Park, CA.

Mikolojski, Andrew. 1997. *Water Plants,* Lorenz Books, New York.

Mills, Dick. 1992. *A Popular Guide to Garden Ponds*, Tetra Press, Blacksburg, VA.

Mills, Dick. 2002. *The Bumber Book of Garden Ponds,* Interpet, Surrey, UK.

Nash, Helen. 1994. *The Pond Doctor,* Sterling Publishing, New York.

Nash, Helen. 1996. *The Complete Pond Builder,* Sterling Publishing, New York.

Nash, Helen. 1996. *Low Maintenance Water Gardens,* Sterling Publishing, New York.

Nash, Helen and C. Greg Speichert. 1996. *Water Gardening in Containers,* Sterling Publishing, New York.

Nash, Helen. 1997. *Fountains and Moving Waterfalls,* Sterling Publishing, New York.

Nash, Helen and Steve Stroupe. 1998. *Aquatic Plants and Their Cultivation,* Sterling Publishing, New York.

Nash, Helen and Steve Stroupe. 1998. *Plants for Water Gardens,* Sterling Publishing, New York.

Nash, Helen and Eamonn Hughes. 1999. *Waterfalls, Fountains, Pools & Streams,* Sterling Publishing, New York.

Nash, Helen. 2000. *Pond Planting,* Sterling Publishing, New York.

Nash, Helen. 2000. *The Living Pond,* Sterling Publishing, New York.

Nash, Helen. 2000. *Water Gardening Basics,* Sterling Publishing, New York.

Nash, Helen. 2001. *Water Features for Every Garden,*

Nash, Helen. 2002. *Landscaping the Pond,* Sterling Publishing, New York.

Ortho Books. 1988. *Garden Pools and Fountains,* The Solaris Group, San Ramon, CA.

Papworth, D. 1984. *A Fishkeeper's Guide to Garden Ponds,* Tetra Press, Blacksburg, VA.

Paul, Anthony and Yvonne Rees. 1986. *The Water Garden,* Penguin Books, New York.

Perry, Frances. *The Garden Pool,* David & Charles,

Pool, David. 1988. *Digest for a Successful Pond,* ADI 52, Tetra Press, Morris Plains, NJ.

Pool, David. 1993. *Hobbyist Guide to Successful Pond Keeping,* Tetra Press, Blacksburg, VA.

Poole. 1986. *Ponds & Water Gardens,* Blanford Press, UK.

Porter, Valerie. 1989. *The Pond Book,*

Quick, Graham. 1999. *An Essential Guide to Choosing Your Pond Fish and Aquatic Plants,* Barron's Educational Series, Hauppauge, NY.

Rees, Yvonne and Peter May. 2001. *The Water Garden Design Book,*

Reid, George K. 1987. *Pond Life,* Western Publishing, Racine, WI.

Reid, Jeffrey. 1997. *How to Build Ponds and Waterfalls,* Tetra Press, Blacksburg, VA.

Rhudy, Robyn. 2002. *Robyn's Pond Book,*

Roberts, Debbie and Ian Smith. 2001. *Creating Garden Ponds and Water Features,*

Robinson, Brian. 1985. *Howell Beginner's Guide to Garden Ponds*, Howell Book House, New York.

Robinson, Peter. 1993. *Pool and Waterside Gardening*, Timber Press, Portland, OR.

Robinson, Peter. 1995. *The Water Garden*, Sterling Publishing, NY.

Robinson, Peter. 1997. *The American Horticultural Society Complete Guide to Water Gardening,* Dorling-Kindersley, London, UK.

Robinson, Peter. 2000. *Pond Basics,*

Robinson, Peter. 2001. *Rock & Water Gardening: A Practical Guide to Construction and Planting,*

Robinson, Peter. 2001. *Water Gardens in a Weekend,* Hamlyn, UK.

Rockwell, Jane. 1989. *All About Ponds: Question and Answer Book,*

Russell, Stanley. 1986. *The Stapeley Book of Water Gardens,*

Sandford, Gina. 2000. *Essential Guide to Choosing Your Pond Fish & Aquatic Plants,* Barron's Educational Series, Hauppauge, NY.

Sandford, Gina. 2000. *Practical Guide to Creating a Garden Pond,* Barron's Educational Series, Hauppauge, NY.

Schimana, Walter. 1994. *Garden Ponds for Everyone*, T.F.H. Publications, Neptune, NJ.

Sera. 1993. *Pond Guide: How to Build My Garden Pond,* Sera GmbH, Heinsberg, Germany.

Sera. 1993. *Pond Guide: How to Maintain and Cultivate My Garden Pond,* Sera GmbH, Heinsberg, Germany.

Shaffer, Marcella. 2001. *10 Steps to Better Water Gardens,* Storey Communications, Pownal, VT.

Skinner, Archie and David Arscott. 1996. *The Stream Garden*, Ward Lock, London, UK.

Slocum, Perry D., et al. 1993. *Water Gardening: Water Lilies and Lotuses,* Timber Press, Portland, OR.

Smith, Charles. 2000. *Easy-Care Water Garden Plants,* Storey Communications, Pownal, VT.

Speichert, C. Greg, 2001. *Ortho's All About Water Gardening,* The Solaris Group, San Ramon, CA.

Sperling, Alan. 1995. *Pondscapes Fax Digest,* Happy Pondering Products, Roswell, GA.

Sperling, Alan. 1995. *Pondscapes Journal,* Happy Pondering Products, Roswell, GA.

Sperling, Alan. 1997. *Glossary of Pond Terms,* Happy Pondering Products, Roswell, GA.

Sperling, Alan. 1999. *National Pond Society Pond Hobbyist's User Guide & Reference Handbook,* Happy Pondering Products, Roswell, GA.

Sperling, Alan. 1999. *Truths About Pond Care,* National Pond Society, Roswell, GA.

Spier, Carol. 1993. *For Your Garden: Water Gardens,* Michael Friedman Publishing Group, New York.

Stadelmann, Peter. 1992. *Water Gardens,* Barron's Educational Series, Hauppauge, NY.

Stetson, Paul. 1963. *Garden Pools,* T.F.H. Publications, Neptune, NJ.

Stevens, David. 2001. *Water Features,* Soma Basics,

Stroupe, Steve, et al. 1999. *Plants for Water Gardens,* Sterling Publishing, New York.

Swift, Penny and Janet Szymanowski. 1996. *Step-by-Step Ponds, Pools and Rockeries,*

Swindells, Philip. 1984. *The Overlook Water Gardener's Handbook,*

Swindells, Philip. 1985. *Book of the Water Garden,* Salem House,

Swindells, Philip. 1990. *The Complete Book of the Water Garden,*

Swindells, Philip. 1991. *At the Water's Edge: Gardening With Moisture-Loving Plants,*

Swindells, Philip. 1991. *Small Garden Pools,*

Swindells, Philip. 1994. *Water Gardens,* Ward Lock, London.

Swindells, Philip. 1994. *Waterside Planting,*

Swindells, Philip. 1999. *Quick and Easy Container Water Gardens,* Storey Communications, Pownal, VT.

Swindells, Philip. 2000. *Popular Pond Plants,* Interpet, UK.

Swindells, Philip. 2001. *Container Water Gardens,*

Swindells, Philip. 2001. *Pond Features and Decorations,*

Swindells, Philip. 2001. *Pond Plants and Cultivation,*

Swindells, Philip. 2002. *Formal Ponds and Water Gardens,* Barrons Educational Series, Hauppauge, NY.

Swindells, Philip. 2002. *The Master Book of the Water Garden,*

Swindells, Philip. 2002. *Natural Water Gardens,*

Thimes, Joseph Lee. 1999. *Planting a Water Garden,* T.F.H. Publications, Neptune, NJ.

Thomas, Charles B. 1988. *Water Gardens for Plants and Fish,* T.F.H. Publications, Neptune, NJ.

Thomas, Charles B. 1991. *Creating Your Own Water Garden,* Storey Communications, Pownal, VT.

Thomas, Charles B. 1997. *Water Gardens: How to Plan & Plant a Backyard Pond,* Houghton Mifflin, New York.

Thomas, Charles. 2002. *Ortho's All About Building Waterfalls, Ponds, and Streams,* The Solaris Group, San Ramon, CA.

Thomas, G. L., Jr. 1965. *Goldfish Pools, Water-Lilies, and Tropical Fishes,* T.F.H. Publications, Neptune, NJ.

Thompson, Gerald. 1984. *The Pond,*

Time Life. 1980. *Rock and Water Gardens*, Time Life, NY.

Time Life. 2001. *Water Gardens: Simple Steps for Adding the Beauty of Water to Your Garden,* Time Life, NY.

Tomocik, Joseph. 1996. *Water Gardening,* Pantheon Books, New York.

Tucker, Craig S., et al. 1993. *Water Quality & Pond Soil Analyses for Aquaculture,* University of Alabama Press, Auburn, AL.

Tucker, Craig S., et al. 1998. *Pond Aquaculture Water Quality Management,* Kluwer Academic Publishers,

Uber, William C. 1995. *The Basics of Water Gardening,* Dragonflyer Press, Upland, CA.

Ulrich, Tim. 1999. *Creating Ponds, Brooks, and Pools: Water in the Garden,* Schiffer Design,

Van Der Horst, Arend. *Garden Ponds and Water Features Installing,*

Van Sweden, James. 1995. *Gardening with Water*, Random House, New York.

Walter, Ken. 1998. *Water Gardening in Containers*, Storey Communications, Pownal, VT.

Warring, R. *Garden Pools and Fishponds,*

White, Hazel. 1998. *Water Gardens: Simple Projects. Contemporary Designs,*

Wieser, K. H. and P.V. Loiselle. 1992. *Your Garden Pond*, Tetra Press, Morris Plains, NJ.

Wilson, Andrea. 1995. *The Creative Water Gardener*, Ward Lock, London.

Wittstock, Greg. 1998. *Succeeding & Prospering with Water Features,* Aquascape Designs, Batavia, IL.

Koi and Water Gardening Magazines:

Aquascape Designs, Aquascapes Designs, 1119 Lyon Rd. Batavia, IL 60510.

Aquascape Lifestyles, Pond Guy Publications, PO Box 638, West Chicago, IL 60186.

British Koi Keepers Society monthly magazine, UK.

Garden Ponds Quarterly, T.F.H. Publications, 1 TFH Plaza, Neptune, NJ 07753.

Koi-Bito, Kotsubo 1-26-20, Zushi-shi, Kanagawa-ken, 249-0008, Japan.

Koi Carp, Freestyle Publications, Dorset, UK.

Koi Health Quarterly, Koi Health Group, UK.

Koi Ponds and Gardens, Origin Publishing, Bristol, UK.

Koi USA, AKCA, PO Box 1, Midway City, CA 92655.

Koi World, Fancy Publications, 3 Burroughs, Irvine, CA 92618.

KSA News, Koi Society of Australia, Balgownie, Australia.

Mid-Atlantic Koi, 3290 Shaker Ct., Montclair, VA 22026.

Nichirin, Zen Nippon Airinkai, Japan.

Nishikigoi International, Lowton, Warrington, Cheshire, WA3 1BG, UK.

Nishikigoi Monthly, Kinsai Publishing, Toshima-ku, Tokyo, 170-0013, Japan.

Pond & Garden, 1670 S. 900 E., Zionsville, IN 46077.

Pond Keeper, Garden Pond Promotions, 1000 Whitetail Ct., Duncansville, PA 16635.

Ponds USA, Fancy Publications, 3 Burroughs, Irvine, CA 92618.

Pondscapes Magazine, The National Pond Society, 3933 Loch Highland Pass, Roswell, GA 30075.

Pondscapes Journal, The National Pond Society, 3933 Loch Highland Pass, Roswell, GA 30075.

Rinko, Shin Nippon Tosho, Shimonoseki, Japan.

The Journal of Japanese Gardening, Roth Tei-en, PO Box 159, Orefield, PA 18069.

Water Garden Journal, 1401 Johnson Ferry Rd., Marietta, GA 30062.

Water Garden News, Fancy Publications, PO Box 6050, Mission Viejo, CA 92690.

Water Gardening, PO Box 607, St. John, IN 46373.

Aquarium Fish Magazines:

Aquarium Digest International, Tetra Press, 201 Tabor Road, Morris Plains, NJ 07950.

Aquarium Fish, Fancy Publications, 3 Burroughs, Irvine, CA 92618.

Freshwater and Marine Aquarium, PO Box 487, Sierra Madre, CA 91024.

Practical Fishkeeping, PO Box 500, Leicester, LE99 0AA, UK.

The Aquarist and Pondkeeper, 9 Tufton Street, Ashford, Kent, TN23 1QN, UK.

Tropical Fish Hobbyist, T.F.H. Publications, 211 Sylvania Ave., Neptune, NJ 07753.

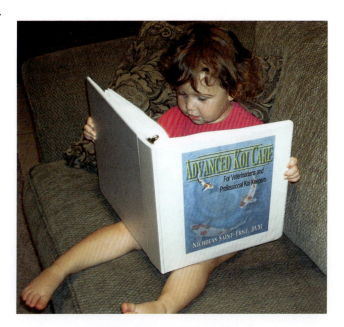

Proofreading the final draft!

Periodic Table of the Elements

Group	1	2	3		4	5	6	7	8	9
	I A	II A	III B		IV B	V B	VI B	VII B	VIII B	VIII B

Period	Alkali Metals	Alkaline Earth Metals			Transition Metals					

KEY:
Atomic Number
Element Symbol
Element Name
Atomic Weight*

* The Atomic Weight is the element's Molar Mass measured in grams/mole. Hydrogen weighs approximately 1 gram per mole, while Carbon weighs approximately 12 grams per mole. A mole is 6.0221367×10^{23} atoms of the element. This number, called Avogadro's Number after the Italian physicist Amedeo Avogadro (1776-1856), is based on the number of Carbon atoms necessary to weigh 12 grams, and serves as a reference point for comparing the mass of the elements. Each molecule of the elements gets progressively heavier as the atomic number increases. Numbers in parentheses indicate the mass of the most stable isotope.

Period	1	2	3		4	5	6	7	8	9
1	1 H Hydrogen 1.008									
2	3 Li Lithium 6.941	4 Be Beryllium 9.012								
3	11 Na Sodium 22.99	12 Mg Magnesium 24.31								
4	19 K Potassium 39.1	20 Ca Calcium 40.08	21 Sc Scandium 44.96		22 Ti Titanium 47.88	23 V Vanadium 50.94	24 Cr Chromium 52	25 Mn Manganese 54.94	26 Fe Iron 55.85	27 Co Cobalt 58.47
5	37 Rb Rubidium 85.47	38 Sr Strontium 87.62	39 Y Yttrium 88.91		40 Zr Zirconium 91.22	41 Nb Niobium 92.91	42 Mo Molybdenum 95.94	43 Tc Technetium (98)	44 Ru Ruthenium 101.1	45 Rh Rhodium 102.9
6	55 Cs Cesium 132.9	56 Ba Barium 137.3	57 La Lanthanum 138.9	** Lanthanide Series	72 Hf Hafnium 178.5	73 Ta Tantalum 180.9	74 W Wolfram 183.9	75 Re Rhenium 186.2	76 Os Osmium 190.2	77 Ir Iridium 190.2
7	87 Fr Francium (223)	88 Ra Radium (226)	89 Ac Actinium (227)	*** Actinide Series	104 Rf Rutherfordium (257)	105 Db Dubnium (260)	106 Sg Seaborgium (263)	107 Bh Bohrium (262)	108 Hs Hassium (265)	109 Mt Meitnerium (266)

Classification of the elements in a periodic table was first suggested by Russian chemist Dmitri Ivanovich Mendeleev in 1869.

** Lanthanide Series	58 Ce Cerium 140.1	59 Pr Praseodymium 140.9	60 Nd Neodymium 144.2	61 Pm Promethium (147)	62 Sm Samarium 150.4	63 Eu Europium 152	64 Gd Gadolinium 157.3
*** Actinide Series	90 Th Thorium 232	91 Pa Protactinium (231)	92 U Uranium (238)	93 Np Neptunium (237)	94 Pu Plutonium (242)	95 Am Americium (243)	96 Cm Curium (247)

APPENDIX

10 VIII B	11 I B	12 II B	13 III A	14 IV A	15 V A	16 VI A	17 VII A	18 VIII A
				Metals			Non Metals	Noble Gases
								2 He Helium 4.003
			5 B Boron 10.81	6 C Carbon 12.01	7 N Nitrogen 14.01	8 O Oxygen 16	9 F Fluorine 19	10 Ne Neon 20.18
			13 Al Aluminum 26.98	14 Si Silicon 28.09	15 P Phosphorus 30.97	16 S Sulfur 32.07	17 Cl Chlorine 35.45	18 Ar Argon 39.95
28 Ni Nickel 58.69	29 Cu Copper 63.55	30 Zn Zinc 65.39	31 Ga Gallium 69.72	32 Ge Germanium 72.59	33 As Arsenic 74.92	34 Se Selenium 78.96	35 Br Bromine 79.9	36 Kr Krypton 83.8
46 Pd Palladium 106.4	47 Ag Silver 107.9	48 Cd Cadmium 112.4	49 In Indium 114.8	50 Sn Tin 118.7	51 Sb Antimony 121.8	52 Te Tellurium 127.6	53 I Iodine 126.9	54 Xe Xenon 131.3
78 Pt Platinum 195.1	79 Au Gold 197	80 Hg Mercury 200.5	81 Tl Thallium 204.4	82 Pb Lead 207.2	83 Bi Bismuth 209	84 Po Polonium (210)	85 At Astatine (210)	86 Rn Radon (222)
110 Uun Ununnulium (269)	111 Uuu Unununium (272)	112 Uub ununbium (277)	113 Uut ununtrium ( )	114 Uuq ununquadium (289)	115 Uup ununpentium ( )	116 Uuh ununhexium (289)	117 Uus ununseptium ( )	118 Uuo ununoctium (293)

65 Tb Terbium 158.9	66 Dy Dysprosium 162.5	67 Ho Holmium 164.9	68 Er Erbium 167.3	69 Tm Thulium 168.9	70 Yb Ytterbium 173	71 Lu Lutetium 175
97 Bk Berkelium (247)	98 Cf Californium (249)	99 Es Einsteinium (254)	100 Fm Fermium (253)	101 Md Mendelevium (256)	102 No Nobelium (254)	103 Lr Lawrencium (257)

Nick
Saint-Erne
2002

CONSTRUCTION OF A KOI POND USING EPDM LINER

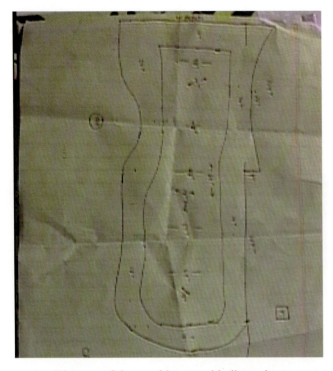

Diagram of the pond layout with dimensions.

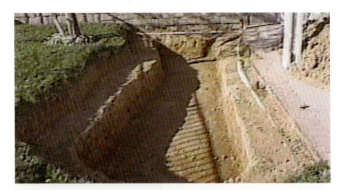

The pond is dug and protrusions in the soil from rocks, pebbles, and roots are removed as much as possible to keep the surface smooth.

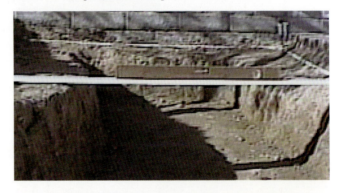

A level is used on a board across the pond to be sure the shelf and edges are level.

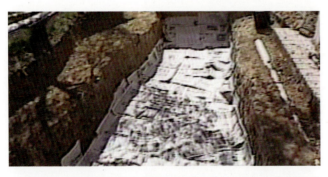

A thick layer of newspaper is used to smooth out the pond bottom. Cloth pond liners or carpeting can also be used.

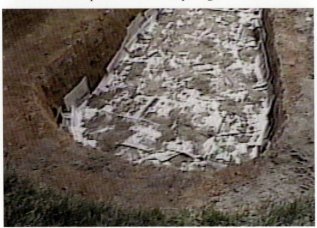

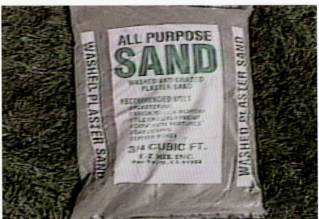

Sand is used to weigh down the newspaper, and to smooth the surface of the shelf at the edge of the pond. The sand is also used to cover the irrigation pipe that was exposed in digging the pond. Then this will all be covered by the pond liner.

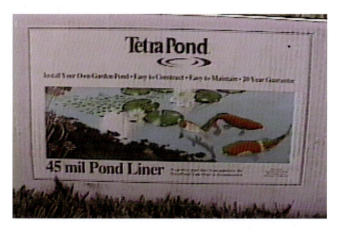

This pond was built from a kit that came with a liner, filter, and other supplies. It was assembled in two days by two people.

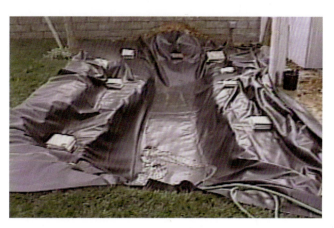

The EPDM liner was stretched across the hole, and then fitted to the pond's contours. The edges were weighted down and it was filled with water.

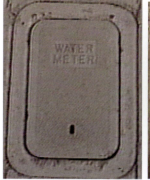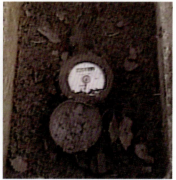

Check the reading on the water meter before filling the pond to get the initial reading. If no other water is being used, the meter will be stationary.

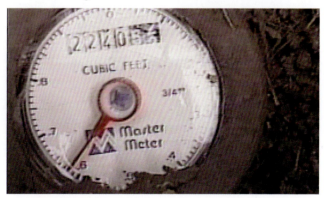

Get a second reading after the pond is full. Subtracting the first reading from the second reading will give the amount of water in the pond.

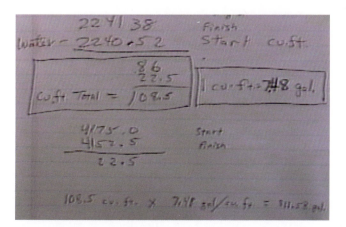

If the meter reads in cubic feet, rather than in gallons, multiply the volume in cubic feet by 7.48 gal/ cu. ft. to get the volume in gallons. Write down the pond volume and save it for future reference!

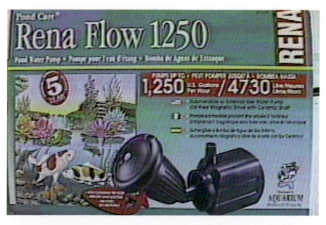

Assemble the filtration system. This 811 gallon pond will use a submersible pump that flows 1250 gallons per hour (1.5 times the pond volume) and an in-pond filter chamber.

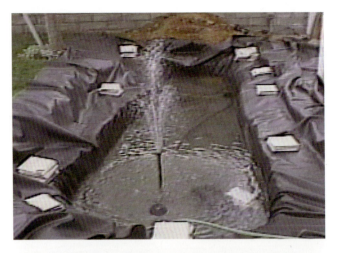

The water is drawn through the in-pond filter chamber by the submerged pump, and out a fountain head.

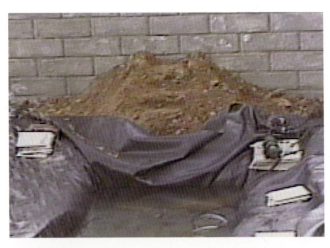

A dirt mound is piled at one end of the pond against the block wall to make a waterfall.

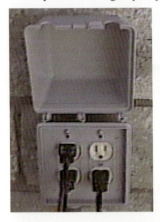
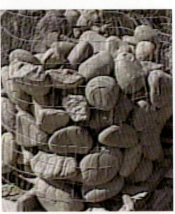

A covered, water-proof outlet box should be used on a GFCI circuit for the pumps and UV filter.

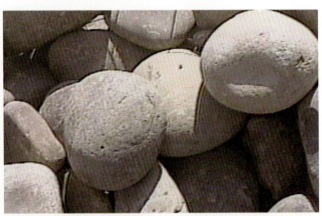

Rocks from a landscaping supply company will be used around the edge of the pond.

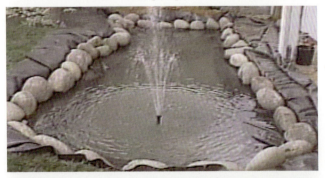

Rocks are placed on the shelf around the pond's edge.

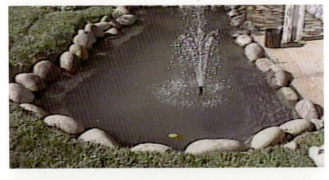

The liner is trimmed and its edges are folded over and tucked down behind the rocks. Smaller rocks and sand are used to fill in the gaps and cover the liner.

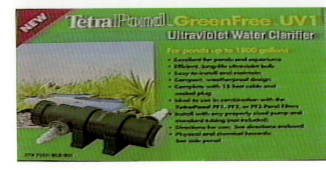

LEFT: The UV sterilizer is placed outside the pond near the waterfall. Water from a second submersible pump will flow through it and then down the waterfall.

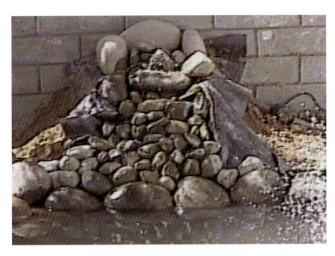

Smaller rocks are placed over the extra
liner used to form the waterfall.

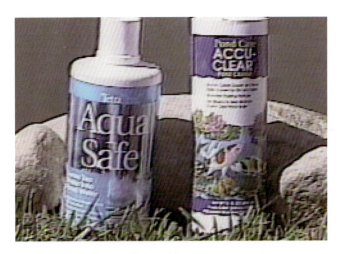

Dechlorinator is used to remove chlorine
from the tap water before adding any fish.

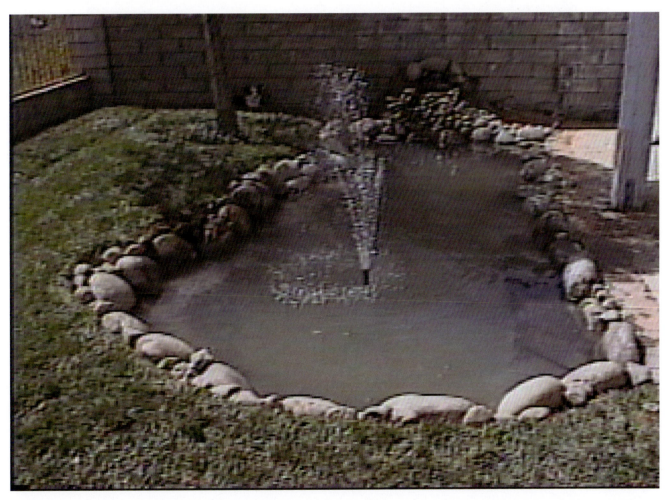

The pond construction is complete! Now it will be landscaped by adding potted aquatic plants on the underwater shelf and terrestrial plants around each side of the waterfall. Salt is added at a rate of 1 pound per 100 gallons of water to reach a 0.1% salinity. The filter will run a few days to clear the pond water and start the establishment of bacteria in the biological filter before any koi are added. Then the fish will slowly be introduced over the next 3-6 weeks. Daily water tests are necessary with new ponds to monitor for ammonia or nitrite spikes. Partial water changes are needed if these levels rise. Even the dog enjoys watching the new pond!

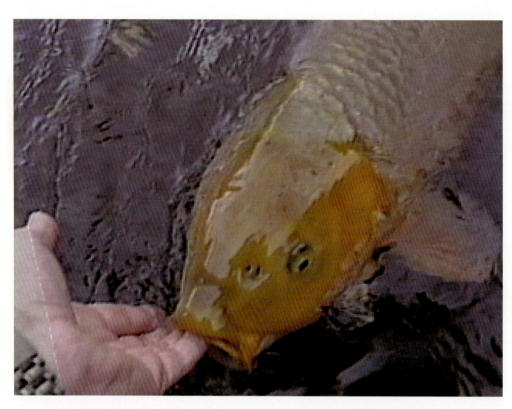
A Chagoi literally eating out of my hand - or biting the hand that feeds it!

INDEX

A

Achlya 19, 69
activated carbon 101-102, 106, 110-111, 115, 132, 148
aeration 18, 38-39, 52, 57, 98, 101, 105-106, 116-117, 128, 131-132, 142, 144, 148-150, 156
Aeromonas 65, 67-68, 70, 74, 92, 118, 120, 131, 139-140, 154
alcohol 44, 50
algae 20, 89, 92, 98-99, 106, 114-115, 118, 124, 141-143, 150, 156-158
alkalinity 39, 94, 98-101, 103, 106-108, 137, 150
ammonia 30-31, 33, 38-40, 46, 70, 89-90, 92, 94-96, 98-99, 101-102, 105, 108, 110-113, 118-119, 122, 125, 130-131, 137-138, 140, 142-144, 157-158, 160, 188
anatomy 27, 29-30, 34-35, 53, 93
anchor worms 83, 131, 139, 162
anemia 78, 82, 91-92
anesthetic 20, 41, 50-53, 55, 59, 137-138
annelid worm 78-79, 81
anoxia 156, 166
antibiotic 43, 54, 65, 67, 73, 118, 123, 137-140, 161
Argulus 72, 83-84, 135, 139, 162
artificial respiration 121
ascorbic acid 77, 90-91
aspirin 130
auction 129
autumn 14, 93, 119-120, 170

B

bacterial hemorrhagic septicemia 65
baking soda 59, 100
barbel 27
barley straw 114
biochemical oxygen demand 98, 105
biofilter 111-113, 116, 120, 156
biological filter 106, 111, 113, 116, 118, 136, 140-142, 188
biopsy 40-42, 44, 49, 70, 74, 76, 78-79, 82, 86, 123, 139-141
blood cells 30, 42-43, 45-47, 78, 96, 167
bog filter 114
Branchiomyces 69-70
breeding 7-8, 18-22, 24, 33, 59, 64, 79, 103, 116, 141, 173-174
buffer 50, 100-101
buoyancy 32, 53, 66, 68

C

calcium bicarbonate 100-102
calcium carbonate 95, 99-103, 106, 111
Capillaria 82
carbohydrates 89-90, 92
carbon dioxide 30-31, 46, 50, 59, 90, 94, 98, 100-101, 119, 123, 125
carbon filter 110-111
carotenoids 92
carp 2, 4-8, 11, 13-14, 17, 20, 24, 34, 60, 63-65, 79, 81, 89, 126, 168-169, 172-174, 181
carp pituitary extract 20
carp pox 63-64
Caryophyllaeus 81
cestodes 81
Chilodonella 73, 150-152
chloramine 96, 101-102, 160
Chloramine-T 67, 80, 148-149, 163
chlorhexidine 70, 131
chlorine 40, 94, 96, 101-102, 108, 110-111, 119, 137, 143, 160, 188
chromatophores 29
chromosome 22
cilia 73, 75, 77
clams 85, 162
clinoptilolite clay 102, 111
clove oil 50
coccidia 161
conductivity 103, 106, 109
copper 5, 67, 73, 76, 85, 92, 94, 99, 111, 125, 137, 150, 164
copper toxicity 125
copper sulfate 67, 73, 76, 85, 125, 150
Costia 77
culling 21-22
culture and sensitivity testing 65, 161

D

Dactylogyrus 72, 79-80, 86, 135, 140, 143-144, 162, 190
Daphnia 19, 190
dechlorinator 119, 125-126, 131, 143, 149, 188

Dimilin 83-84, 140, 163
disinfection 65, 67, 132
dissolved organic carbon 110, 116
dolomite 111
dropsy 64-66, 137

E

eggs 7, 18-22, 33, 64, 69-70, 74, 79, 81, 83-84, 89, 118-119, 153, 163, 167
Eimeria 73
electrocardiogram 57
electrocution 121
endoscopy 49
English-style koi show 131
Enterobacter 139-140
epidermis 28-29, 54, 64, 74-75, 77, 123, 138, 166
Epistylis 73-74
epithelium 28, 42, 63-64, 74-75, 77, 80, 86, 96, 135, 143, 166
Ergasilus 83
erythrocytes 45-46
erythrophores 29
euthanasia 50, 59, 135
eye 27, 65, 122, 149-162, 168

F

fall 8, 16, 64, 119
fat 64, 90-92, 119, 122, 170
fatty acids 90, 92, 129
fecal exam 44
feces 20, 44, 64, 73, 77, 82, 118
feeding 42, 48, 65, 74-75, 78, 81-82, 84-85, 89-92, 96, 118, 122, 125, 129, 131, 168
fenbendazole 82, 163
filtration 20, 38-40, 96-97, 102, 104-106, 108-115, 117, 119-120, 122, 125, 128-129, 131-132, 144, 147-148, 186
fin rot 67
fish handler's disease 67
fish lice 64-65, 83-84, 131, 135-136, 139-140, 156, 162
flagella 77-78
flashing 74, 79, 101, 119
Flexibacter 67, 150
fluke 79, 148
fluorescein stain 40
formalin 18, 56, 64, 69, 73-74, 76-78, 80, 96, 98, 106, 118-119, 125, 131, 135, 139-140, 149, 151-153, 163-164

fountains 98, 116, 119, 144, 175-178
fry 7, 18-22, 24, 119, 122, 170
fungus 19, 69-70, 125, 131
furuncles 65-66

G

gallbladder 31-32
gas bubble disease 123
genotype 20-22, 166
gill flukes 79, 135-136, 142-144, 149, 162
gills 19, 28, 30-31, 33, 40, 42, 44, 46, 49, 51, 53, 55-57, 63-65, 69-70, 73-74, 77-81, 85, 90, 92, 95-97, 101-102, 106, 115, 119, 121, 123, 137, 140-144, 154, 156, 166
glochidia 85
goldfish 6, 24, 65, 70, 79, 126, 141-144, 172, 174, 181
Goussia 73
Gyrodactylus 79-80, 139, 143, 162

H

hardness 39, 94, 99-100, 103, 106-108, 111, 137-138, 143, 148-149
heart rate 57
heaters 119
heavy metals 94, 110-111, 125
hematocrit 45, 166
hematopoietic 31-33, 63
Henneguya 78
hepatic lipidosis 64, 90, 122
hermaphroditic 79-82
Herpesvirus cyprini 63
heterophils 45-46
Hexamita 77, 155
histopathology 44, 56, 79, 135, 136, 138
Hoferellus 78-79, 137
hormones 32-33, 90
hospital tank 38, 121, 138, 159
hydrogen peroxide 19, 69-70, 99, 106, 153, 163
hydrogen sulfide 103, 105, 113, 116, 142, 156
hyperplasia 42, 54, 63, 70, 74, 79, 91, 95-96, 106, 139, 143-144, 166
hypoxia 42, 63, 70, 74, 79, 96, 98, 101, 120, 132, 141-144, 153, 166

I

Ichthyobodo necator 77, 139-140, 143, 150-152

Ichthyophthirius multifiliis 42, 72-75, 86, 114, 139-140, 143, 150-152
infusoria 19
injection 20, 58, 64, 67, 81, 137
iodine 53-54, 65, 92, 154, 163
iridocytes 29
iridophores 29
iroage 92, 168

J

Japanese-style koi show 63, 131
jumping out of pond 121

K

kidneys 30, 32-33, 46, 79, 137, 142
Klebsiella 140
Koi Herpesvirus 63-64
koi shows 5, 16, 131, 168, 172
koi varieties 14, 16, 165, 168

L

leeches 64, 78, 82
Lernaea 83, 139, 162
leukocytes 29, 45-46, 136
lice 64-65, 83-84, 131, 135-136, 139-140, 156, 162
limestone 99-100, 111
liver 31-32, 43, 89-91, 122, 126, 129, 141-142
lufenuron 84, 163
lymphocytes 45, 47, 129, 141

M

magnesium 46, 92, 99, 102-103, 106, 111, 119
malachite green 18-19, 69-70, 73-74, 76-78, 80, 118-119, 131, 135, 139-140, 152, 163
manganese 92, 156
mechanical filters 110, 112
melanophores 29, 54
metal poisoning 125
methemoglobinemia 96, 159
methylene blue 19, 69-70, 163
metronidazole 77, 155, 163
microchip transponder 20, 22, 59

microscope 39-41, 44-45, 73, 78
minerals 89, 92, 99, 109, 119, 143, 159
mirror 6, 8, 60, 169
monocytes 45, 47
mucus 29, 40-42, 63-64, 73, 77, 80, 82, 95, 119, 129, 138, 159, 166
muscle 33, 50, 53-54, 57-59, 66, 68, 81, 91, 121, 125
Mycobacterium 67, 70, 135-137
mycotoxins 125
Myxobolus 78

N

necropsy 31, 34, 43-44, 49, 60, 64, 66, 79, 135-137, 140-141, 144
nematodes 82, 143
neoplasia 125, 135
nets 40, 63, 130-132
neutrophils 45-46, 129, 135, 141
nitrate 39, 94, 96, 98, 102-103, 107-108, 111-112, 118, 131-132, 140, 142, 144, 157-158
nitrite 39-40, 94, 96-98, 102, 107-108, 111-113, 118, 131, 137-138, 140, 142, 144, 157-159, 188
nitrogen cycle 97
nuptial tubercles 18

O

oil 50, 125-126
Oodinium 150
ORP 106, 108-109
overcrowding 63, 73, 77, 98-99, 106, 129, 153
overfeeding 73, 89, 106, 119, 122
overstocking 122
oxygen 8, 30-31, 38-40, 42, 46, 50, 52, 55, 57, 63, 69, 90, 94-99, 101, 103, 105-106, 108, 111-113, 115-119, 122, 124-125, 129-130, 132, 142-143, 148, 150-153, 156-158, 166
oxytetracycline 92, 163
ozone 106, 115, 117

P

pancreas 32
paraformaldehyde 151-152
peritonitis 66-67, 136
pH 19, 39, 50, 59, 69, 94-96, 98-103, 105-109, 112, 115, 119, 125, 131, 137, 142-144, 148-149,

162
phenotype 21-22, 24, 167
phosphate 96, 100, 103
photosynthesis 98, 101, 115, 119, 124
physical examination 41, 138
pigment 29, 54
piping 99
pituitary 20, 34, 190
plant filter 114
plants 5, 7, 18, 40, 69, 79, 82, 89-90, 92, 98, 100-102, 105, 110, 113-114, 118-119, 123, 125, 142, 157-159, 172, 175, 177-180, 188
platelets 47
poison 124, 150
population density 39, 142
potassium permanganate 80, 105-106, 125, 142, 153, 156, 163-164
praziquantel 80-81, 163
predators 122-123
prefilter 110
protein 18, 46, 89-90, 92, 115, 119, 136, 141, 161, 166
protein skimmer 115
Pseudomonas 67, 139

Q

quarantine 39, 63-64, 125, 131-132, 140-141, 155, 161, 167

R

radiographs 35, 47-49, 137
red blood cells 30, 45-47, 78, 96, 167
redox potential 106
respiration 40, 50, 55, 59, 64, 98, 100-101, 115, 119, 121, 125, 142, 190
Rhabdovirus 64
roe 20-21, 33, 48, 167, 174
rotifers 19

S

salinity 69, 94-95, 97-98, 102-104, 118, 131, 147-148, 188
salt 18, 21, 33, 59, 65, 67, 70, 73-74, 76-78, 82-83, 85, 96-97, 102-104, 111, 118-119, 121, 130-131, 140, 147-150, 159, 163-164, 188
sand filter 110, 136, 141, 143

Sanguinicola 81
Saprolegnia 19, 69, 74
scales 6-8, 13-16, 28-29, 40, 53, 58, 60, 65, 68, 123, 129-130, 138, 166, 168-170
scoliosis 90
seasonal variations 63, 79, 118
seizures 125
Sekoke disease 90-91, 170
septicemia 65-66, 92, 136, 140, 144, 167, 190
settling chamber 113-114
shrimp 19, 92
Siemens 103
simazine 157-158
skin 28-29, 40-41, 43-44, 49-50, 53-54, 56-58, 63-70, 73-75, 77-80, 82-84, 90-91, 102, 115, 119, 121, 123, 129-131, 135-140, 142-143, 149-152, 154-163, 166, 168, 170
snails 81-82, 85, 162
sodium 45-46, 59, 92, 97, 99-103, 106, 111, 130, 149, 154, 159-160, 163
sodium bicarbonate 59, 100
sodium chloride 97, 102-103, 106, 111, 154, 159-160, 163
sodium thiosulfate 101, 160
sonogram 49, 53
spawning 4, 7, 18-20, 24, 69, 118, 121, 153
specific gravity 103, 136, 141
spinal injury 125
Spironucleus 77, 155
spleen 32, 46
spring 8, 63-65, 83, 118, 120
spring viremia of carp 64
stress 39-41, 47, 50, 65, 77, 94-95, 109, 118-121, 129, 132, 139, 142, 147, 159, 167
sulphates 105
summer 63-64, 118-119, 141-143
sunburn 123, 143
supersaturation 110, 115-116, 123-124
surgery 1, 49-50, 52-53, 55-56, 60, 135, 137-138

T

tapeworms 81
taxonomy 5, 11
teeth 7, 27, 30
telangiectasis 42, 70, 86, 167
temperature 7, 18-21, 39, 43, 50, 57, 63-65, 67, 74-75, 78-79, 83-84, 89, 94-96, 98, 100, 103, 105, 107-109, 112, 115, 118-120, 124-125, 129-131, 137, 142-144, 162
tetracycline 65, 73, 92, 138-140, 161, 163, 193
total dissolved solids 103, 106
total particulate matter 106

toxins 42, 124
transporting koi 130
trematodes 79, 81, 140, 149, 151-153
trichlorfon 80-85, 125, 131, 135, 139-140, 144, 162-163
Trichodina 77, 143, 151-152
trickle filter 113
Trypanosoma 78
tube-feeding 65
Tubifex 78-79, 81
tumors 35, 48, 50, 53, 135-138

U

ulcer 65-66, 139
ultrasound (sonography) 49, 53
ultraviolet light 64, 76, 101, 114-115, 117, 132, 148
urea 21, 30, 46, 90

V

vacation 89, 122
vaccine 64
venturi 116, 141
Vibrio 140
viruses 62-63, 114-115, 153, 167
vitamins 89-92, 129

W

water quality 1, 38-40, 63, 65, 67, 73, 77, 88, 94, 105, 108-109, 115, 118, 122, 125, 127, 129, 131-132, 137, 139, 141-142, 181
waterfalls 98, 116, 119, 175, 178, 180
Weber's ossicles (Weberian apparatus) 5, 33-36
white blood cells 42, 45-47
winter 8, 20, 73, 79, 83, 118-120, 139

X

xanthophores 29
xanthophylls 92

Y

yellow prussic acid 159

Z

zeolite 102, 111
zinc 73, 92, 99, 125, 152
zoonotic disease 67